Fetal
Alcoho
Syndro

DATE DUE

APR 16 2005

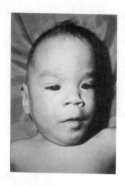 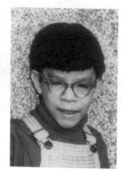 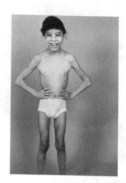

With deep appreciation, I dedicate this book to all my patients and friends with FAS/FAE and to their parents and families. My understanding of this often hidden disability has been enriched beyond all imagination by the hopes and dreams and sorrows that you have shared with me over the past 25 years.

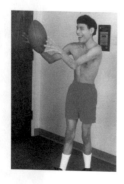 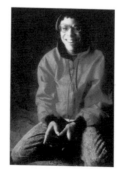 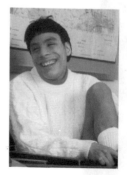

Fetal Alcohol Syndrome

A Guide for Families and Communities

by

Ann Streissguth, Ph.D.
University of Washington
Fetal Alcohol and Drug Unit
Seattle

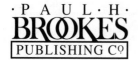
·P·A·U·L·H·
BROOKES
PUBLISHING C?

Baltimore • London • Toronto • Sydney

Paul H. Brookes Publishing Co.
Post Office Box 10624
Baltimore, Maryland 21285-0624

Typeset by Brushwood Graphics, Inc., Baltimore, Maryland.
Manufactured in the United States of America by
Versa Press, East Peoria, Illinois.

All of the vignettes in this book are based on the author's actual experiences. In all instances, names have been changed; in some instances, identifying details have been altered to protect confidentiality.

All royalties from this book will be donated to the Fetal Alcohol Research Fund at the University of Washington Medical School.

Library of Congress Cataloging-in-Publication Data

Streissguth, Ann Pytkowicz.
   Fetal alcohol syndrome : a guide for families and
   communities / Ann Streissguth.
        p.   cm.
      Includes bibliographical references and index.
      ISBN 1-55766-283-5
      1. Fetal alcohol syndrome.   I. Title.
RG629.F45S78   1997
618.3′268—DC21   96-47826
                                                                      CIP

British Library Cataloguing in Publication data are available from the British Library.

Contents

List of Tables and Figures ix
List of Photographs xiii
About the Author xv
Foreword   *Godfrey P. Oakley, Jr.* xvii
Foreword   *Kenneth R. Warren* xxi
Preface xxiii
Acknowledgments xxv

I   THE DISEASES OF FETAL ALCOHOL

1   Overview of Fetal Alcohol Syndrome   3

Prenatal Alcohol Exposure Can Cause a
    Spectrum of Effects
Problems with Getting a Diagnosis
Incidence of FAS
Problems with Studying FAS Populations
Overview of Sections

2   Diagnosing Fetal Alcohol Syndrome 17

Fetal Alcohol Syndrome
Documenting Exposure
The Diagnostic Process
Physical Findings in FAS
Age-Related Changes in FAS Features
Fetal Alcohol Effects and Alcohol-Related
    Neurodevelopmental Disorder
Measuring CNS Dysfunction

3   From Awareness to Public Policy 35

The Path to Clinical Recognition
The Path to Scientific Validation
Tracking the Long-Term Effects of FAS
The Path to an Effective Public Policy on
    Alcohol and Pregnancy

II   THE SCIENCE OF FETAL ALCOHOL SYNDROME

4   Alcohol as a Teratogen 55

Understanding Teratology
Neurobehavioral Teratology of Alcohol

5 Alcohol's Impact on Children.. 71

Children of Alcoholic Mothers
How a Mother's Alcoholism Affects Her Children
    and Her Health
Children of Alcoholic Fathers and Families
Alcohol and Children When Mothers Drink
    Socially
Conclusions

6 Primary and Secondary Disabilities............................ 95

Primary Disabilities Arise from Organic Brain
    Damage
Brain–Behavior Relationships that Contribute
    to Primary Disabilities
Measuring Primary Disabilities in Groups of
    Individuals with FAS/FAE
Measuring Secondary Disabilities in Groups of
    Individuals with FAS/FAE
Risk and Protective Factors Associated with
    Secondary Disabilities
Conclusions

**III A LIFE-SPAN APPROACH TO FETAL ALCOHOL
SYNDROME**

7 Living with Fetal Alcohol Syndrome...............................119

Seven Common Misconceptions About FAS/FAE
Problems, Concerns, and Recommendations
Identifying the Behavioral Phenotype of FAS/FAE
Focusing on the Individual
Understanding People with FAS/FAE
    Throughout the Life Span
Four Wishes

8 The Advocacy Model...145

What Is an Advocate?
Who Can Be an Advocate?
What Makes an Advocate Successful?
Preventing Secondary Disabilities Through
    Advocacy
Advocating for Advocates

9 Families Speak Out..165

Families Have Diverse Backgrounds
Families Illustrate Important Issues
Families Reveal Similar Needs
Conclusions

**IV PREPARING PEOPLE WITH FAS FOR LIFE IN THE
COMMUNITY**

10 Preparing Children with FAS/FAE for Adulthood 185
Problems Encountered by People with FAS/FAE
Recognizing and Accepting Disabilities
Planning Early for a Healthy Life
Building Personal Strengths at Home
How Society Can Help

11 Guidelines for Schools...207
An FAS/FAE Plan for School Districts
School–Parent Collaboration
FAS Overview for Classroom Teachers
Guidelines for Using the Advocacy Model with
    a Student with FAS/FAE at School
Summary

12 Guidelines for Human Services..................................227
Identifying and Serving Individuals with
    FAS/FAE with Community Services
Alcohol and Other Drug Treatments
Mental Health Treatment
Juvenile Justice and Corrections
Conclusions

V PREVENTING FETAL ALCOHOL DAMAGE

13 Education, Training, and Public Policy 249
Public Education
Professional Training
Public Policy
Conclusions

**14 Effective Prevention Programs for
High-Risk Mothers**...263
Intervening in Alcohol Abuse During Pregnancy
Intervening After Delivery

Epilogue 279

Resource Appendix 281

Permissions..291

Index 293

List of Tables and Figures

I: THE DISEASES OF FETAL ALCOHOL

1: Overview of Fetal Alcohol Syndrome

Figure 1.1: Ethanol crosses the placenta freely 5
Figure 1.2: Mothering begins before birth 13

2: Diagnosing Fetal Alcohol Syndrome

Table 2.1: CNS structural and functional effects by
age that can be alcohol related 19
Figure 2.1: Alcohol equivalencies of common
beverages 20
Figure 2.2: Useful topics for a retrospective prenatal
alcohol exposure history 21
Figure 2.3: Diagram of FAS facial characteristics in
young child 24
Figure 2.4: Two girls born to alcoholic mothers 28

3: From Awareness to Public Policy

Figure 3.1: Pauline "Kallikak" 37
Figure 3.2: The first child diagnosed with FAS at
birth 39
Figure 3.3: Three babies born with fetal alcohol
syndrome 40

II: THE SCIENCE OF FETAL ALCOHOL SYNDROME

4: Alcohol as a Teratogen

Table 4.1: Teratogens can cause four distinct types
of outcomes in exposed offspring 57
Figure 4.1: Malformations and growth deficiency in
pup and chick produced by heavy
prenatal alcohol exposure 59
Figure 4.2: Exencephaly in mouse produced by
heavy prenatal alcohol exposure 60
Figure 4.3: How prenatal alcohol produces the face
of FAS in boy and mouse 61
Figure 4.4: Alcohol chick fails detour learning test 62
Table 4.2: Behavioral effects following prenatal alcohol
exposure in humans and animals 65

5: Alcohol's Impact on Children

Figure 5.1: Birth weight of successive offspring of five mothers who have chronic alcoholism 78

Figure 5.2: Alcohol and other drug use among women of childbearing age 84

6: Primary and Secondary Disabilities

Figure 6.1: MRI showing normal corpus callosum (a) compared with a thin (b) and absent (c) corpus callosum in individuals with FAS, respectively 98

Figure 6.2: IQ distributions for FAS and FAE compared with the normal curve 103

Table 6.1: Maladaptive behaviors and symptoms in people with FAS/FAE that indicate or suggest possible organic etiology 104

Table 6.2: Clinical implications of characteristic FAS/FAE cognitive impairments 106

Figure 6.3: Secondary disabilities in FAS/FAE 108

III: A LIFE-SPAN APPROACH TO FETAL ALCOHOL SYNDROME

7: Living with Fetal Alcohol Syndrome

Table 7.1: Psychosocial needs associated with FAS and FAE 124

8: The Advocacy Model

Table 8.1: Behavioral and emotional consequences of fetal alcohol–associated brain damage and advocate strategies 152

Table 8.2: Advocacy strategies for preventing secondary disabilities in people with FAS/FAE 161

IV: PREPARING PEOPLE WITH FAS FOR LIFE IN THE COMMUNITY

11: Guidelines for Schools

Table 11.1: What students with FAS/FAE need at school 209

Table 11.2: Tasks of the school advocate of a student with FAS/FAE 215

Table 11.3: A 10-step school plan for students suspected of having FAS/FAE 216

Figure 11.1: Dolly's test scores over time 217

Table 11.4: Guidelines for the classroom teacher
working with students with FAS/FAE....................221

12: Guidelines for Human Services

Figure 12.1: *Au salon de la rue des Moulins* [In the Moulins
Street salon] by Henri de Toulouse-Lautrec...........243

V: PREVENTING FETAL ALCOHOL DAMAGE

13: Education, Training, and Public Policy

Figure 13.1: Washington State warning sign about
prenatal alcohol exposure.......................................259

**14: Effective Prevention Programs
for High-Risk Mothers**

Figure 14.1: Decrease in maternal alcohol use after
intervention during pregnancy 266

Epilogue

Figure 1: *La Buveuse* [The Hangover] by Henri de
Toulouse-Lautrec..279

List of Photographs

On the Cover

Three babies born with fetal alcohol syndrome

In the Text

Frontispiece: Collage of boy with FAS across the life span   ii
Photograph of the Author (by Rob Casey).....................................   xv

I: Boy with FAS across the life span....................................   1
1:    Newborn with FAS...   3
2:    Infant with FAS   17
3:    Toddler with FAS..   35

II: Girl with FAS across the life span....................................   53
4:    Preschool girl with FAS...   55
5:    Young boy with FAS and his mother   71
6:    Boy with FAS   95

III: Girl with FAS across the life span....................................117
7:    Girl with FAS and her mother..119
8:    Girl with FAS and her mother..145
9:    Mother with FAS/FAE and her two children 165

IV: Boy with FAS across the life span.....................................183
10:   Boy with FAS and his mother...185
11:   Girl with FAS...207
12:   Boy with FAS and his brother 227

V: Girl with FAS across the life span....................................247
13:   Man with FAS..249
14:   Boy with FAS and his mother...265

About the Author

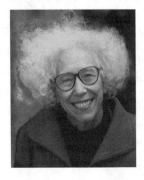

Ann Streissguth, Ph.D., is a professor in the Department of Psychiatry and Behavioral Sciences at the University of Washington School of Medicine. She received her master's degree in child development from the University of California at Berkeley and her doctoral degree in clinical psychology from the University of Washington. Dr. Streissguth is a licensed clinical psychologist with a specialty in behavioral teratology. She has 25 years of experience working with individuals with fetal alcohol syndrome (FAS) and fetal alcohol effects (FAE), as well as with their families and communities.

Researchers at the University of Washington Fetal Alcohol and Drug Unit, which Dr. Streissguth directs, have investigated many types of prenatal influences on later development in offspring, including alcohol, tobacco, cocaine, aspirin, and acetaminophen. Prior to her position at the Fetal Alcohol and Drug Unit, Dr. Streissguth studied the impact of poverty, preschool experience, caregiving experiences, and the rubella virus on child development. In all, she has published more than 150 scientific papers, two books, and a slide-teaching curriculum on alcohol and pregnancy.

Dr. Streissguth and her colleagues have been actively involved in research on preventing FAS/FAE since these conditions were identified. In 1978, she collaborated with Dr. Ruth Little in a 3-year project (The Pregnancy and Health Program) funded by the National Institute on Alcohol Abuse and Alcoholism (NIAAA) to develop methods to intervene in female alcohol abuse during pregnancy and to prevent FAS/FAE. More recently, Dr. Streissguth and colleagues developed and evaluated the impact of a model advocacy program (Seattle Birth to 3) for helping high-risk women who are abusing alcohol and drugs during pregnancy and not receiving prenatal care. At the conclusion of the 5-year research program funded by the Center for Substance Abuse Prevention (CSAP), a local philanthropist provided funding to continue the program; then the governor of Washington State provided funds to develop a second site in another city. As of 1997, the Washington State legislature has funded the two sites for the biennium.

Dr. Streissguth has been principal investigator of the Pregnancy and Health Study, a longitudinal prospective study of the relationship between early experiences and child development, funded by NIAAA since 1974. She has completed a major research project funded by the Centers for Disease Control and Prevention (CDC) on secondary disabilities in individuals with FAS/FAE and associated risk and protective factors, which culminated in an international conference in Seattle in September 1996. Since 1983, Dr. Streissguth has worked with Native American communities and the Indian Health Service to provide FAS training workshops, screening clinics, research findings, and direct consultations to Native Americans and Alaskan Natives. With her colleagues, she has also initiated a 5-year study of magnetic resonance imaging and neuropsychological functioning in people with FAS/FAE, funded by NIAAA.

Along with Dr. Paul Lemoine of France, Dr. Streissguth was co-recipient of the 1985 International Jellinek Memorial Award for Advancement of the Field of Alcohol Studies. In 1987, along with Dr. Ruth Little, she received the annual award for outstanding contribution from the American Medical Society on Alcoholism and Other Drug Dependencies. In 1992, the National Council on Alcoholism and Drug Dependence presented the Silver Key Award to Dr. Streissguth on behalf of her "outstanding contribution and research on FAS/FAE." In 1997, she received the Outstanding Public Service Award from the University of Washington for her efforts to help individuals with FAS/FAE and their families.

Foreword

I spent the academic years of 1970–1972 as a birth defects fellow in Seattle, where I had the privilege of seeing patients with Dr. David Smith. I remember that he and I once saw a patient with a developmental delay, but we were not able to determine the cause. David kept a file on such unknown diagnoses, however, and within 18 months he and his then-current fellow, Ken Jones, determined that the cause of that child's developmental delay was a previously unrecognized syndrome that they had recently defined: fetal alcohol syndrome (FAS). In June 1997, a new survey conducted by the March of Dimes showed that almost all women of reproductive age now know that drinking alcohol during pregnancy can harm the developing embryo and fetus. Thus, in the space of 25 years, we have gone from a situation in which one of the best clinical experts of our time did not recognize a child with FAS to one in which almost all American women know that drinking during pregnancy can seriously damage the embryo and fetus. This is a tremendous accomplishment, but it is far from sufficient. Despite the widespread knowledge of the damage that alcohol can cause to a developing fetus, we continue to have many babies born with damage caused by prenatal exposure to alcohol. We must find a way to prevent this major cause of disability among children and adults.

We do not know the causes for most birth defects and developmental disabilities among children born today, and we all agree that much more research is needed to recognize these causes so that we can develop appropriate prevention strategies. We sometimes forget, however, that finding the causes of any disease is just the first step toward preventing that disease. For example, N.M. Gregg made the causal association between rubella and birth defects in 1941, yet it was not until the late 1960s that we had an effective vaccine, and only recently have vaccine programs in this country been sufficiently effective to virtually eliminate the birth defects and developmental disabilities caused by the rubella virus. Even with an effective vaccine available, there are still many parts of the world without rubella immunization programs; hence, these birth defects continue to occur unnecessarily. Similarly, in spite of widespread knowledge that two micronutrients, iodine and the B-vitamin folic acid, are essential to the normal development of a fetus, millions of women worldwide still do not consume enough of these micronutrients, and as a result, countless children are unnecessarily born with birth defects and developmental disabilities.

David Smith was a remarkable man, and he had the good judgment to ask Ann Streissguth to join him in studying FAS. I don't know if he had any conception at the time of where that collaboration would lead, but I believe that if he were alive today he would say that asking Ann to work with him on FAS was one of the best decisions he ever made. He certainly could not have predicted how an academic psychologist would become a "Renaissance woman" in the battle against alcohol damage in children. Although Ann began with an academic interest in whether drinking during pregnancy could damage an embryo or fetus, she has also worked to prevent women from drinking during pregnancy and to develop intervention programs to help parents, communities, and affected individuals ameliorate or cope with the adverse effects of the in utero damage.

Alcohol has been available for human consumption for thousands of years and has probably had an adverse affect on millions of human beings through in utero exposure. Putting an end to this unnecessary human tragedy by preventing such prenatal damage and promoting healthy lives among people affected by maternal drinking is a very tall order. Fortunately, anyone wanting to join these efforts will have this book to help him or her. I know that as difficult as these tasks will be, they have been made easier because Ann gave us this book. Thousands of unborn children will benefit from it.

We have eradicated smallpox and are about to eradicate polio worldwide. These great public health achievements should encourage us to envision a world in which no children are damaged by maternal drinking. It took 200 years after the development of an effective intervention to rid the earth of smallpox. Let's hope we can get to the total prevention of prenatal alcohol damage much more quickly. Because alcohol is a legal addicting drug, finding and implementing effective prevention strategies is a herculean task. A very practical first step, as Ann points out, is to identify the women at highest risk and ensure that they have access to programs that reduce alcohol consumption and encourage them to make responsible decisions concerning reproductive choices.

Even as we attempt to save future generations from the tragically unnecessary effects of prenatal alcohol exposure, we should help Ann in working for the best possible life for people already affected by such exposure. Ann's research has shown us that although there is no cure for the irreversible damage that alcohol inflicts upon a developing fetus, people affected by that damage can, in Ann's words, "function fairly well when their needs are understood and met."

In the 1990s, we have learned much about what FAS means to affected individuals, their families, and their communities. No one has contributed more to this understanding than Dr. Ann Streissguth. She has given of her intellect and talents as a researcher, but she has given even more of herself as a warm, caring human being. She has answered the early-morning and late-night calls of countless parents and clinicians over the years, listening to their struggles and helping as only she is able. Ann, thank you for all that you have done to help us understand the serious consequences of this preventable cause of disabilities. Keep up the good work.

Godfrey P. Oakley, Jr., M.D.
Director, Division of Birth Defects and
Developmental Disabilities
National Center for Environmental Health
Centers for Disease Control and Prevention
Atlanta, Georgia

Foreword

Twenty-five years ago, the first reports identifying a pattern of birth defects that appeared attributable to alcohol appeared in the English language medical journals. Understandable skepticism regarding the existence of this serious birth defect that David Smith, the eminent scholar of genetic and environmental birth defects, named the fetal alcohol syndrome (FAS) greeted the 1973 reports by Jones and Smith and Jones, Smith, Ulleland, and Streissguth. With the advances that had been made in our understanding of health and disease prior to the 1970s and a history of human alcohol use spanning millennia, how could such a major consequence of alcohol exposure in pregnancy have gone undetected for so many years? In fact, the view that alcohol, at any exposure level, was an innocuous agent with respect to the developing embryo or fetus and, indeed, could be helpful in alleviating some conditions associated with pregnancy had been touted in texts for both medical professionals and expectant mothers through the 1960s.

Within a short time span, a major change in the medical perspective on alcohol use and pregnancy occurred. By June 1977, only 4 years after the initial naming of FAS, the then U.S. Department of Health, Education, and Welfare issued its first health advisory on alcohol and pregnancy. This first advisory was a cautiously phrased medical alert, taking care not to exceed the knowledge accrued at that point in time, stating that heavy drinking was dangerous and that the risks of drinking at lower levels were then, as yet, unclear. In May of 1981, the Surgeon General of the United States updated the initial medical alert based on new knowledge. In the landmark *Surgeon General's Advisory on Alcohol and Pregnancy*, the nation's senior health official for the first time advised women to avoid all alcohol during pregnancy.

The scientific and medical community's acceptance of alcohol use as a risk factor in pregnancy was due in no small measure to the rigorous scientific research that had been initiated shortly after the initial reports by Jones et al. But research requires funding, and that funding was undoubtedly facilitated by another significant event of the 1970s. In 1970, Congress passed a law creating the National Institute on Alcohol Abuse and Alcoholism (NIAAA) with a mission to address health issues relating to alcohol abuse and alcoholism. NIAAA began to support both clinical and basic research on alcohol and pregnancy outcomes shortly after the first published case reports on FAS.

Of particular importance in the early years of investigation were basic research studies with animal models. Animal research enabled researchers to separate alcohol from other potential harmful factors in demonstrating that alcohol could cause the pattern of birth defects seen in FAS, an important confirmation of the existence of FAS.

Since its initial recognition, Ann Streissguth has been a central figure in FAS research, clinical care, and prevention. As a researcher, she initiated a longitudinal investigation on the effects of alcohol exposure on pregnancy outcomes and development, a study that has been ongoing for 23 years. As a clinician, she was the developmental psychologist who characterized the neurobehavioral deficits among the first children recognized with FAS and fetal alcohol effects (FAE). Her accomplishments also include the development of one of the first FAS prevention programs, the characterization of the secondary disabilities in FAS and FAE, the development of an advocacy-based approach to aid children and adults with FAS/FAE, and the development of parent support groups. But most important, Ann Streissguth has willingly and graciously shared her knowledge of alcohol and pregnancy with professionals and with families of those affected by prenatal alcohol use.

We have come a long distance in understanding FAS and other alcohol-related birth defects in the past 25 years, as Ann Streissguth describes so well in this book. But there is much yet to be learned, and this knowledge will be obtained only through further research. Through continued research, we will learn how to more effectively intervene with women of childbearing age who have alcohol abuse or dependence problems. We will learn how to reduce the potential for injury to the fetus who is exposed to alcohol. And we will learn how to more effectively address the cognitive and behavior problems in children and adults with FAS/FAE, helping them to improve their quality of life and their potential for human achievement.

Kenneth R. Warren, Ph.D.
Director, Office of Scientific Affairs
National Institute on Alcohol Abuse and Alcoholism
National Institutes of Health
Bethesda, Maryland

REFERENCES

Jones, K.L., & Smith, D.W. (1973). Recognition of the fetal alcohol syndrome in early infancy. *Lancet, 2*(836), 999–1001.

Jones, K.L., Smith, D.W., Ulleland, C.N., & Streissguth, A.P. (1973). Pattern of malformation in offspring of chronic alcoholic mothers. *Lancet, 1*(815), 267–1271.

Preface

Millions of words have been written about alcohol's effects on the developing fetus since fetal alcohol syndrome (FAS) was first defined and recognized as a birth defect in 1973. Most of these words have focused on describing the syndrome and defining alcohol as a drug that can cause birth defects. Very few of these words have been in books focused on developmental disabilities, mental retardation, learning problems, and mental health or psychiatric disabilities or in books on how to teach, treat, or help affected children.

I want to go on record at the outset of this volume, stating my belief that children with FAS and fetal alcohol effects (FAE) are not hopeless, deplorable, or wretched. Diagnosing children with FAS/FAE does *not* thwart their development, limit their horizons, or assign them to life as second-class citizens. Ignorance is seldom therapeutic.

This book was written because the world can't wait for all the studies to be carried out, for every professional to read every scientific publication, or for the best solutions to be stumbled upon in each community. Our children, our families, our schools, and our communities are suffering because of FAS/FAE. They are suffering from lack of understanding and awareness, and, even as they suffer, the problems FAS/FAE generates are compounding. Misunderstood children with FAS/FAE are dropping out of school and often having babies for whom they can't care. Their parents are unable to cope with their problems, which go beyond the demands for normal parenting. Professionals are still confused because needed research hasn't been carried out yet. Communities are uncertain about how to respond.

This book was written because it is essential and urgent that we as a society spend resources to attack this problem. Research on recommended practices and model programs must be carried out and replicated in community after community throughout the United States if we are to save future children from prenatal alcohol damage and prevent secondary disabilities in children already born with prenatal alcohol effects.

It is my hope that this book will be a vehicle for parents and professionals to use in working together to help children with FAS/FAE. If you know of a child you think might have FAS or FAE, whether in a familial, a professional, or a community relationship—this book is for you. If you feel it is unjust and unproductive to send young people with brain damage to prison or to relegate them to life in the shadows because society never recognized their disabilities, taught them in a way they could understand, or helped them gain appropriate job skills so they could lead productive lives and value work like other citizens—this book is for you. If you care about public policy, public health, the welfare of children, and educational and care systems as mechanisms to enhance personal competence and productivity and to prevent debilitating secondary disabilities—this book is for you.

This book is addressed to families in the hope that it will help them to work more effectively with their own children and neighbors with FAS/FAE and to advocate more effectively for them in the community. This book is addressed to professionals and community leaders in the hope that they will each do their part to bring understanding and opportunity to this underserved but large population of people of all ages who are prenatally affected by alcohol. This book is addressed to students and researchers in the hope that their knowledge and insight will help us solve the many problems of effective prevention, intervention, and treatment of FAS/FAE that still remain unsolved.

Acknowledgments

In the 25 years it has taken to prepare this book, my own ideas and those of my colleagues have become inextricably linked, as together we have sought to bring meaning to the tapestry of information that was increasingly spread before us. Many thanks are due.

To the late David W. Smith, the founding father of the field of dysmorphology, and to his fellow, Kenneth Lyons Jones, my gratitude is boundless. Along with other Smith fellows (Jon Aase, Sterling Clarren, James Hanson, and John Graham), they taught me dysmorphology—how the body can reflect the intrauterine experience and how the face can reflect the earliest maldevelopment of the brain.

To Sterling Clarren, special gratitude is due for being able and willing to diagnose FAS after Smith's death in 1981. Dr. Clarren's diagnostic acumen and accessibility provided a steady stream of diagnosed patients of all ages who have been affiliated with our Fetal Alcohol and Drug Unit over these many years.

To Paul Lemoine, of Nantes, France, and Philippe Dehaene, of Roubaix, France, I express my personal appreciation for sharing their experiences and their pediatric patients with me in 1981 in my quest to understand the impact of prenatal alcohol in the cross-cultural context. I discovered that French children with FAS were exactly like American children with FAS, except that they spoke better French.

I thank Carrie Randall, Jim West, and Ed Riley, three scientists whose early animal models of FAS clearly demonstrated the teratogenic effects of alcohol on physical malformations, on brain damage, and on brain-related behaviors. Their work provided the necessary biological underpinnings for our work with children.

I thank Ruth Little and Therese Grant, cherished colleagues instrumental in the development and implementation of two successful prevention models developed on our unit for the prevention of fetal alcohol damage in children, in 1977–1981 and in 1991–1997, respectively. In addition, I commend the courage and enthusiasm of the birth-to-3 advocates: Roberta Wright, Liz Morales, Gail Haynes, Carryn Johnson, and Anna Ximines; Beth Gendler, social worker; Cara Ernst, evaluator; and Pam Phipps, recruiter/interviewer. These women have truly demonstrated that the mothers the community thought were "untouchable" are indeed reachable.

I thank Helen Barr and Paul Sampson, statisticians, and Fred Bookstein, consultant at the Fetal Alcohol and Drug Unit, whose care and nurturing of data, whose respect and understanding of numbers, and whose continuing ability to forge new methods for our very large human behavioral teratology studies have truly made our joint research endeavors a reality.

I thank Julia Kogan, Mike Hampton, and Kaylin Anderson, colleagues on the FAS Secondary Disabilities Study, Project Director, Psychometrist, and Outreach Worker, respectively, whose clinical skills so greatly facilitated the research.

I thank my five postdoctoral fellows who have brought their own expertise to the research endeavors of our unit, thereby enriching our understanding of FAS/FAE: Robin LaDue (Native American clinical psychologist), Heather Carmichael Olson (early intervention psychologist), Karen Kopera-Frye (inner-city developmental psychologist), Natalie Novick (sexual deviancy specialist and clinical psychologist), and Paul Connor (neuropsychologist).

I thank the hundreds of students and staff on our unit whose dedicated work and enthusiasm have pushed us forward over the years. Special thanks are extended to three interns (Jana Carr, Sara Noble, and Audrey Don) and eight medical students (Ellen Wilbur, Lisa Jabolay, Caitlin Cadena, Annalisa Gorman, Chris Famy, Shoshanna Press, Jennifer Porter, and Shane Holloway) who worked on FAS projects.

I thank Pam Phipps and Cara Ernst, grants manager and publications manager, respectively, at the Fetal Alcohol and Drug Unit, who have been instrumental in keeping our research funded and our scientific papers rolling out. I express my deep appreciation to them, as without their skillful collaboration, the work of our unit would not have been successfully accomplished or disseminated. To Craig Borowiak, John Anzinger, Gunnel Tanimoto, Joan Sienkiewicz, Jonathan Kanter, Shari Jackson, Kristi Covell, Tomarra LeRoy, and Lisette Womack, I extend thanks for invaluable technical assistance.

I thank the four governmental agencies that have funded major components of the research at our unit during these past 25 years: The National Institute on Alcohol Abuse and Alcoholism (Grant No. AA01455-01-22), and in particular, Kenneth Warren, Laurie Foudin, and Mary Dufour; the Indian Health Service (Contracts 240-83-0053 through 282-92-009), especially Eva Smith; the Centers for Disease Control and Prevention (Grant No. RO4-CCROO8515), and especially Godfrey Oakley, Robert L. Burt, Karen L. Hymbaugh, and Joe Smith; and the Center for Substance

Abuse Prevention (Grant No. 6H86 SP02897-01-05), especially Jeanette Bevett-Mills.

I thank some important Washington State supporters of FAS work, former Governor Michael Lowry and his wife, Mary; Kenneth Stark, Head of the Division of Alcohol and Substance Abuse; Maxine Hayes, Assistant Secretary, Community and Family Health; Nancy White, formerly with the March of Dimes; and the Washington FAS Family Resources Institute, in particular Jocie DeVries, Linda LaFever, Vickie McKinney, and Ann Waller, who have been important sources of parental support and public advocacy.

I thank the five colleagues with whom I have worked most closely on FAS/FAE in the clinical realm—Sandra P. Randels, Robin LaDue, Sterling Clarren, Donna Burgess, and Marceil Ten Eyck—it is with great humility that I acknowledge your contributions to my thinking and to this volume. To my editors at Brookes, Jennifer Kinard and Lisa Rapisarda, and to Fred Bookstein (who read and critiqued this book twice), I extend gratitude for help and support in turning my thoughts into a book. To Daphne Phelps, whose tranquil Casa Cuseni in Sicily provided me a refuge for writing, I extend a hearty "grazie."

Finally, I gratefully acknowledge my strongest resource: my family. I thank my parents, Agnes Roth and the late Arie Roth, immigrants who believed in the value of education and in the freedom of thought and investigation, whose characteristics of hard work, perseverance, and fortitude in the face of adversity gave me the personal attributes to carry on with this work when the obstacles seemed insurmountable. I thank my dear husband, Daniel Streissguth, and our fine son, Benjamin Streissguth, for living and breathing fetal alcohol syndrome with me at a time when the words were scarcely known. Without their loving support, neither the research of the past 25 years nor this volume would have been possible.

To Abel Dorris,
brave son of Michael Dorris and Louise Erdrich,
whose story helped the world
to understand fetal alcohol syndrome

and

to Danny Simpson,
whose presence made many of our early studies
of individuals with fetal alcohol syndrome possible

I

The Diseases
of Fetal Alcohol

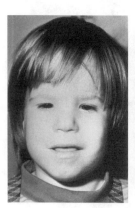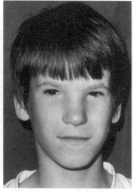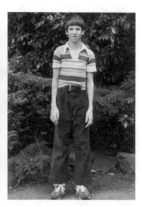

1

Overview of Fetal Alcohol Syndrome

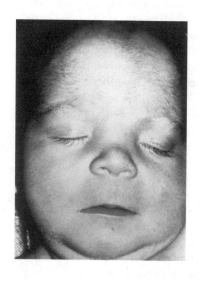

It was January 1973. I was in shock. I had just finished administering a psychological examination to the seventh young child in the group that Jones and Smith, my dysmorphology colleagues (physicians with expertise in congenital malformations), had asked me to see. Although the seven children represented three racial groups and were not themselves related, they looked eerily alike: small, sparkly eyes; small heads; and an appearance about the mouth that appeared as though they were pursing their lips even when they weren't smiling. Except for the two who were still infants and the one who was so flaccid she was carried in the arms of her mother, the other children had a wispy, flighty quality. I thought to myself that these children who were so curiously and surprisingly unafraid of me were like butterflies.

These children clearly had brain damage. To an experienced clinician, their neurological insults were as obvious as the aftereffects of meningitis or encephalitis. Each of these children had experienced damage to his or her central nervous system (CNS) that was apparent in his or her erratic movements, poor coordination, flighty attentional states, and poor performance on psychological tests, despite a captivatingly alert and bright-eyed manner.

"You think that alcohol causes this?" I asked incredulously of Jones and Smith. "Well, we think so; their mothers were all alcoholic and drinking heavily throughout pregnancy," they explained. "But, wouldn't someone have written about this? Wouldn't someone have studied the effects of alcohol on the unborn child?" I asked in disbelief. "Not that we know of," they replied.

I dashed to the medical library, expecting to find information on alcohol and pregnancy but found nothing. After weeks of intensely searching the national and international citations, I realized that Jones and Smith were right— the available medical literature in 1973 contained no information whatsoever about the effects of alcohol on pregnancy and the unborn child.

I imagined the myriad of pregnant women consuming alcohol throughout the world. If this carried even the slightest risk of damaging their infants, didn't they have the right to know? I decided to spend 10 years of my professional life examining this unsettling question. Twenty years later, I decided to write this book.

People with fetal alcohol syndrome (FAS) are born with it. FAS is a birth defect that has its primary effect on the brain. Some people with FAS are slightly affected and manifest only mildly dysfunctional behavior; others are severely affected, devastatingly disabled in their ability to cope with even simple day-to-day interactions. Each child with FAS has his or her own special needs, problems, and capabilities. FAS is a birth defect whether or not it is noticeable at birth. One does not outgrow FAS, although the manifestations may change with age. A bad environment (e.g., one in which there is abuse, neglect, or poverty) cannot cause FAS, just as a good environment (e.g., one with loving, caring parents) cannot fully undo it. A good environment and proper community supports, however, can protect the person with FAS from secondary disabilities, which can also be debilitating.

FAS is caused by prenatal alcohol exposure (see Figure 1.1) and is characterized by growth deficiency, a specific pattern of facial features, and some signs of CNS dysfunction.

PRENATAL ALCOHOL EXPOSURE
CAN CAUSE A SPECTRUM OF EFFECTS

Prenatal alcohol exposure does not always result in FAS. Depending on the dose, timing, and conditions of exposure as well as on the individual characteristics of the mother and fetus, prenatal alcohol exposure can cause a range of disabling conditions. Some children

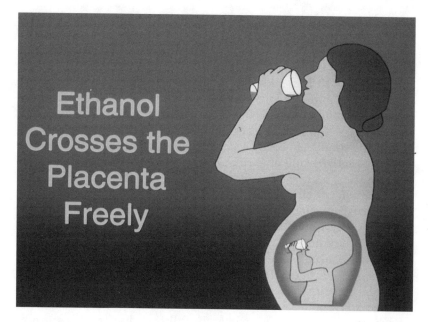

Figure 1.1. When a pregnant woman drinks alcohol, the blood-alcohol levels in mother and fetus are approximately equal within minutes after consumption. (From Streissguth & Little, 1994; reprinted by permission.)

are diagnosable with the full FAS; others have only partial manifestations, usually the CNS effects without the characteristic facial features or growth deficiency. Children who have only some of the characteristics of FAS (i.e., not enough for a full diagnosis) are often said to have fetal alcohol effects (FAE) or possible fetal alcohol effects (PFAE). These terms, although useful descriptively, have no specific differentiating criteria that would warrant their own diagnoses, even though these conditions can be just as debilitating as FAS. In 1996, the term alcohol-related neurodevelopmental disorder (ARND) was introduced by the Institute of Medicine (IOM, Stratton, Howe, & Battaglia). Focusing on the CNS characteristics (rather than on the growth deficiency and characteristic face), ARND is used congruently with FAE in this book. As these CNS effects can be caused by alcohol but are not unique to alcohol, the terms FAE, PFAE, and ARND are not appropriately used in the absence of a prenatal alcohol exposure history.

Research has shown that people with both FAS and those with FAE/PFAE/ARND experience many of the same kinds of problems growing up. Their families and communities also face many of the same kinds of challenges raising them. Therefore, this book frequently refers to these terms in the collective (i.e., FAS/FAE) in tacit recognition of the fact that it is the behavior problems caused by the prenatal damage from alcohol that present the primary challenge to treatment and management.

People with FAS/FAE, like everyone else, have a variety of talents and capabilities. They exhibit a wide range of intellectual levels and functional disabilities that probably reflect differing sites and degrees of prenatal brain damage due to different levels, patterns, and timing of prenatal alcohol exposure and individual differences in mothers and offspring. Despite their wide array of talents and abilities, many people with FAS exhibit some of the same general behavioral characteristics. They are usually trusting (even overly trusting), loving, and naive despite their years. They can also be grumpy, irritable, and rigid. As a result of their prenatal brain damage, they may have difficulty, especially as they mature, in evaluating a situation and using their past experiences to cope with the problems at hand. They seem to need more protection, supervision, and structure for a longer period of life than usual. Individuals with both FAS and FAE also vary widely in their ultimate outcomes and in the number of secondary disabilities that they acquire as they mature. In 1996, research from the University of Washington indicated that these secondary disabilities become more and more observable in people with FAS/FAE as they mature (Streissguth, Barr, Kogan, & Bookstein, 1996). Extremely high rates of mental illness as well as high rates of disrupted school experiences, trouble with the law, and alcohol and other drug problems are alarming. These secondary disabilities can be as debilitating as the primary disability—the brain damage—with which they were born. Many individuals with FAS/FAE need ongoing help across the life span—anything from a protective environment to a trusted friend, spouse, or advocate to help them stay grounded and focused.

Research, however, has also shown that there are risk and protective factors associated with these secondary disabilities. In other words, there are things that families and communities can do that can truly make a difference in what happens to children with FAS/FAE as they mature. But orchestrating these (i.e., mobilizing the protective factors and diminishing the risk factors) hinges on understanding the cause of the child's problems (i.e., getting a diagnosis).

PROBLEMS WITH GETTING A DIAGNOSIS

A diagnostic evaluation is the starting point for understanding, treating, and managing any medical condition. Yet, surprisingly, despite 2 decades of research and clinical observations, it remains difficult for families to find diagnosticians and clinicians specializing in FAS/FAE. An appropriate diagnosis and an understanding of that diagnosis can help families set realistic expectations, plan for some successes in their children's lives, and build a network of support and structure (see the discussion of an advocacy network in Part III). Diagnostic information about FAS not only helps people to better understand the syndrome's accompanying challenges but also facilitates appropriate treatment, intervention, and planning.

Experienced parents and teachers know that the everyday behaviors of children with FAS/FAE can be "unexpected," "perplexing," and even "unusual." Yet, because these particular behaviors have not yet been clearly linked to structural anomalies in the human brain and because they have not yet been described in the authoritative listing of mental disorders (*Diagnostic and Statistical Manual of Mental Disorders, Fourth Edition* [DSM-IV], American Psychiatric Association [APA], 1994), many professionals do not yet have the nomenclature to fully understand the syndrome and its implications or really "hear" what parents are saying. Although the field has grown dramatically since the mid-1980s, much confusion still exists, and there remains a gap between scientific knowledge and general clinical information. Often, parents have had to advocate for children whom they suspected had been prenatally affected by alcohol—searching out diagnosticians willing to diagnose this often unheard-of condition, searching out teachers willing to be instructed in appropriate educational methods, and searching out mental health and social services professionals willing to offer their children the extra support and understanding their condition requires.

As I was packing for an extended trip, the frantic mother of a 16-year-old boy with FAS called. She and her husband had just returned from a parent conference with Max's school psychologist. According to her report, the psychologist had indeed heard of FAS, but he thought that children with FAS simply had mental retardation. Therefore, he concluded after examining this adolescent that Max couldn't possibly have FAS because with a performance IQ well into the normal range and a verbal IQ at the lower end of normal, he clearly wasn't mentally retarded. Furthermore, the psychologist was positive that Max had only attention-deficit/hyperactivity disorder and a conduct disorder and warned his parents against putting labels such as FAS on him because they would thwart his development.

The mother begged me to give Max some test that would prove that their son had the brain damage associated with FAS, so that he could get the help and support they knew he needed. Although we did work out a plan, her quest has no easy solution. The tests have not yet been developed, and the research has not yet been done. Understanding the personal consequences of FAS/FAE on children and families and on society at large should accelerate both prevention and intervention efforts once the magnitude of the problem is recognized.

INCIDENCE OF FAS

It is important to outline what is known about prenatal alcohol exposure, which causes FAS/FAE. Alcohol is a teratogen (i.e., any agent or chemical that causes a birth defect). In fact, alcohol is the most frequently ingested teratogen in the world. Alcohol is an addictive but entirely legal drug. According to the Assistant Secretary of Health and Human Services (National Institute on Alcohol Abuse and Alcoholism [NIAAA], 1990), more than 10 million adults in the United States are addicted to alcohol. An additional 7 million abuse alcohol but are not addicted. Many of these 17 million are women in their childbearing years.

Thousands of experiments with laboratory animals have shown conclusively that alcohol can cause birth defects in almost any species, even when it is not coupled with other drug use. Among humans, prenatal alcohol exposure can and does affect children of all races and socioeconomic backgrounds. Researchers at the IOM (1996) estimate that between 0.5 and 3.0 of every 1,000 infants are  born with some degree of FAS. (For additional information, see Cordero, Floyd, Martin, Davis, & Hymbaugh, 1994; Dehaene, 1995; Dehaene et al., 1991; May, Hymbaugh, Aase, & Samet, 1983; NIAAA, 1990.) If this estimate is accurate, 2,000–12,000 of the projected 4 million children born in the United States each year will have FAS.

The most accurate estimates of incidence come from a small number of studies that used expert diagnosticians. Large variations can exist from one study population to another, depending on the rate of maternal alcohol abuse and the study design. The NIAAA (1990) estimated that 1.9 in every 1,000 children are born with FAS or ARND, a rate that is nearly double the incidence of Down syndrome and almost five times that of spina bifida, two of the most commonly recognized birth defects. The NIAAA (1990) also estimated that FAE (as a clinical categorization) occurs three times more often than FAS.

On some Indian reservations, where alcohol abuse is common among women, FAS has been reported in 1 in 100 children (May et al., 1983). In one small Native American community, the incidence of FAS was 1 in 8 (Robinson, Conry, & Conry, 1987). At that frequency, FAS is a community catastrophe that threatens to wipe out any culture in just a few generations. However, FAS is not a Native American problem or a problem of poverty per se. It is an *alcohol* problem, and it is *our* problem.

Because it is caused by alcohol, FAS is completely preventable. Yet, it continues to swell the ranks of people with mental retardation. In fact, FAS is the most common known cause of mental retardation (NIAAA, 1987). In one large study conducted throughout Sweden, more cases of mental retardation resulted from alcohol-related birth defects than from all known genetic causes of mental retardation combined (Hagberg, Hagberg, Lewerth, & Lindberg, 1981).

PROBLEMS WITH STUDYING FAS POPULATIONS

Studying children affected by alcohol involves special problems. Alcohol is a legal drug, openly sold and advertised throughout the United States. Alcohol is primarily a social drug. It is used in American society to celebrate or commemorate every occasion from marriage to death. Just as the alcoholic often uses denial to ward off awareness of impending alcoholism, society seems to use denial to avoid facing the fact that alcohol can be damaging to the next generation. It is more comfortable and easier to wage a war on illegal drugs than to face the not-so-hidden dangers that alcoholic beverages pose to the fetus.

To further complicate the issue, infants and children with FAS/FAE often appear physically quite "normal," which can prevent them from obtaining the help and services they need. Unlike many birth defects, which are identified at birth and often treated surgically, FAS and FAE are usually overlooked at birth and treated later by community professionals—often unknowingly. Because damage to the brain can occur at lower doses of alcohol than those that produce gross physical anomalies or low birth weights, the brain is the organ in the body most vulnerable to the effects of prenatal alcohol. Unfortunately, we don't yet have the technology to see the brain in living people in a manner that distinguishes the subtle disruptions that shape our misperceptions and guide our maladaptive responses.

In fact, the individual features of FAS are subtle enough that many people with this birth defect pass through life undiagnosed.

Certainly, most occurrences of FAS are not recorded on birth certificates, making it useless to try to obtain these data from the usual birth defects surveillance registries that were set up to measure major congenital defects (e.g., club foot, cleft lip or palate). Consider for a moment the difficulty in detecting these subtle features in a newborn in the midst of a busy urban obstetric practice, especially when there is little time to talk with mothers about their drinking. Little and colleagues (1990) have shown a 100% failure rate in detecting FAS in one of the largest maternity hospitals in the country. Unless occurrences of FAS/FAE are associated with gross physical malformations, they often remain undetected in the newborn baby.

FAS and FAE are usually "hidden" birth defects that primarily affect the brain, conditions about which neither medical science nor society has much understanding beyond the general awareness that heavy prenatal alcohol use is bad for the outcome of pregnancy. For example, the 1990 National Health Survey of more than 13,000 representative respondents found that although 89%–92% of all women knew that heavy drinking during pregnancy could increase the chances of miscarriages, mental retardation, low birth weight, and birth defects, only 29% of women of childbearing age could correctly identify FAS as a type of birth defect. Most thought it meant being born addicted to alcohol (Dufour, Williams, Campbell, & Aitken, 1994).

The effects of FAS are difficult to fathom—subtle disruptions in the proliferation and migration of the brain cells that provide the architecture for later problem solving and subtle deviations in the neurochemical balance that permits the transport of messages from one part of the brain to another. When these processes are disrupted, it is difficult to store, retrieve, and transform past experiences into knowledge in order to modify future behaviors—a source of great frustration for those with FAS and a cause of dysfunctional and maladaptive behaviors.

Dysfunctional behavior is difficult to treat effectively, even when its causes are understood. When dysfunctional behavior occurs in children with undiagnosed FAS/FAE, the cause remains unknown and the children's behavior remains an enigma. As a result, the problem behaviors of people with alcohol-related birth defects are being regularly dealt with in schools, community mental health centers, and alcohol and other drug abuse treatment programs as well as through juvenile justice and adult corrections facilities. By failing to diagnose these people as having FAS/FAE and by failing to understand that their unpredictable and often bizarre behaviors stem from the organic brain damage with which they were born, human services providers run the risk of actually causing more of the problem behaviors they are trying to ameliorate.

Much research is needed, particularly on recommended practices for treatment, education, job training, and management; policy change is also needed to reduce barriers to existing services that people with FAS/FAE need but for which they often do not qualify. Every dollar spent on education, prevention, and intervention will reap benefits in future savings. Once the problem is fully understood, effective action is possible. Already, much is known that can benefit the lives of people with FAS/FAE and their families; there is no need for families or communities to wait another minute before putting this knowledge into action. This book seeks to provide the understanding necessary for effective action.

OVERVIEW OF SECTIONS

Preview of Part I: The Diseases of Fetal Alcohol

In most communities around the United States, it is far too difficult to obtain a diagnostic evaluation. This is a huge obstacle to prevention, effective intervention planning, and community awareness and understanding. Part I of this book provides an overview of the spectrum of effects related to prenatal alcohol exposure. Chapter 2 describes the diagnostic process, including the importance of taking relevant prenatal alcohol histories. Chapter 3 gives a brief overview of the remarkable progress of a 25-year period of history in which the country moved from the initial awareness that prenatal alcohol exposure could damage the fetus to scientific validation of alcohol as a teratogen and to the development of an effective and appropriate public policy for prevention.

Preview of Part II: The Science of Fetal Alcohol Syndrome

Part II describes the research evidence produced during the 25-year period in which much of the mystery surrounding FAS/FAE was resolved. Chapter 4 explains why alcohol is a teratogenic drug and reviews the magnificent body of animal studies that have documented the teratogenic properties of alcohol and how these are relevant to the human condition. Chapter 5 documents the impact of alcohol on children, reviewing studies on children born to alcoholic mothers in countries around the world and the impact of alcoholism on families (including fathers and the mothers themselves). It also reviews the population-based studies on the effects on children whose mothers drank socially during pregnancy, especially focusing on the neurobehavioral findings. Chapter 6 describes research on the organic brain damage (the primary disability of FAS) caused by fetal alcohol exposure and the latest findings from a 1996 study of the largest group of people with FAS/FAE ever evaluated. Data on the frequency of secondary disabilities in people with FAS/FAE are useful to parent and community leaders in planning interventions and providing services for this population. For the first time, data are now available on environmental factors that increase the risk of these adverse secondary disabilities as well as those conditions (e.g., an early diagnosis, a stable and nurturing home, appropriate services) that "protect" individuals against secondary disabilities.

Preview of Part III: A Life-Span Approach to Fetal Alcohol Syndrome

Part III presents a life-span look at FAS/FAE, based on data from clinical observations and from the reflections of individuals with FAS/FAE themselves and their parents and caregivers. Chapter 7 describes characteristics and needs of people with FAS/FAE from infancy to childhood. It also gives recommendations for helping people with FAS/FAE and lays to rest some common misperceptions. Chapter 8 describes the advocacy model for helping people with FAS/FAE, answering such questions as, What is an advocate? Who can be an advocate? What makes an advocate successful? and How can effective advocacy prevent or improve secondary disabilities? Chapter 9 is about families, including biological, adoptive, and foster families—virtually anyone involved in raising an individual with FAS/FAE. In telling their own stories, the families express their needs. Community leaders and service providers can learn much from these families in terms of interacting with and designing interventions for people with FAS/FAE.

Preview of Part IV: Preparing People with FAS for Life in the Community

Part IV is about preparing people with FAS/FAE for life in the community. Chapter 10 describes how families can begin early in planning for healthy lives for their young children with FAS/FAE and developing the support systems that communities must have in place in order to respond to the needs of these patients and their families. Chapter 11 gives specific recommendations for school districts and educators in meeting the challenges presented by students with FAS/FAE. A 10-step school plan for students suspected of having FAS/FAE is described, along with guidelines for incorporating the advocacy model into educational plans. Chapter 12 presents strategies for effective management of people with FAS/FAE as they come under the jurisdiction of community institutions providing social services, namely, corrections and juvenile justice, alcohol and drug treatment, and mental health treatment programs. Guidelines are given for screening individuals for FAS/FAE at intake and developing an effective management or treatment plan are provided as are guidelines for after-care and continuing case management and advocacy.

Preview of Part V: Preventing Fetal Alcohol Damage

Part V deals with preventing FAS and FAE, a vital concern for all communities. Effective strategies for educating the public, training professionals, and changing public policy are described in Chapter 13 (see Figure 1.2). The Surgeon General issued a warning on alcohol and pregnancy in 1981, recommending that women refrain from alcohol consumption when pregnant or planning a pregnancy. Chapter 14 presents effective programs to intervene with mothers who abuse alcohol and other drugs during pregnancy. There is even a way to help those who do not obtain prenatal care.

Flying home from a trip, a beautiful older woman seated beside me inquired about my work. When I told her that I was writing a book on FAS, she said she'd never heard of it. As I explained more about FAS, she became intensely interested, asking very perceptive questions. Finally she said, "Well, that must be what's wrong with Carol!"

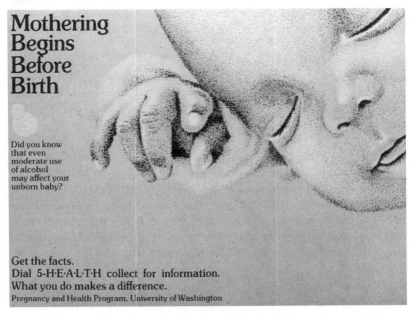

Figure 1.2. Bus sign from the Pregnancy and Health Program, Seattle, Washington, 1978. (From Washington State Liquor Control Board; reprinted by permission.)

"Who's Carol?" I asked.

She told me this story: *"When my husband and I were young, our three children grew up very closely with the three adopted children of our best friends. Carol was the middle child of those three adopted children. From the start, Carol seemed different—as though she were born irritable. She was never a 'bad kid'; she just never seemed to 'get it.' When she was older, she researched her biological family and learned that both parents were alcoholics. Now all of the children are in their 50s, and she's the only one who just never got her life together. She got married all right and had three children, but the marriage fell apart, and now my friends, the grandparents, are raising her three children. Carol can never hold a job—she just goes from one thing to another, always talking these big pipe dreams about what she's going to do but never does. . . ."*

As she spoke, my mind drifted to Johnny, one of my former patients who was fortunate to have been examined at age 3 by David Smith and diagnosed as having FAS. The diagnostic information about FAS, coupled with his own good sense and compassion, was enough to keep Johnny's father (who had custody of him) constantly vigilant to Johnny's needs at every age. The first thing he did was to find "Miss Pearl," an amazing special-needs preschool teacher who worked exclusively with Johnny at first, and later with a handful of other children, to help Johnny find alternate routes to learning in order to work around his cognitive disabilities. It was a long, hard road, but the knowledge he gained after learning of the FAS diagnosis helped him to be able to understand how the world of first grade must have looked to feisty little Johnny when he bit and scratched at kids who teased him when he couldn't remember his lessons.

Now Johnny is a grown man with a fairly responsible job in the armed services. Recently, I met with Johnny and his father, who smiled modestly at Johnny's success. The two explained to me that one of the virtues of his current job is a system of checks and balances: Although Johnny checks on the work of others, there are also people above him checking on his work.

"A lot of the credit goes to Johnny," his father said. "He's really pulled himself up. He's developed a system for doing what he calls 'work arounds.' Because he thinks he's wired a certain way that is different from other people, he finds ways to 'work around' his problems."

Johnny explained, "Everybody's wired one way or another—it's like my brain's not in the same order as everybody else's. It's like I'm wired differently. Most people think in terms of a-b-c-d. I think a-g-y-b-x-c. I have to take a different route to get there. My route takes me longer but doesn't mean I can't get there. It's like I learn slower. I can't remember eight numbers; maybe I can do only four or five. But I just use a Post-It note. I find a way to solve the problem; I write it all down. I had to learn how to do lots of abbreviations to write it all down."

When I asked Johnny what he'd like me to tell other families about raising people with FAS/FAE, he said, "People like me need lots of love and sup-

port and a good moral system. Teach us right and wrong and build us a web of support and good friends, trusted people we can easily call to back us up. Besides love and attention, we need someone sitting down and telling us when we've done something wrong. Focus on what makes us feel good about ourselves. Self-confidence is a real problem; so is hypersensitivity. Create your personality so you can be like a sponge and a mirror: A mirror to reflect away the things you don't want to become part of yourself, the bad things, and a sponge to soak in the good things that will help you."

Carol's home life was probably as stable as Johnny's (maybe even more so, as Carol had two loving parents), but Johnny was raised knowing the cause of his dysfunctional behavior. His father realized that his actions were a call for help, the manifestation of a subtle birth defect of the brain that required some special planning and support. Working with families like Johnny's over so many years has taught me how effective parents can be as advocates when they're properly informed of the child's diagnosis at an early age and encouraged to put that into the perspective of their own child's individuality.

. . . I returned from my reverie when she stopped talking. "Yes," I replied, "it's a sadly familiar story. That's why I'm writing this book."

REFERENCES

American Psychiatric Association (APA). (1994). *Diagnostic and statistical manual of mental disorders* (4th ed.). Washington, DC: Author.

Cordero, J.F., Floyd, R.L., Martin, M.L., Davis, M., & Hymbaugh, K. (1994). Tracking the prevalence of FAS. *Alcohol Health and Research World, 18*(1), 82–85.

Dehaene, P. (1995). La grossesse et l'alcool [Alcohol and Pregnancy]. *Que Sais-Je?*, 2934. Paris: Presses Universitaires de France.

Dehaene, Ph., Samaille-Villette, C., Boulanger-Fasquelle, P., Subtil, D., Delahousse, G., & Crépin, G. (1991). Diagnostic et prévalence du syndrome d'alcoolisme fœtal en maternité [Diagnosis and prevalence of fetal alcohol syndrome]. *Presse Médicale, 20*, 1002.

Dufour, M.C., Williams, G.D., Campbell, K., & Aitken, S. (1994). Knowledge of FAS and the risks of heavy drinking during pregnancy, 1985 and 1990. *Alcohol Health and Research World, 18*(1), 86–92.

Hagberg, B., Hagberg, G., Lewerth, A., & Lindberg, U. (1981). Mild mental retardation in Swedish school children: I. Prevalence. *Acta Paediatrica Scandinavica, 70*, 441–444.

Institute of Medicine (IOM), Stratton, K.R., Howe, C.J., & Battaglia, F.C. (Eds.). (1996). *Fetal alcohol syndrome: Diagnosis, epidemiology, prevention and treatment.* Washington, DC: National Academy Press.

Little, B.B., Snell, L.M., Rosenfeld, C.R., Gilstrap, L.C., & Gant, N.F. (1990). Failure to recognize fetal alcohol syndrome in newborn infants. *American Journal of Diseases of Children, 144*(10), 1142–1146.

May, P.A., Hymbaugh, K.J., Aase, J.M., & Samet, J.M. (1983). Epidemiology of fetal alcohol syndrome among American Indians of the Southwest. *Social Biology, 30*(4), 374–387.

National Institute on Alcohol Abuse and Alcoholism (NIAAA). (1987). *Sixth special report to the U.S. Congress on alcohol and health.* Washington, DC: U.S. Department of Health and Human Services.

National Institute on Alcohol Abuse and Alcoholism (NIAAA). (1990, January). *Seventh special report to the U.S. Congress on alcohol and health.* (From the Secretary of Health and Human Services, U.S. Department of Health and Human Services, DHHS Publication No. [ADM] 90-1656.) Washington, DC: U.S. Government Printing Office.

Robinson, G.C., Conry, J.L., & Conry, R.F. (1987). Clinical profile and prevalence of fetal alcohol syndrome in an isolated community in British Columbia. *Canadian Medical Association Journal, 137,* 203–207.

Streissguth, A.P., Barr, H.M., Kogan, J., & Bookstein, F.L. (1996). *Understanding the occurrence of secondary disabilities in clients with fetal alcohol syndrome (FAS) and fetal alcohol effects (FAE): Final report to the Centers for Disease Control on Grant No. RO4/CCR008515* (Tech. Report No. 96-16). Seattle: University of Washington, Fetal Alcohol and Drug Unit.

Surgeon General's Advisory on Alcohol and Pregnancy. (1981). *FDA Drug Bulletin, 11*(2), 9–10. Rockville, MD: U.S. Department of Health and Human Services.

2

Diagnosing Fetal Alcohol Syndrome

It was January of 1973. I was examining the daughter of a majestic African American mother. "This puny little runt," she said disdainfully of her tiny child who raced about the room, "doesn't even seem to know how to nurse. I've had six other kids. They all knew what to do. I can tell you," she exclaimed, "there's something wrong with this one!"

Experienced mothers often do know that there is "something wrong" with children with fetal alcohol syndrome (FAS). Although they may have a hard time specifying the exact nature of the problem, they often sense that something is just not right, as in the case of this young girl whose mother began abusing alcohol later in life after bearing six healthy and unaffected children. There was indeed "something wrong" with this child—she had FAS. Her poor suckling ability was only one of the many manifestations of central nervous system (CNS) damage caused by alcohol. Her mother's alcohol abuse would leave this child with mental retardation—unable to care for herself long after her beautiful mother was dead of alcoholism.

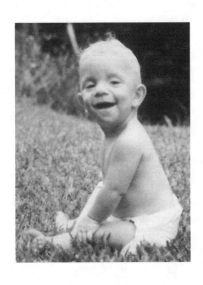

Alcohol can have a direct toxic effect on the rapidly developing cells of the embryo and fetus. Prenatal alcohol exposure can damage the developing embryo and fetus in many different ways, causing a whole spectrum of effects. In a broad sense, this damage is referred to as "prenatal effects of alcohol" or as "fetal alcohol effects." Some of these effects are observable in the newborn baby (e.g., poor suckling ability, heart defects, low birth weight). Others, however, are detectable only within the framework of an appropriate developmental stage or a specific environment. For example, hyperactivity is contingent on walking ability; attentional and learning problems become apparent in the classroom.

Most individual fetal alcohol effects are not unique to alcohol in the sense that only alcohol can cause them. But they are justifiably called "fetal *alcohol* effects" because research has shown that prenatal alcohol exposure significantly increases the rate of their occurrence. In fact, a large body of scientific literature, including experimental studies with laboratory animals, case/control studies of children of alcoholic mothers, and well-controlled epidemiological studies with large cohorts of children, has substantiated the existence of many specific fetal alcohol effects that can be traced to prenatal alcohol in both experimental animal studies and in studies on groups of children (see Chapters 3–6).

When certain fetal alcohol effects cluster in a specific way, in a given individual, and in a way that is *unique* to alcohol, it is called FAS. These features are growth deficiency, a specific pattern of facial features, and some CNS damage. FAS involves a specific *pattern* of fetal alcohol effects occurring in unison, a pattern of features that has not, as a group, been associated with any other prenatal condition.

FETAL ALCOHOL SYNDROME

FAS, a birth defect caused by prenatal exposure to alcohol, is diagnosed when children meet the following three criteria:

1. Growth deficiency, prenatally or postnatally, for height or weight or both
2. A specific pattern of minor anomalies that includes a characteristic face, generally defined as short palpebral fissures (eye slits), a flat midface, a short upturned nose, a smooth or a long philtrum (the ridges running between the nose and the lips), and a thin upper lip
3. Some CNS damage, including microcephaly (small size of the brain), tremors, hyperactivity, fine or gross motor problems, at-

tentional deficits, learning disabilities, intellectual or cognitive impairments, or seizures. Mental retardation and developmental delays also qualify as CNS criteria but, like the other single items listed here, are not necessary for diagnosis. (Table 2.1 provides a more complete list of the range of CNS effects observed in individuals with FAS at various ages.)

A diagnosis of FAS also requires some presumed history of significant prenatal alcohol exposure. In 1996, the Institute of Medicine (IOM, Stratton, Howe, & Battaglia, 1996) suggested two classifications of FAS: one with and one without confirmed maternal alcohol exposure.

DOCUMENTING EXPOSURE

In reaching a determination that an individual has been affected by fetal alcohol exposure, two pieces of information are necessary: an examination of the individual and some historical information relative to prenatal alcohol exposure. Except in unusual circumstances, both are necessary. Of the two, the exposure history is often the most difficult to obtain. Taken months or years after the exposure actually took place, in many cases the informant is actually a foster or adoptive parent, a social services worker, or even the adult with FAS. Because some women drink at a level that is harmful for their fetuses without

Table 2.1. CNS structural and functional effects by age that can be alcohol related

Age	Effects
Newborn:	Microcephaly, jitteriness, opisthotonus (hyperextension of body with arched back) seizures, tremors, weak suck, unpredictable and disrupted sleep/wake cycles, hypotonia, hypertonia, poor state regulation, decreased vigorous bodily activity, hyperacusis (low hearing threshold), failure to thrive (given adequate opportunity), poor habituation (difficulty tuning out redundant stimuli), EEG abnormalities
Infancy:	Delayed development in one or more area, head banging and/or body rocking, poor fine motor or gross motor control, neurological dysfunction (including cerebral palsy)
Preschool:	Hyperactivity, poor eye–hand coordination, poor balance, poor tandem gait, central auditory dysfunction, delayed or perseverative language, mental retardation
Early school age:	Attentional impairments, learning disabilities, arithmetic disabilities, specific cognitive disabilities, deficits in higher order receptive and expressive language, poor impulse control
Later school age and adolescence:	Memory impairments, difficulties with judgment, difficulties with abstract reasoning, poor adaptive functioning

Sources: Bingol et al., 1987; Church, 1996; Clarren & Smith, 1978; Hanson, Streissguth, & Smith, 1978; Ioffe & Chernick, 1988; Jones, Smith, Ulleland, & Streissguth, 1973; Streissguth, Aase, et al., 1991; Streissguth, Bookstein, Sampson, & Barr, 1993.

Note: Items are listed at the age at which they might be observed for the first time.

acknowledging alcohol problems themselves, and because women taking illicit drugs may downplay their alcohol use, it is important to ask about alcohol use patterns (especially binge drinking and peak drinks per occasion) as well as about alcohol problems. Figure 2.1 is provided, which indicates that a standard "drink" of most alcoholic beverages contains about the same amount of absolute alcohol.

Studies show that many women lose their appetite for alcohol after their pregnancy is well established and spontaneously decrease alcohol use as pregnancy progresses (Little, Schultz, & Mandell, 1976). Therefore, it is important to ask about alcohol use and binge drinking not only during the pregnancy but also during the general period of time before the pregnancy. These boundaries get blurry with time, and different techniques of retrospectively establishing prenatal alcohol exposure may be needed. In addition to collateral interviews, records from medical care, adoption, social services, and schools can all provide useful information. Figure 2.2 lists questions found to be useful in eliciting a retrospective alcohol exposure history. It may be that only a few of them are needed in a given situation.

As denial is a well-known accompaniment to alcohol abuse, a negative maternal report is not necessarily definitive. Furthermore, the absence of a notation about prenatal alcohol exposure in the medical records should not necessarily be interpreted to mean "no exposure." The clearer the documentation of exposure, the easier the diagnostic process will be. For diagnosing FAS or other alcohol-related effects, the IOM identifies "excessive" intake as "substantial regular intake or heavy episodic drinking" (IOM et al., 1996, p. 5).

THE DIAGNOSTIC PROCESS

Like other clinical birth defect syndromes, FAS can be diagnosed at birth (Jones & Smith, 1973) and is described in the recognized authoritative source, *Recognizable Patterns of Human Malformations* (Jones, 1988; Smith, 1982). FAS is also included in the *International Classification of Diseases* by the World Health Organization (1989) as Code 760.71. Yet, unlike most birth defects, it is often overlooked in newborns (Little, Snell, Rosenfeld, Gilstrap, & Gant,

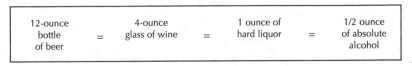

Figure 2.1. Alcohol equivalencies of common beverages. One serving each contains about the same amount of alcohol and has about the same effect on the fetus.

I. Alcohol/drug abuse history of biological mother
- Did the individual's mother have a problem with alcohol?
- Did the individual's mother ever receive treatment for an alcohol problem?
- Did the individual's mother have any alcohol-related health problems (e.g., liver cirrhosis)?
- Did the mother have any alcohol-related social or family problems?
- Did the mother have any alcohol-related job or legal problems?
- Did the mother ever receive a ticket for driving while intoxicated (DWI) or driving under the influence (DUI)?
- Did the mother use alcohol in conjunction with illegal drugs (e.g., cocaine)?
- Were people ever concerned about the mother's drinking?
- Did the mother ever try to cut down on her drinking?
- Did the mother take a drink when she got up in the morning?
- Did the mother say or do things when she was drinking that she was unable to remember later?

II. Alcohol use pattern of biological mother
- Was the individual's mother a binge drinker (i.e., consuming four or five or more alcoholic drinks on occasion)?
- Could the mother drink more than four or five drinks without falling asleep or passing out?
- Did the mother drink to get drunk, even if she only drank occasionally?
- Did the mother drink heavily and/or regularly? If yes, describe the nature of her use.

III. Red flags to obtain more information
- * Is there a family history of alcoholism or drug abuse?
- * Did the individual's father have a problem with alcohol?
- * Did the individual's mother start drinking quite young?
- * Did the individual's mother receive little or no prenatal care?
- * Did the individual's mother have a history of successively poorer pregnancy outcomes (e.g., low birth weight babies, miscarriages, stillbirths)?
- * Did the individual's mother relinquish the care of her children because she was unable to care for them?
- * Did the individual's mother have children removed from her home by authorities due to neglect or abuse?
- * Did the individual's mother have an early death?

IV. Questions for an adult regarding his or her own mother's alcohol abuse history (when no other source is available)
- * Do you think your biological mother had alcohol problems?
- * For how much of your life were you raised by your biological mother?

Figure 2.2.   Useful topics for a retrospective prenatal alcohol exposure history. Any one of the bulleted items is suggestive of a significant alcohol history; it is not necessary to ask all questions. After establishing a significant history, try to determine generally when this occurred in relation to the target pregnancy. Precise estimates of either exposure or timing are seldom possible retrospectively. Red flags (*) are useful for lead-ins or to indicate that further searching is warranted when the current source is not informative regarding an alcohol history.

1990). FAS is not diagnosed by the presence or absence of any single major malformation that would be recognizable at birth, although the frequency with which all major malformations appear is increased in children with FAS. (See Clarren & Smith, 1978, and

Jones, 1986, for a description of the range of malformations observed in individuals with FAS.)

The FAS diagnosis is made only by clinical examination; at this time, there are no confirming laboratory tests and no validated checklists. Thus, the diagnosis is dependent on the clinical expertise of the diagnostician. Traditionally, dysmorphologists or clinical geneticists are most skilled at detecting birth defects. However, many infants and children with FAS have been diagnosed and described in the medical literature by astute neonatologists, pediatricians, and others who may work with populations at high risk for FAS. Although FAS is definitely not confined to the lower social classes, it is more visible there. Clinicians who work with the children of mothers who abuse alcohol—particularly in settings where poverty, poor housing, high unemployment, and alcohol and other drug abuse are rampant—have surely seen people of all ages with FAS. But seeing is not recognizing. The clues to recognition lie in a subtle interplay of physical and psychosocial characteristics, maternal alcohol history, and the child's own behavioral history. The initial recognition of FAS for an individual clinician often involves the "A ha" phenomenon:

I can still remember bracing myself for the experience the first time I spoke with a patient about having FAS. After rehearsing the words in my mind, I finally spoke them aloud to a sweet child of about 12 years. I'll never forget her engaging smile and ingenuous manner as she exclaimed, "Oh, is that what I've got? I always knew I had something, but I never knew what!"

Often after a lecture I've given in which I've shown slides of people with FAS and described their behaviors, someone from the audience will tell me "Why, I've seen people who were just like that—I just never knew what they had!"

The diagnostician is an extremely important part of the diagnostic process. In *Diagnostic Dysmorphology*, Jon Aase (1990) likened the process of diagnosing birth defect syndromes to the work of a detective—every available physical clue must be examined, along with the testimony of witnesses. As in all clinical diagnoses, FAS necessitates that the clinician possess the ability to perform a painstaking physical examination and to obtain a meticulous history, both of which are usually highly complicated in cases of FAS.

The "painstaking physical exam" involves not only what the diagnostician sees in terms of the size, positioning, and subtle interrelationships of minor physical anomalies, but also what significance the diagnostician attributes to them in relation to the pattern of FAS features. It is, therefore, valuable to obtain a diagnosis from someone who has had specific experience with birth defects syndromes in general and with FAS in particular. To assist diagnosticians, Aase (1994b) has developed a useful video on the FAS diagnosis, and Astley and Clarren (1997) have produced a screening guide.

The "meticulous history" involves not only the history of the child's development in the postnatal period but, more important, the history of prenatal alcohol exposure, which is woefully underreported in most intake settings. Obtaining brief histories for each member of the family, particularly for those who have had difficulties with alcohol, is also important. Sometimes the mother of a child with FAS has FAS herself (see Grant, Ernst, Streissguth, & Porter, 1997), which may have major implications for her parental coping skills and complicate the examination and diagnosis. If both mother and child are affected by prenatal alcohol, they both may have short stature or learning disabilities and attentional deficits. This may mislead the diagnostician into thinking of possible genetic influences on the child rather than teratogenic influences on both—a big mistake in terms of prevention and intervention.

PHYSICAL FINDINGS IN FAS

The face has become the hallmark of FAS: the small eyes, the smooth philtrum, and the thin upper lip. In addition to these characteristics, several disproportions also give the FAS face its unique appearance. In fact, diagnosticians have increasingly emphasized the relationship *between* facial features. For example, not only the palpebral fissure lengths but also the inner canthal distance (the space between the eyes) are measured. In the typical face, the width of each eye slit is the same as the distance between the eyes. In individuals with FAS, the width of each eye slit is often smaller than the distance between the eyes. The length of the nose in relation to the midfacial length is another disproportion sometimes studied. In young children with FAS, the nose length may be short, only 50%–60% of the midfacial length, making the length of the philtrum proportionately longer. (See Aase, 1994a, and Clarren & Astley, 1995, for in-depth discussions of these relationships.)

In addition to these primary facial effects, there are secondary effects that also appear with increased frequency in the faces of people with FAS but do not carry the same diagnostic significance. For example, epicanthal folds (folds in the small flaps of skin that drape the inner corner of the eye) are present in many children with FAS but are also characteristic of most Asians and Native Americans.

Figure 2.3 depicts both the discriminating and the associated facial features of FAS.

Children with FAS also have an increased occurrence of other physical problems that can be traced to their prenatal alcohol exposure and can contribute to their overall disability. Additional eye anomalies can include ptosis (drooping eyelid), strabismus (deviation of the eye), and myopia (nearsightedness), as well as hypoplasia (underdevelopment) of the optic nerve and tortuosity (twistedness) of the retinal vessels and blindness. Strömland (1996) emphasizes the importance of the ophthalmologist in making the FAS diagnosis, noting that 90% of children with FAS have ocular signs or symptoms, of which optic nerve hypoplasia is the most frequent, reflecting the vulnerability of the CNS to alcohol exposure during embryonic and fetal development. The high occurrence of hearing disorders in children with FAS is associated with alcohol-induced developmental delays including sensorineural hearing loss, recurrent serous otitis media, and central auditory processing disorders associated with abnormalities of the brain stem, auditory cortex, or corpus callosum. Malaligned and misshapen secondary teeth are also common—all part of the early prenatal disruption of craniofacial development. (These characteristics are described in more detail in Church, 1996; Jones, 1986; Streissguth, Clarren, & Jones, 1985; and Strömland, Miller, & Cook, 1991.)

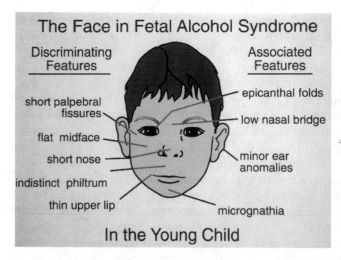

Figure 2.3. Diagram of FAS facial characteristics in young child. (From Streissguth & Little, 1994; reprinted by permission.)

Skeletal anomalies occur with increased frequency in children with FAS, particularly minor anomalies of the hands, fingers, toes, and arms. These include altered palmar crease patterns (longitudinal palmar creases and the "hockeystick" crease, in which there is an abrupt angulation of the distal transverse crease, exiting between the index and middle fingers); camptodactyly or clinodactyly (crooked fingers or shortened little finger); tapering fingers; and hypoplastic finger- and toenails. Some individuals with FAS experience limitation of movement in certain joints, including joint anomalies of the fingers and elbows and radioulnar synostosis (fusion of bones in the arm). Lemoine and Lemoine (1992) and Smith et al. (1981) demonstrated the usefulness of radiographic studies to detect these skeletal anomalies in individuals with FAS, but these usually are not part of a clinical diagnosis. In one study of 54 individuals with FAS in British Columbia and the Yukon Territory, radiographic studies revealed that 72% had tapering terminal phalanges (the last bone of the fingers), a finding that was not age related. Cervical spine abnormalities were found in 43% of individuals (Smith et al., 1981). Renal anomalies as well as anomalies of the genitals and thoracic cage also occasionally accompany FAS. (For further details, see Aase, 1994a; Clarren & Smith, 1978; Lemoine & Lemoine, 1992; and Smith et al., 1981.)

Heart defects occur in about 30% of the individuals with FAS, particularly ventricular septal defects. Although some of these are serious, others are reflected in heart murmurs that disappear spontaneously as the children mature (see Clarren & Smith, 1978; Dupuis et al., 1978; Jones, 1986; Smith et al., 1981; Streissguth et al., 1985).

AGE-RELATED CHANGES IN FAS FEATURES

When I hosted the National Institute on Alcohol Abuse and Alcoholism–funded International Workshop on FAS in Seattle in 1980, 49 scientists and clinicians from six countries came together for the first time to discuss their findings and their patients (see Streissguth et al., 1981, for selected papers). We all used different words and systems to describe the diagnostic process. For instance, David W. Smith from Seattle described his global clinical approach to diagnosing FAS, while Frank Majewski from Germany shared his scoring system based on a long list of associated characteristics. But when we projected the pictures of our patients onto the big screen, the children all looked alike. Blond, blue-eyed children from Sweden and Germany (where the FAS patients were all Caucasian) had FAS as clearly as our multi-ethnic children from Seattle. As we talked about the behaviors of our patients, we realized they also had similar behaviors. (In those days, they were almost all young children.) Even before the end of the first decade of clinical identification, there was unanimity among experienced clinicians about the clinical characteristics of FAS in young children.

Because the initial FAS diagnosis was based on the examinations of 11 children, all of whom were younger than 5 years, historically the characteristic "look" of FAS became immortalized as the face of the young child. As I watched these children grow in the 1970s, it became apparent that children outgrow the classic FAS face (as well as the FAS body). In the early days, caregivers of preschool and young school-age children with FAS commonly complained that they could not get their children with FAS "fattened up." The image of a rather emaciated child (the 8-year-old boy shown in the frontispiece is typical in this regard), reflecting significantly decreased adipose tissue, has become the hallmark physical phenotype for FAS. These features, however, may be characteristic only for the early stage of development (during infancy and early childhood). For young children, the growth deficiency for weight is most pronounced. For adolescents and adults, the growth deficiency for height (i.e., short stature) is often more pronounced.

As children with FAS approach puberty, they often gain a disproportionate and unexpected amount of body weight. Their faces, also, may undergo changes that make them appear less characteristic. Noses and chins can show disproportionate growth with the onset of puberty; changes have even been noted in the degree to which philtral ridges and thin upper lips are altered over time (Spohr, Willms, & Steinhausen, 1994; Streissguth et al., 1985). As individuals with FAS reach adulthood, they usually display a shortness of stature. In a study my colleagues and I conducted of 61 adolescents and adults (Streissguth, Aase, et al., 1991), only 16% of the individuals with FAS were within the normal range for height, but 25% were within the normal range for weight—some were actually overweight. In FAS, there is an extremely broad distribution in individuals' weight-to-height age percentiles, from 3% (very thin) to 98% (very heavy). The average weight-to-height age percentile for these adolescents and adults with FAS was 48%, whereas studies with younger children with FAS show a distribution of 1%–15%. (See the photographs on the section openers, which depict changes in facial dimensions and body shapes in five children with FAS/FAE as they grew; see also Majewski, 1993).

Changes in growth deficiency and facial features tend to obscure the classic FAS characteristics, which makes many diagnosticians cautious about diagnosing adolescents and adults. Childhood photographs are recommended as an accompaniment to the diagnostic evaluation in older people, but even these present difficulties as smiling faces can distort the appearance of the upper lip and philtrum. Other diagnostic problems that can be accentuated with age revolve around racial differences in facial phenotypes. African American children, because of their racial heritage, often do not have a thin upper lip; but the absence of this characteristic should not preclude a positive diagnostic evaluation.

FETAL ALCOHOL EFFECTS AND ALCOHOL-RELATED NEURODEVELOPMENTAL DISORDER

Alcohol's impact on embryonic and fetal development follows the principles of teratology and is influenced by the dose, timing, and conditions of exposure, as well as by the individual characteristics of both mother and offspring. Although it is widely recognized that prenatal alcohol exposure can cause a spectrum of prenatal alcohol effects, of which FAS is only a part, confusion surrounds the diagnosis and terminology of any effects that do not constitute full-blown FAS but are still observable in individual children (see Figure 2.4). In the last publication before his death, David W. Smith (1981) wrote, "One extremely important concept is to speak and to write of fetal alcohol effects rather than fetal alcohol syndrome. One finds every gradation from FAS to milder effects of alcohol on the developing fetus. Of greatest concern are the effects on brain development and function" (p. 127). If he had lived, he might have led the way to solving the conundrum of classification that has resisted resolution for more than 20 years: namely, how to clinically classify those individuals who are exposed to significant alcohol in utero and have clear CNS manifestations but lack the characteristic facial features or the growth deficiency of FAS.

Molly brought her daughter, Heather, in to see me because of her attentional problems, although she believed this lovely child didn't have FAS because she wasn't growth deficient and never had been. Heather had been a large baby at birth and now at 6 years was a strapping young girl, without a trace of the skinniness that often characterizes children with FAS at this age. Her head was normal in size, and she tested in the normal range on standardized IQ tests. She was talkative, bright-eyed, and charming—the apple of her mother's eye.

a 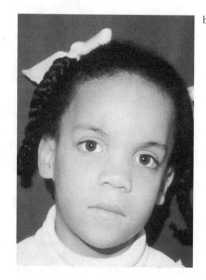 b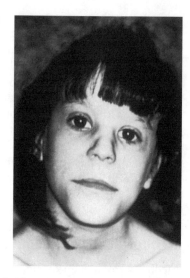

Figure 2.4.   Two girls born to alcoholic mothers. a) Girl without FAS and without growth deficiency whose mother stopped drinking early in life; b) girl with FAS (including classic facial features, microcephaly, and growth deficiency) whose mother drank heavily throughout pregnancy.

But Molly was an alcoholic, drinking heavily at the time she probably became pregnant. She had heard about FAS and stopped drinking altogether when she had a positive pregnacy test (see Chapter 13) and hadn't drunk since.

Molly said she knew her daughter didn't have FAS, not only because of the girl's size but because of her certainty that Heather wasn't mentally retarded. Her daughter was overactive, but Molly interpreted her daughter's sprightliness as a sign of vigor and her bright eyes and open manner as a sign of curiosity. It wasn't until Molly enrolled her daughter—whom she believed to be precocious—in kindergarten that she realized that Heather wasn't exactly like other children: There was a flightiness to her manner and a fleetingness to her attention spans that the other children didn't exhibit. What had seemed like an avid curiosity at home took on a quality of distractibility that prevented her from focusing on the simple kindergarten learning tasks at school, tasks that other children who seemed less "bright-eyed" were mastering without difficulty. A perplexed Molly knew her child didn't have FAS, but what did she have?

Since 1978, the term fetal alcohol effects (FAE) has been used to describe conditions that are presumed to be caused by prenatal alcohol exposure (Clarren & Smith, 1978; Hanson, Streissguth, & Smith, 1978) but do not follow the exact configuration of the three characteristics that uniquely identify FAS (growth deficits, CNS damage, and the distinctive pattern of facial anomalies). Typically, children with FAE are of normal size and have some but not all of the facial anomalies and CNS dysfunctions associated with FAS (see Figure 2.4 on page 28). Because there are no specific criteria for FAE, FAE is not officially recognized as a "diagnosis." In fact, the term has even been criticized (Aase, Jones, & Clarren, 1995). Nonetheless, FAE is widely used and has gained popularity among parents and clinicians, probably for lack of a better term.

The term possible fetal alcohol effects (PFAE) has also been suggested (Clarren & Smith, 1978). This term, however, presents its own problems, as it does not specify what the "possible" modifies—the "alcohol" or the "effects." It seems paradoxical to term some effects as possibly caused by alcohol in situations in which prenatal alcohol exposure is confirmed but the facial features are too subtle for an FAS diagnosis. And it seems unnecessary to refer to certain conditions as "possible effects," for, in most cases, the effects, however slight they may appear to be to clinicians, are what prompt families to bring their children into clinics to be diagnosed. When a diagnosis of PFAE is given, parents seem to drop the "possible" as soon as they leave clinic. However, it can become problematic if the official documents listing the word must be submitted as evidence for the need for services. Often, the "possible" serves as a major deterrent to appropriate service delivery. The term alcohol-related birth defects (ARBD) has also been suggested (Sokol & Clarren, 1989), but this has not proven clinically useful either, as it is also an umbrella term without specific criteria.

The IOM (IOM et al., 1996) suggested a five-category system to describe the spectrum of prenatal alcohol effects on offspring. In addition to "FAS" (Categories 1 and 2, with and without confirmed maternal alcohol exposure, respectively), a category of "partial FAS" (Category 3) is suggested, which includes confirmed exposure; evidence of some components of the pattern of characteristic facial anomalies; and one of the following: 1) "growth retardation; 2) evidence of CNS neurodevelopmental abnormalities (including decreased cranial size at birth, structural brain abnormalities, including microcephaly, and neurological hard or soft signs, such as impaired fine motor skills, neurosensory hearing loss, poor tandem gait, poor eye–hand coordination); or 3) evidence of a complex pattern of behavior or cognitive abnormalities that are inconsistent with developmental level and cannot be explained by familial background or environment alone, such as learning difficulties; deficits in school performance; poor impulse control; problems in social perception; deficits in higher-level receptive and expressive language; poor capacity for abstraction or metacognition; specific deficits in mathematical skills; or problems in memory, attention, or judgment" (p. 4). The IOM also suggests two additional diagnostic categories using the term "alcohol-related effects." Both categories require a history of maternal alcohol exposure and involve a clinical condition that has been linked to maternal alcohol ingestion in clinical or animal research. The first, "alcohol-related birth defects (ARBD)" (Category 4), includes a range of congenital anomalies (both malformations and dysplasias) including those described previously in this chapter. The other, "alcohol-related neurodevelopmental disorder (ARND)" (Category 5), includes criteria 2 and 3 from "partial FAS" (Category 3). For general purposes, the term FAE, as used in this book, includes IOM categories 3 and 5, "partial FAS" and "ARND."

MEASURING CNS DYSFUNCTION

Age-related changes in the physical phenotype of maturing children with FAS led some observers to suggest that the syndrome went away as the children grew older, which is simply not true. Like most birth defects, FAS is a lifetime condition. Growth and facial features are not really the essence of FAS—they are just early markers that, in combination with CNS effects, embody the constellation of features that characterize the syndrome. The real long-term disability in FAS is the CNS dysfunction—the brain damage—that compromises the development of the affected person. It is the identification of the CNS dysfunction that is critical in the diagnosis of the older individual, for whom the growth and facial features may be less noticeable.

One of the easiest aspects of CNS impairment to measure is head circumference. The exterior size of the head is produced by the growing brain and so is strongly correlated with the size of the brain. Microcephaly (small brain size) can be caused by prenatal alcohol exposure and is often noted in children with FAS; however, it is not a necessary condition for an FAS diagnosis. In one study, the average head circumference of adolescents and adults with FAS was almost 2 standard deviations below the age/sex norms (Streissguth, Aase, et al., 1991). Almost half of the group was identified as having microcephaly. Sometimes infants with FAS are not born with microcephaly but then do not undergo the typical postnatal brain growth spurt, which results in their being microcephalic by 8–12 months of age. Seizures or convulsions are also uncomplicated to measure but characterize only about 10% of individuals with FAS. Many of the CNS dysfunctions listed in Table 2.1 are assessed in clinical examination.

Another easily measured aspect of CNS development is an IQ score. In general, the IQ scores of individuals with FAS/FAE remain fairly stable from early childhood to adolescence and adulthood (Streissguth, Herman, & Smith, 1978; Streissguth, Randels, & Smith, 1991). However, IQ scores alone often fail to give an adequate picture of either organic brain damage or dysfunctional and maladaptive behaviors. Children with FAS who have IQ scores in the normal range can still have specific cognitive or neuropsychological impairments or problems with adaptive behaviors that do not register on IQ test scores. The demands of coping with real-life problems are both more complicated and more demanding of sustained attention than answering questions on an IQ test, particularly as one gets older and has less help and support from the community. Many neuropsychological, cognitive, and information-processing impairments associated with FAS/FAE have been assessed in a laboratory or a clinical context (Streissguth, 1986; see Chapter 6). At this time, however, no single type of CNS damage or pattern of dysfunction has been identified that characterizes all children with FAS/FAE.

Understanding these age-related changes in CNS functioning that accompany FAS/FAE will facilitate both the diagnostic examination and the care and nurturing of the child. Trying to define the essential CNS features of FAS/FAE is like taking aim at a moving target as our understanding of these concepts continues to evolve. Nevertheless, because understanding the cause of the disability is invaluable—both for prevention and for intervention—no effort should be spared in obtaining a diagnostic evaluation and using this to develop an appropriate action plan for each affected individual, regardless of age.

REFERENCES

Aase, J.M. (1990). *Diagnostic dysmorphology*. New York: Plenum.

Aase, J.M. (1994a). Clinical recognition of FAS: Difficulties of detection and diagnosis. *Alcohol Health and Research World, 18*(1), 5–9.

Aase, J.M. (1994b). *The clinical diagnosis of fetal alcohol syndrome* [Videotape]. (Available from Flora & Company Multimedia, P.O. Box 8263, Albuquerque, New Mexico 87198; 505-255-9988.)

Aase, J.M., Jones, K.L., & Clarren, S.K. (1995). Do we need the term "FAE"? *Pediatrics, 95*(3), 428–430.

Astley, S.J., & Clarren, S.K. (1997). Diagnostic guide for FAS and related conditions. Seattle: University of Washington. (Available by calling 206-526-2522.)

Bingol, N., Schuster, C., Fuchs, M., Iosub, S., Turner, G., Stone, R.K., & Gromisch, D.S. (1987). The influence of socioeconomic factors on the occurrence of fetal alcohol syndrome. *Advances in Alcohol and Substance Abuse, 6*(4), 105–118.

Church, M.W. (1996). The effects of prenatal alcohol exposure on hearing and vestibular function. In E.L. Abel (Ed.), *Fetal alcohol syndrome: From mechanism to prevention* (pp. 85–111). Boca Raton, FL: CRC Press.

Clarren, S.K., & Astley, S. (1995). A screening guide for fetal alcohol syndrome. (Sponsored by U.S. Department of Health and Human Services, U.S. Public Health Service, National Centers for Disease Control and Prevention, Cooperative Agreement U59-CCU006992-2 and Washington State Department of Health, Parent–Child Health Services.)

Clarren, S.K., & Smith, D.W. (1978). The fetal alcohol syndrome. *New England Journal of Medicine, 298*(19), 1063–1067.

Dupuis, C., Dehaene, P., Deroubaix-Tella, P., Blanc-Garin, A.P., Rey, C., & Carpenter-Courault, C. (1978). Les cardiopathies des enfants nés de mère alcoolique. *Archives des Maladies du Coeur et des Vaisseaux, 71*(5), 656–672.

Grant, T.M., Ernst, C.C., Streissguth, A.P., & Porter, J. (1997). An advocacy program for mothers with FAS/FAE. In A. Streissguth & J. Kanter (Eds.), *The challenge of fetal alcohol syndrome: Overcoming the secondary disabilities* (pp. 97–106). Seattle: University of Washington Press.

Hanson, J.W., Streissguth, A.P., & Smith, D.W. (1978). The effects of moderate alcohol consumption during pregnancy on fetal growth and morphogenesis. *Journal of Pediatrics, 92*(3), 457–460.

Ioffe, S., & Chernick, V. (1988). Development of the EEG between 30 and 40 weeks' gestation in normal and alcohol-exposed infants. *Developmental Medicine and Child Neurology, 30*, 797–807.

Institute of Medicine (IOM), Stratton, K.R., Howe, C.J., & Battaglia, F.C. (Eds.). (1996). *Fetal alcohol syndrome: Diagnosis, epidemiology, prevention and treatment.* Washington, DC: National Academy Press.

Jones, K.L. (1986). Fetal alcohol syndrome. *Pediatrics in Review, 8*, 122–126.

Jones, K.L. (1988). *Smith's recognizable patterns of human malformation* (4th ed.). Philadelphia: W.B. Saunders.

Jones, K.L., & Smith, D.W. (1973). Recognition of the fetal alcohol syndrome in early infancy. *Lancet, 2*(836), 999–1001.

Jones, K.L., Smith, D.W., Ulleland, C.N., & Streissguth, A.P. (1973). Pattern of malformation in offspring of chronic alcoholic mothers. *Lancet, 1*(815), 1267–1271.

Lemoine, P., & Lemoine, Ph. (1992). Avenir des enfants de mères alcooliques (étude de 105 cas retrouvés à l'âge adulte) et quelques constatations d'intérêt prophylactique. *Annales de Pédiatrie (Paris), 39*, 226–235.

Little, B.B., Snell, L.M., Rosenfeld, C.R., Gilstrap, L.C., & Gant, N.F. (1990). Failure to recognize fetal alcohol syndrome in newborn infants. *American Journal of Diseases of Children, 144*(10), 1142–1146.

Little, R.E., Schultz, F.A, & Mandell, W. (1976). Drinking during pregnancy. *Journal of Studies on Alcohol, 37*(3), 375–379.

Majewski, F. (1993). Alcohol embryopathy: Experience with 200 patients. *Developmental Brain Dysfunction, 6*, 248–265.

Smith, D.F., Sandor, G.G., MacLeod, P.M., Tredwell, S., Wood, B., & Newman, D.E. (1981). Intrinsic defects in the fetal alcohol syndrome: Studies on 76 cases from British Columbia and the Yukon Territory. *Neurobehavioral Toxicology and Teratology, 3*(2), 145–152.

Smith, D.W. (1981). Fetal alcohol syndrome and fetal alcohol effects. *Neurobehavioral Toxicology and Teratology, 3*, 127.

Smith, D.W. (1982). *Recognizable patterns of human malformation: Genetic, embryologic, and clinical aspects* (3rd ed.). Philadelphia: W.B. Saunders.

Sokol, R.J., & Clarren, S.K. (1989). Guidelines for use of terminology describing the impact of prenatal alcohol on the offspring. *Alcoholism: Clinical and Experimental Research, 13*(4), 597–598.

Spohr, H.L., Willms, J., & Steinhausen, H.C. (1994). The fetal alcohol syndrome in adolescence. *Acta Paediatrica, 404*, 19–26.

Streissguth, A.P. (1986). The behavioral teratology of alcohol: Performance, behavioral and intellectual deficits in prenatally exposed children. In J.R. West (Ed.), *Alcohol and brain development* (pp. 3–44). New York: Oxford University Press.

Streissguth, A.P., Aase, J.M., Clarren, S.K., Randels, S.P., LaDue, R.A., & Smith, D.F. (1991). Fetal alcohol syndrome in adolescents and adults. *Journal of the American Medical Association, 265*(15), 1961–1967.

Streissguth, A.P., Bookstein, F.L., Sampson, P.D., & Barr, H.M. (1993). *The enduring effects of prenatal alcohol exposure on child development: Birth through 7 years, a partial least squares solution.* Ann Arbor: University of Michigan Press.

Streissguth, A.P., Clarren, S.K., & Jones, K.L. (1985). Natural history of the fetal alcohol syndrome: A ten-year follow-up of eleven patients. *Lancet, 2*, 85–91.

Streissguth, A.P., Herman, C.S., & Smith, D.W. (1978). Stability of intelligence in the fetal alcohol syndrome: A preliminary report. *Alcoholism: Clinical and Experimental Research, 2*(2), 165–170.

Streissguth, A.P., & Little, R.E. (1994). *Alcohol, pregnancy, and the fetal alcohol syndrome: Unit 5. Biomedical education: Alcohol use and its medical consequences* (slide lecture series, 2nd ed.). Hanover, NH: Dartmouth Medical School, Project Cork. (Available by calling 1-800-432-8433.)

Streissguth, A.P., Noble, E.P., Randall, C.L., Rosett, H.L., Schenker, S., Smith, D.W., & Tabakoff, B. (Eds.). (1981). Fetal alcohol syndrome research: Selected papers from the fetal alcohol syndrome workshop, Seattle, Washington, May 2–4, 1980. *Neurobehavioral Toxicology and Teratology, 3*(2), 1–248.

Streissguth, A.P., Randels, S.P., & Smith, D.F. (1991). A test–retest study of intelligence in patients with the fetal alcohol syndrome: Implications for care. *Journal of the American Academy of Child and Adolescent Psychiatry, 30*(4), 584–587.

Strömland, K. (1996). Present state of the fetal alcohol syndrome. *Acta Ophthalmologica Scandinavica, 219*(Suppl.), 10–12.

Strömland, K., Miller, M., & Cook, C. (1991). Ocular teratology. *Survey of Ophthalmology, 35*(6), 429–446.

World Health Organization. (1989). *International classification of diseases: Vol. 1. Clinical modification* (9th Rev. ed.). Ann Arbor, MI: Commission on Professional and Hospital Activities.

3

From Awareness to Public Policy

Behold, thou shalt conceive and bear a son: and now drink no wine or strong drinks (Judges 13:7)

Foolish, drunken, and harebrained women most often bring forth children like unto themselves, morose and languid. (Aristotle)

A ritual that forbade the drinking of wine by the bridal couple so that a defective child would not be conceived. (Ancient Carthage)

Parental drinking is a cause of weak, feeble, and distempered children. (Report by the College of Physicians to the British Parliament, 1726)

Infants born to alcoholic mothers sometimes had a starved, shriveled, and imperfect look. (British House of Commons, 1834)

(These historical references are cited in Jones & Smith, 1973, and Warner & Rosett, 1975.)

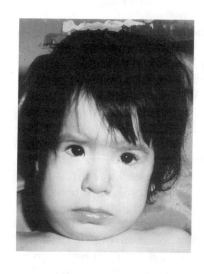

Since ancient times, people have warned of the dangers of drinking alcohol during pregnancy, perhaps without knowing the exact nature or reasoning of their cautions. Then, in a remarkable 25-year period, fetal alcohol syndrome (FAS) was recognized, named, and confirmed; a coherent body of scientific data surrounding the condition was assembled; and an appropriate public policy for prevention was established. Here's how it happened and what was achieved.

THE PATH TO CLINICAL RECOGNITION

Early Studies

At the turn of the 20th century, reports began to appear on children of alcoholics in many countries. For the most part, there was no attempt to localize the effect to one parent or another. In 1899, Dr. William Sullivan, a prison physician, published a study of 120 female "drunkards" at the Liverpool prison in Liverpool, England. He found that the pregnancies of these women resulted in stillbirths and infant deaths 2½ times more often than those of their sober female relatives. These rates, Sullivan found, were completely unrelated to paternal sobriety or the mothers' parental history of alcoholism. Sullivan believed these findings clearly contradicted a hereditary cause and instead pointed to maternal intoxication as the main source of damage to the fetus.

However, for the next few decades, Sullivan's brilliant early study on the direct effects of alcohol on the fetus was apparently largely unheeded. Only two out of hundreds of studies reviewed by Fretz (1931) in the 50-year interim between 1870 and 1930 appear to have even attempted to distinguish children of alcoholic mothers from those of alcoholic fathers. In 1910, Pearson and Elderton did note, after studying several hundred school children in Edinburgh, Scotland, that short stature was associated only with maternal, not paternal, alcoholism. In 1931, Fretz concluded, "The germ injurious effect of alcohol is accepted by most authors, doubted by some, and denied by a few" (p. 145). As late as 1942, alcoholism experts Haggard and Jellinek attributed the greater incidence of feeblemindedness, mental disorder, idiocy, and epilepsy found among offspring of alcoholics during the first half of the 20th century to the "poor stock" and social upheaval in alcoholic families. Only in the 1990s, in a startling revision of history, have researchers (the first was Karp, 1993; Karp, Quazi, Moller, Angelo, & Davis, 1995) demonstrated that the Kallikak children (see Figure 3.1)—who at the turn of the 20th century were used as examples of the hereditary nature of mental retar-

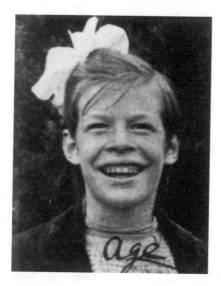

Figure 3.1.   Pauline "Kallikak." (From Karp, R.J. [Ed.]. [1993]. *Malnourished children in the United States: Caught in the cycle of poverty* [p. xxii]. New York, 10012: Springer Publishing Company, Inc.; reprinted by permission of the publisher.)

dation, poverty, and antisocial behavior (Goddard, 1912)—almost certainly had FAS and fetal alcohol effects (FAE).

In France, at the turn of the 20th century, Nicloux (1900) documented in dogs, sheep, and humans that alcohol consumed by a mother passed through to her milk and then on to her suckling offspring. In a turn-of-the-century doctoral thesis, Paul Ladrague (1901) reported from personal observation that alcoholic mothers had a high proportion of spontaneous abortions, weak and poorly developed infants, early infant demise and epilepsy, and idiocy among their children. He also presented 10 cases in which infants who were breast-fed by mothers or wet nurses who were alcoholic exhibited diarrhea, vomiting, extreme agitation, and convulsions. In all cases, the symptoms disappeared when the wet nurse was discharged or when nurse or mother curtailed her alcohol use (Ladrague, 1901). Almost 30 years later, Sullivan's (1899) results were replicated in Zurich, Switzerland. Offspring of female drinkers had twice as many spontaneous abortions and stillbirths and three times as great an infant mortality rate as offspring of nondrinking women. There were no such outcomes from drinking fathers (Boss, 1929). After another 30 years, a medical thesis from Paris described 100 foundling home children born to alcoholic mothers and fathers who had malformations very similar to those now recognized as constituting FAS (Rouquette, 1957). She concluded that maternal alcoholism, in particular, posed very grave dangers for the developing fetus and child.

Clinical Recognition: France and Seattle

In 1968, Dr. Paul Lemoine and co-workers in Nantes, France, described 127 children born to alcoholic mothers who exhibited a similar pattern of physical anomalies, growth deficiency, and problems of comportment (e.g., too lively, ceaselessly agitated, irritable). According to their report, which was published in a local French journal and not translated into English, these children also had very peculiar faces, especially in profile, including protruding foreheads; sunken nasal bridges; short, upturned noses; retracted upper lips; receding chins; and deformed ears (Lemoine, Harousseau, Borteyru, & Menuet, 1968).

In Seattle, in the late 1960s, work was under way at the King County Hospital on infants with "failure to thrive." A pediatric resident, Dr. Christy Ulleland, noted that there was one environmental factor shared by all of the infants: Each of their mothers was an alcoholic. The fact that these infants continued to fail to thrive even when hospitalized and given proper care suggested to Ulleland that the prenatal impact of the mothers' alcoholism might be a more significant factor in their failure to thrive than the actual care provided by the mothers after delivery. Through a medical records search, Ulleland identified 12 children of alcoholic mothers born within an 8-month period, all of whom had growth deficiencies at birth and later showed delayed development (Ulleland, 1972; Ulleland, Wennberg, Igo, & Smith, 1970), which further confirmed her suspicions.

In 1973, David W. Smith (who wrote the definitive text on recognizable patterns of human malformations [Smith, 1970, 1976] and is considered the "father of dysmorphology") saw one of the children in Ulleland's study. He was struck by the lad's unusual face, particularly his short palpebral fissures. He asked to see other children in Ulleland's study all at one time, and eight were brought in. When Smith and his dysmorphology fellow, Kenneth Lyons Jones, examined the eight children of alcoholic mothers, they identified four who looked very much alike and appeared to have the same condition. Quickly they searched their records and located three more similar-looking children—all of whom were also children of alcoholic mothers. By now they knew they were on to something. A short time later, Smith lectured in Ohio about this new condition, and colleagues produced another child of an alcoholic mother who looked like the seven in Seattle.

By June of 1973, a careful description of the constellation of physical features; growth deficiency; and intellectual, motor, and adaptive behavior impairments of these eight children of alcoholic mothers, whose appearance was so strikingly similar, was published in *Lancet,* an international medical journal (Jones, Smith, Ulleland, & Streissguth, 1973). This article brought worldwide attention to the condition as a birth defect. In a 25th anniversary publication commemorating the establishment of the National Institute on Alcohol Abuse and Alcoholism (NIAAA), Jones et al.'s article was listed as one of the 16 seminal papers in the field of alcohol studies, cited more than 1,000 times in the literature between 1973 and 1993 (Randall & Riley, 1994).

Later, in November 1973, Jones and Smith identified three more children of alcoholic mothers: a 7-month-old infant and two newborns, one who lived (see Figure 3.2) and one who died. The latter provided the remarkable first opportunity for direct examination of a baby with FAS whose brain (in autopsy) disclosed serious dysmorphogenesis. This paper also introduced the name "fetal alcohol syndrome" for this constellation of features. The name had the ring of authority. An expert in birth defects syndromes conferred this term, and alcohol seemed like a reasonable "causative agent": All 11 mothers in these first two papers had been consuming large quantities of alcohol during pregnancy, none of the children were related, they represented three racial groups, and they had no other recognizable pattern of malformation.

After the 1973 papers, Smith received a letter from Lemoine in France, congratulating Smith on his work on FAS and announcing his joy that his own work had been confirmed. At the University of Washington, we eagerly reviewed the characteristics that Lemoine had found in children of alcoholic mothers in Nantes; they were stun-

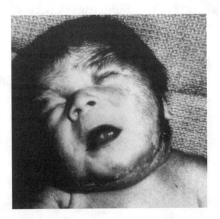

Figure 3.2.   The first child diagnosed with FAS at birth. (From Jones, K.L., & Smith, D.W. [1973]. Recognition of the fetal alcohol syndrome in early infancy. *Lancet, 2*[836], 999, © by The Lancet, Ltd. 1973; reprinted by permission.)

ningly similar to ours. At the time, Smith noted that we should be sure to recognize the important discovery of Dr. Lemoine in our next paper. Dr. Lemoine and colleagues' (1968) article included the startling comment "Ces enfants se ressemblent tous (au point qu'il nous arrive fréquemment d'affirmer l'ethylisme maternal à la vue d'un enfant et que l'enquête sociale a toujours confirmé les faits)" [The infants all looked alike (to the degree that alcoholism in the mother could be determined by observing the children)] (p. 477).

The two reports from Nantes, France, and Seattle, Washington, were met with both excitement and disbelief. The excitement rang around the world, where, in country after country, clinicians recognized that they, too, had patients who looked like this—and that their patients, too, had alcoholic mothers. Isolated cases were soon reported from places such as Iceland, South Africa, Canada, and Australia. Within 4 years, there were 41 reported cases of FAS in Seattle (Hanson, Jones, & Smith, 1976); 65 in southern Germany (Majewski et al., 1976); and 16 in northern France (Dehaene et al., 1977) (see Figure 3.3). By 1978, Clarren and Smith reported 245 cases of FAS in the Western world; then, in 1979, just 6 years after the identification of FAS, 618 individuals with FAS were identified from various centers around the world (D.W. Smith, 1979). The clinical confirmation was exhilarating: The "FAS face" appeared to be unique to alcohol.

THE PATH TO SCIENTIFIC VALIDATION

Three kinds of studies were soon undertaken in response to the clinical recognition of FAS: 1) comparisons between children of alcoholic mothers and children whose mothers were not alcoholic;

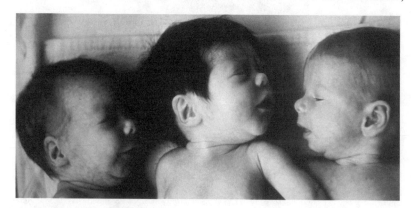

Figure 3.3.   Three babies born with fetal alcohol syndrome.

2) longitudinal prospective studies of the children of large groups of women who were not necessarily alcoholic but who drank varying amounts of alcohol (as documented during the pregnancy); and 3) experimental studies in the animal laboratory, where dose, pattern, and timing of exposure could be tightly controlled (see also Chapters 4 and 5).

The Case/Comparison Group Study

In 1974, Smith, Jones, and I flew to Bethesda, Maryland, with great anticipation to embark on the first case/comparison group study of children of alcoholic mothers, made possible through access to a large national database from the Collaborative Perinatal Project of the National Institute on Neurologic Diseases and Stroke. This was the most comprehensive study ever conducted on the causes of neurological impairment in children. Multidisciplinary teams of specialists systematically examined the children of 55,000 women from 12 sites across the United States for 7 years after birth. In 1960, when the study began, there was no hint in the contemporary medical literature that prenatal alcohol could be damaging to the developing fetus. Therefore, not a single question about alcohol was even included in the otherwise thorough interviews given to mothers both before and after the birth of their children. Fortunately, though, in some instances, clinicians had noted in the medical records that a mother appeared to have alcoholism when she came in for prenatal care. These women became the focus of our study.

Smith examined the maternal records of all mothers who had been flagged in the clinical notes as having signs of alcoholism. He examined them "blindly" (i.e., without any knowledge of child outcomes) and identified 23 women with reasonable evidence of chronic alcoholism before and during pregnancy. Each of these 23 women was then matched (on seven factors that affect child outcomes) with two comparison mothers selected from the other 55,000 mothers in the study. Jones and I then conducted a blind examination of the 69 child records (he the pediatric records, and I the psychological records).

This fortuitous study (Jones, Smith, Streissguth, & Myrianthopoulos, 1974) was published just a year after the naming of FAS. It provided a remarkably quick answer to questions raised about the potentially confounding effects of socioeconomic background, maternal education, race, maternal age, parity, marital status, and regional affiliation. Compared with nonalcoholic mothers from very similar backgrounds, the children of alcoholic mothers had much worse outcomes, including a 4-fold increase in low IQ scores (12 out of 16 children born to alcoholic mothers versus 7 out of 32 children born to nonalcoholic mothers had borderline to moderate mental retardation). Alcoholic mothers also had an 8-fold increase in perinatal mortality (4 out of 23 versus 1 out of 46), and 43% of the pregnancies of mothers with chronic alcoholism resulted in death or in a child who appeared to have FAS. Only 2% of the comparison-group pregnancies resulted in similar outcomes (1 death out of 46 and no apparent FAS). (See Streissguth, 1976, for details of the psychological data from this study.)

The Longitudinal Prospective Study

Almost as soon as FAS was identified and confirmed, questions arose about the necessary dose: How much alcohol was enough to damage the fetus? Could women drink during pregnancy if they were not alcoholics? and How is prenatal alcohol exposure related to the traditional outcomes that epidemiologists use to assess the success of a pregnancy (e.g., stillbirths, birth weight)? A different kind of study was needed to examine these questions—a longitudinal prospective study. The longitudinal prospective studies on alcohol and pregnancy, which emerged in the mid- to late 1970s, began with large groups of women who drank varying amounts of alcohol during pregnancy. Careful study design and statistical adjustments for possible confounding influences (e.g., smoking, poor diet, other drugs) permitted the effects of prenatal alcohol exposure on pregnancy and child outcomes to be thoroughly evaluated.

The first longitudinal prospective study was published in France in 1976 and showed a 2½-fold increase in the rate of stillborn babies from mothers who reported drinking three or more drinks per day, on average (Kaminski, Rumeau-Rouquette, & Schwartz, 1976). The next year, Little (1977) reported significantly lower birth weights in infants born to primarily middle-class mothers who drank but received good prenatal care. This finding was statistically significant even after adjustment for other traditional risk factors for low birth weight. Infants born to mothers who reported having two or more drinks per day in late pregnancy had an average birth-weight reduction of 160 grams. That same year, Ouellette, Rosett, Rosman, and Weiner (1977) published findings from the first prospective alcohol study in which the babies were examined clinically (in this case, by a child neurologist). This study, conducted in inner-city Boston, showed that heavy alcohol use during pregnancy was related to significantly more congenital anomalies, minor anomalies, microcephaly, growth deficiency, and prematurity as well as some CNS effects including increased jitteriness and hypotonia and a weak suck (Ouellette et al., 1977). The following year, the first paper from another longitudinal prospective study appeared, showing "fetal alcohol effects" in some newborns of mothers who drank moderately or socially. Fetal alcohol effects were defined as the following: small size at birth, microcephaly, short palpebral fissures, and two or more dysmorphic features judged by clinical observation (Hanson, Streissguth, & Smith, 1978).

The Experimental Animal Research

A rich literature of animal research on the effects of prenatal alcohol exposure was also stimulated by the identification of FAS. These studies proliferated at a rapid rate, and by 1977 there were already animal models of FAS in chickens, mice, rats, guinea pigs, and zebrafish, and some semblance of a crude dose–response curve that related different types of outcomes to different levels of alcohol exposure (Streissguth, 1977). Elegant animal studies (see Chapter 4, which reviews the experimental animal literature within the context of teratogenic theory) definitively established alcohol as a teratogen. Scientists continue to document the role of increasingly lower and more discrete doses of alcohol in producing various types of damage to the developing brain and to clarify the brain–behavior relationships disrupted by prenatal alcohol.

Additional Research

Published research on alcohol and pregnancy proliferated in the 1980s. The spectrum of fetal alcohol damage was expanded by additional studies on children of alcoholics and by a broadening base of longitudinal prospective studies (see Chapter 5). Two books published in 1986 were influential in focusing the growing scientific literature and stimulating future directions. *Alcohol and Brain Development* edited by West brought together animal and human studies and highlighted the vulnerability of many parts of the brain to prenatal alcohol exposure. *Handbook of Behavioral Teratology* edited by Riley and Vorhees laid out for the first time the principles of behavioral teratology and the key role of alcohol studies in delineating this field.

TRACKING THE LONG-TERM EFFECTS OF FAS

Meanwhile, children diagnosed with FAS in the early 1970s were growing up. As a result of concern that FAS was not being recognized in adolescence and the fact that our adolescent patients were having more life adjustment problems than anticipated, the first 11 children diagnosed with FAS in 1973 were re-examined at our Fetal

Alcohol and Drug Unit 10 years later. This first systematic follow-up study of a discrete group of children with FAS indicated a surprising rate of premature death, early school dropout, and major adjustment problems (Streissguth, Clarren, & Jones, 1985). IQ scores were broadly distributed 10 years after diagnosis, and only half of the surviving children technically had mental retardation (an IQ score less than 70). It is interesting to note that the only children who seemed appropriately placed in special school programs were those who *did* have mental retardation. (An IQ score less than 70 qualifies you for special education.) Observed changes in facial features and body shape accompanying the onset of puberty answered the question about why so few adolescents around the world had been identified—they no longer had the same characteristic features of FAS as they did when they were 7.

In 1991, my colleagues and I conducted a larger follow-up evaluation of 61 adolescents and adults with FAS/FAE (as diagnosed by dysmorphologists in either the Pacific Northwest or on Indian reservations of the Southwest) (Streissguth et al., 1991). At this time, public awareness of the long-term implications of FAS increased rapidly. For example, the Indian Health Service distributed 30,000 copies of its *Manual on Adolescents and Adults with FAS/FAE, with Special Reference to American Indians* (Streissguth, LaDue, & Randels, 1988), which describes the characteristics and needs of adolescents and adults with FAS/FAE. Families and communities were beginning to realize that FAS was not just a childhood disability.

Publication of *The Broken Cord* (Dorris, 1989) riveted public opinion on FAS. Here, a father, already an award-winning author, documented his experiences raising Adam, an adopted son—first his attempts to make sense out of his son's unusual behaviors; then after learning that his son had FAS, his quest for knowledge about FAS; and finally his struggles to obtain appropriate services even after knowing what the problem was. Adam has become a symbol to families the world over, a symbol of the dangers of abusing alcohol during pregnancy.

> My son will forever travel through a moonless night with only the roar of wind for company. Don't talk to him of mountains, of tropical beaches. Don't ask him to swoon at sunrises or marvel at the filter of light through leaves. He's never had time for such things, and he does not believe in them. He may pass by them close enough to touch on either side, for his hands are stretched forward, grasping for balance instead of pleasure. He doesn't wonder where he came from, where he's going. He doesn't ask who he is, or why. Questions are a luxury, the province of those at a distance from the periodic shock of rain. Gravity presses Adam so hard

against reality that he doesn't feel the points at which he touches it. A drowning man is not separated from the lust for air by a bridge of thought—he is one with it—and my son, conceived and grown in an ethanol bath, lives each day in the act of drowning. For him there is no shore. (p. 264)

Adam died less than 2 years after these words were written. Only 21 years old, he walked in front of a moving car that he never looked for and never saw.

In the 1990s, about 5 years after Dorris published *The Broken Cord*, four scientific papers from three countries were published describing the adolescent and adult manifestations of FAS (Lemoine & Lemoine, 1992; Spohr, Willms, & Steinhausen, 1994; Steinhausen, Willms, & Spohr, 1993; Streissguth et al., 1991). The findings of these studies (conducted with hundreds of individuals with FAS/FAE), discussed more fully in Chapter 5, confirmed the experiences of Michael and Adam Dorris. In general, the long-term picture that emerged was distressing and consistent.

> Fetal alcohol syndrome is not just a childhood disorder; there is a predictable long-term progression of the disorder into adulthood, in which maladaptive behaviors present the greatest challenge to management. (Streissguth et al., 1991, p. 1961)

The longest of these long-term follow-up studies was conducted by Lemoine in his retirement. With the help of his physician son, he tracked down 99 of his former patients with FAS 30 years after his original contact. Lemoine concluded that mental problems constituted the most severe manifestations of FAS in adulthood, including both intellectual mental retardation and behavior problems (Lemoine & Lemoine, 1992). He found that persisting behavior problems often prevented these individuals from effectively using their intellectual potential and even their manual skills. He reported from his clinical observations that individuals with FAS often could not focus on their work or their work environments because of their immaturity, considerable instability, and refusal to cooperate. Restlessness and hyperactivity concealed their lack of assurance and initiative as well as their need for assistance and protection. Although apparently euphoric and excited, they also were fearful, anxious, and depressed. Some were jokesters and comics; others were irritable and aggressive (Lemoine & Lemoine, 1992). (An English account of Lemoine's paper is included in Streissguth, 1994.)

In 1996, the final report to the Centers for Disease Control and Prevention on a research study of the secondary disabilities in over 400 individuals with FAS/FAE in the Pacific Northwest revealed the long-term social and societal consequences of the primary disabilities associated with FAS/FAE (Streissguth, Barr, Kogan, & Bookstein, 1996).

THE PATH TO AN EFFECTIVE PUBLIC POLICY ON ALCOHOL AND PREGNANCY

During the 25-year period in which FAS was identified, named, and confirmed, public policy was also being defined in accordance with the accruing scientific knowledge. Prior to the identification of FAS, public policy about drinking during pregnancy reflected the state of the research and the prevailing public opinion that prenatal alcohol was not hazardous. A couple of pre-1973 examples follow:

The old notions about children of drunken parents being born defective can be cast aside, together with the idea that alcohol can directly irritate and injure the sex glands (Yale Center for Alcohol pamphlet, How Alcohol Affects the Body, 1955 [as cited in Rosett, 1976]).

It can now be categorically stated, after hundreds of studies covering many years, that no matter how great the amounts of alcohol taken by the mother— or the father for that matter—neither the germ cells nor the development of the child will be affected... (Montagu, 1965, p. 114).

The research and media attention on FAS and other prenatal alcohol effects, however, quickly reached influential writers, such as Montagu, who began to change their advice to prospective mothers. Some of the influential findings included the following: Dehaene, a neonatologist in northern France in charge of a high-risk newborn nursery in Roubaix, began identifying and tracking the prevalence of FAS almost as soon as it was identified. Dehaene (like Majewski in Germany) classified his FAS patients in terms of severity, in early recognition of the spectrum of impairment associated with prenatal alcohol. By 1977, Dehaene had identified 39 babies with FAS out of 8,284 births, for a rate of 1 FAS birth per 212 births for all levels of FAS and 1 per 690 births for the most severe form (Dehaene, 1995). These figures were quickly replicated in a U.S. study in which two newborns with FAS were identified out of approximately 1,430 births by a dysmorphologist conducting "blind" examinations (without knowledge of maternal exposure) on a subset of infants born to the heaviest drinking mothers and nonexposed or lightly exposed babies born on the same day (Hanson et al., 1978). The following year, Olegård reported an incidence of FAS in Göteborg, Sweden, of 1 per 600 births, and estimated the incidence of FAE at twice that of FAS (Olegård et al., 1979).

By the late 1970s, there was enough consensus from all types of studies to establish that alcohol was teratogenic. The deleterious effects of prenatal alcohol exposure were observed clinically in the faces of individuals with FAS; empirically through epidemiological studies; and experimentally in the findings of a number of well-controlled studies in animal laboratories where both alcohol and other salient factors were under explicit control. Furthermore, it was apparent that there were many more adverse effects of alcohol than just FAS. Some of these were the adverse pregnancy outcomes of traditionally studied epidemiological research (e.g., fetal wastage, low birth weight, decreased viability); others were partial clinical manifestations of the FAS.

Public policy also kept pace with the scientific advancements researchers were making with FAS, and in June 1977 the Secretary of the U.S. Department of Health, Education, and Welfare issued a warning in which women were advised that drinking six or more drinks per day constituted a clear risk to the fetus (*Health Caution on Fetal Alcohol Syndrome,* 1977). In 1978, the federal government, through the NIAAA, funded two demonstration projects to develop methods to prevent FAS. One grant went to develop an alcohol awareness campaign in California, the other to the University of Washington Medical School to develop a 3-year demonstration program to intervene in female alcohol abuse during pregnancy and to prevent FAS (Little, Streissguth, & Guzinski, 1980). Local efforts to identify obstetric patients at high risk for alcohol abuse and to counsel them against drinking were also under way in Boston, Buffalo, Cleveland, and Detroit (see Chapter 13).

Public education efforts concerning risks associated with alcohol use during pregnancy have also been actively pursued since the mid-1970s. National public health advisories with broad media coverage were undertaken by NIAAA, the American Medical Association, and the March of Dimes (NIAAA, 1983).

In 1979, hearings were held by the Bureau of Alcohol, Tobacco, and Firearms (BATF, the government agency that regulates alcohol) regarding the proposal that warning labels be placed on alcoholic beverage containers. This plan was opposed by some feminist groups who viewed it as an infringement on women's personal liberty. Although the BATF decided against imposing warning labels (R.J. Smith, 1979), the alcohol industry was instructed to inform the public of the risks to the fetus.

It was clear by 1980 that FAS was one of the most frequently occurring known causes of mental retardation and certainly the only one that was preventable (Eckardt et al., 1981; Shepard, 1980;

Streissguth, Landesman-Dwyer, Martin, & Smith, 1980). Public health concerns were being raised. Prevention efforts demanded attention. The times were ripe for a more comprehensive public policy. In recognition of the lower-dose studies converging from both epidemiological and animal research, the marked individual differences in outcome to prenatal exposure, and the vulnerability of the embryo and fetus even before a woman knows she is pregnant, the Acting U.S. Surgeon General Dr. Edward N. Brandt, Jr., issued a health warning that women should abstain from alcohol not only when pregnant but also when planning a pregnancy as well (Surgeon General's Advisory on Alcohol and Pregnancy, 1981; see Chapter 13).

The United States, 82 years after the first scientific study of the effects of prenatal alcohol exposure and 8 years after the identification of FAS as a birth defects syndrome, was the first country to have a national policy recommending that women not drink during pregnancy or when planning a pregnancy, although major prevention efforts were also under way in the 1980s in Sweden (Larsson & Bohlin, 1987; Olegård, 1988); British Columbia (Robinson & Armstrong, 1988); and Roubaix, France (Dehaene, 1995). In fact, Roubaix is the only site in the world where systematic annual FAS birth prevalence figures have been maintained. Dehaene (1995) has noted that the prevalence of severe FAS has declined from 1 child in 690 in 1977–1979 to 1 child in 1,004 in 1989–1990; Olegård (1988) estimated that the prevalence of FAS in Sweden dropped from 1 in 600 in the mid-1970s to 1 in 2,400 live-born infants in the mid-1980s.

In 1989, the Anti-Drug Abuse Act of 1988, PL 100-690, was passed by the Congress of the United States requiring that every alcoholic beverage container carry a warning about not drinking during pregnancy on its label. The 1990s brought an increasing restlessness among families with alcohol-affected children in the United States—families concerned with the lack of services for diagnosis, treatment, and intervention. Parent activist and support groups organized to demand services for their children.

Information disseminated through books such as *The Broken Cord* (Dorris, 1989) and television programs such as *20/20* (Wenner, 1990) has educated parents on the prevalence, symptoms, and dangers associated with FAS. As parents have increasingly realized that their children might be affected by prenatal alcohol exposure, they have pressed for diagnostic and remediation services, greater professional understanding, and more research. The success of these efforts remains to be evaluated.

REFERENCES

Anti-Drug Abuse Act of 1988, PL 100-690, 21 U.S.C. 1501 § *et seq.*

Boss, M.Z. (1929). Frage der erbbiologischen: Bedeutung des Alkohols [Regarding the question of the genetic significance of alcohol]. *Monatssüchrift fur Psychiatrie und Neurologie, 72,* 264–292..

Clarren, S.K., & Smith, D.W. (1978). The fetal alcohol syndrome. *The New England Journal of Medicine, 298*(19), 1063–1067.

Dehaene, P. (1995). La grossesse et l'alcool [Alcohol and pregnancy]. *Que Sais-Je?, 2934.* Paris: Presses Universitaires de France.

Dehaene, P., Samaille-Villette, C., Samaille, P.-P., Crépin, G., Walbaum, R., Deroubaix, P., & Blanc-Garin, A.-P. (1977). Le syndrome d'alcoolisme fœtal dans le nord de la France. *La Revue de l'Alcoolisme, 23*(3), 145–158.

Dorris, M. (1989). *The broken cord.* New York: HarperCollins.

Eckardt, M.J., Harford, T.C., Kaelber, C.T., Parker, E.S., Rosenthal, L.S., Ryback, R.S., Salmoiraghi, G.C., Vanderveen, E., & Warren, K.R. (1981). Health hazards associated with alcohol consumption. *Journal of the American Medical Association, 246*(6), 648–666.

Fretz, G.P. (1931). *Alcohol and the other germ poisons.* The Hague, the Netherlands: Martinus Nijhoff.

Goddard, H.H. (1912). *The Kallikak family: A study in the heredity of feeblemindedness.* New York: Macmillan.

Haggard, H.W., & Jellinek, E.M. (1942). *Alcohol explored.* New York: Doubleday.

Hanson, J.W., Jones, K.L., & Smith, D.W. (1976). Fetal alcohol syndrome: Experience with 41 patients. *Journal of the American Medical Association, 235*(14), 1458–1460.

Hanson, J.W., Streissguth, A.P., & Smith, D.W. (1978). The effects of moderate alcohol consumption during pregnancy on fetal growth and morphogenesis. *Journal of Pediatrics, 92*(3), 457–460.

Health caution on fetal alcohol syndrome. (1977, June). Washington, DC: U.S. Department of Health, Education & Welfare.

Jones, K.L., & Smith, D.W. (1973). Recognition of the fetal alcohol syndrome in early infancy. *Lancet, 2*(836), 999–1001.

Jones, K.L., Smith, D.W., Streissguth, A.P., & Myrianthopoulos, N.C. (1974). Outcome in offspring of chronic alcoholic women. *Lancet, 1*(866), 1076–1078.

Jones, K.L., Smith, D.W., Ulleland, C.N., & Streissguth, A.P. (1973). Pattern of malformation in offspring of chronic alcoholic mothers. *Lancet, 1*(815), 1267–1271.

Kaminski, M., Rumeau-Rouquette, C., & Schwartz, D. (1976). Consommation d'alcool chez les femmes enceintes et issue de la grossesse. *Revue Epidemiologique Médicale Sociale Santé Publique, 24*(1), 27–40.

Karp, R.J. (1993). Introduction: A history and overview of malnourished children in the United States. In R.J. Karp (Ed.), *Malnourished children in the United States: Caught in the cycle of poverty* (pp. xix–xxviii). New York: Springer-Verlag.

Karp, R.J., Quazi, Q.H., Moller, K.A., Angelo, W.A., & Davis, J.M. (1995). Fetal alcohol syndrome at the turn of the 20th century: An unexpected explanation of the Kallikak family. *Archives of Pediatrics and Adolescent Medicine, 149*(1), 45–48.

Ladrague, P. (1901). *Alcoolisme et enfants.* Thèse pour le doctorat en Médêcine. [*Alcoholism and infants.* Doctoral dissertation, University of Paris, Faculty of Médicine.] Paris: Université de Paris, Faculté de Medêcine.

Larsson, G., & Bohlin, A.-B. (1987). Fetal alcohol syndrome and preventative strategies. *Pediatrician, 14,* 51–56.

Lemoine, P., Harousseau, H., Borteyru, J.-P., Menuet, J.-C. (1968). Les enfants de parents alcooliques: Anomalies obervées, à propos de 127 cas. [Children of Alcoholic Parents: Abnormalities observed in 127 cases.] *Ouest Medical, 21,* 476–482. Selected Translations of International Alcoholism Research (STIAR). Rockville, MD: National Institute on Alcohol Abuse and Alcoholism. (Available from the National Clearinghouse for Alcohol and Drug Information, P.O. Box 2345, Rockville, MD 20847–2345.)

Lemoine, P., & Lemoine, Ph. (1992). Avenir des enfants de mères alcooliques (étude de 105 cas retrouvés à l'âge adulte) et quelques constatations d'intérêt prophylactique. *Annales de Pédiatrie (Paris), 39,* 226–235.

Little, R.E. (1977). Moderate alcohol use during pregnancy and decreased infant birth weight. *American Journal of Public Health, 67*(12), 1154–1156.

Little, R.E., Streissguth, A.P., & Guzinski, G.M. (1980). Prevention of fetal alcohol syndrome: A model program. *Alcoholism: Clinical and Experimental Research, 4*(2), 185–189.

Majewski, F., Bierich, J.R., Löser, H., Michaelis, R., Leiber, B., & Bettecken, F. (1976). Zur klinik und pathogenese der alkohol-embryopathie: Bericht über 68 fälle. *Münchener Medizinische Wochenschrift, 118*(50), 1635–1642.

May, P.A., Hymbaugh, K.J., Aase, J.M., & Samet, J.M. (1983). Epidemiology of fetal alcohol syndrome among American Indians of the Southwest. *Social Biology, 30*(4), 374–387.

Montagu, A. (1965). *Life before birth.* New York: Signet.

National Institute on Alcohol Abuse and Alcoholism (NIAAA). (1983). *Fifth special report to the U.S. Congress on alcohol and health.* Washington, DC: U.S. Department of Health and Human Services.

Nicloux, M. (1900). Dosage comparatif de l'alcool, dans le sang et dans le lait, après ingestion dans l'estomac. *Comptes Rendus Sociologie Biologique, 295, 297, 620, 622.*

Olegård, R., Sabel, K.G., Aronsson, M., Sandin, B., Johansson, P.R., Carlsson, C., Kyllerman, M., Iversen, K., Hrbek, A. (1979). Effects on the child of alcohol abuse during pregnancy. *Acta Paediatrica Scandinavica, 275*(Suppl.), 112–121.

Olegård, R. (1988). The prevention of fetal alcohol syndrome in Sweden. In G.C. Robinson & R.W. Armstrong (Eds.), *Alcohol and child/family health: The proceedings of a conference with particular reference to the prevention of alcohol-related birth defects.* Vancouver, British Columbia, Canada: B.C. FAS Resource Group. (Available from the B.C. FAS Resource Group. UBC Department of Pediatrics, Sunny Hill Hospital for Children, Vancouver, B.C. V5M 3E8, Canada.)

Ouellette, E.M., Rosett, H.L., Rosman, N.P., & Weiner, L. (1977). Adverse effects on offspring of maternal alcohol abuse during pregnancy. *New England Journal of Medicine, 297*(10), 528–530.

Pearson, K., & Elderton, E.M. (1910). *A first study of the influence of parental alcoholism* (2nd ed.). London: University of London.

Randall, C.L., & Riley, E.P. (1994). Commentary. *Alcohol Health and Research World, 19*(1), 38–39.

Riley, E.P., & Vorhees, C.V. (1986). *Handbook of behavioral teratology.* New York: Plenum.

Robinson, G.C., & Armstrong, R.W. (Eds). (1988). *Alcohol and child/family health: The proceedings of a conference with particular reference to the prevention of alcohol-related birth defects.* Vancouver, British Columbia, Canada: B.C. FAS Resource Group. (Available from the B.C. FAS Resource Group. UBC Department of Pediatrics, Sunny Hill Hospital for Children, Vancouver, B.C. V5M 3E8, Canada.)

Rosett, H.L. (1976). Effects of maternal drinking on child development: An introductory review. In F.A. Seixas & S. Eggleston (Eds.), Work in progress on alcoholism. *Annals of the New York Academy of Sciences, 273,* 115–117.

Rouquette, J. (1957). *Influence de l'intoxication alcoolique parentale sur le developpement physique et psychique des jeunes enfants* [Influence of intoxicated alcoholic parents on the physical and psychological development of their young children]. Thèse, Paris.

Shepard, T.H. (1980). *Catalog of teratogenic agents* (3rd ed.). Baltimore: Johns Hopkins University Press.

Smith, D.W. (1970). *Recognizable patterns of human malformations: Genetic, embryologic, and clinical aspects* (1st ed.). Philadelphia: W.B. Saunders.

Smith, D.W. (1976). *Recognizable patterns of human malformations: Genetic, embryologic, and clinical aspects* (2nd ed.). Philadelphia: W.B. Saunders.

Smith, D.W. (1979). Fetal drug syndromes: Effects of ethanol and hydantoins. *Pediatrics in Review, 1*(6), 165–172.

Smith, R.J. (1979, March 2). BATF decides against liquor warning label. *Science, 203,* 858–859.

Spohr, H-L., Willms, J., & Steinhausen, H-C. (1994). The fetal alcohol syndrome in adolescence. *Acta Paediatrica, 83*(404), 19–26.

Steinhausen, H-C., Willms, J., & Spohr, H-L. (1993). Long-term psychopathological and cognitive outcome of children with fetal alcohol syndrome. *Journal of the American Academy of Child and Adolescent Psychiatry, 32*(5), 990–994.

Streissguth, A.P. (1976). Psychologic handicaps in children with the fetal alcohol syndrome. *Annals of the New York Academy of Sciences, 273,* 140–145.

Streissguth A.P. (1977). Maternal drinking and the outcome of pregnancy: Implications for child mental health. *American Journal of Orthopsychiatry, 47*(3), 422–431.

Streissguth, A.P. (1994). A long-term perspective of FAS. *Alcohol Health & Research World, 18*(1), 74–81.

Streissguth, A.P., Aase, J.M., Clarren, S.K., Randels, S.P., LaDue, R.A., & Smith, D.F. (1991). Fetal alcohol syndrome in adolescents and adults. *Journal of the American Medical Association, 265*(15), 1961–1967.

Streissguth, A.P., Barr, H.M., Kogan, J., & Bookstein, F.L. (1996). *Understanding the occurrence of secondary disabilities in clients with fetal alcohol syndrome (FAS) and fetal alcohol effects (FAE): Final report to the Centers for Disease Control and Prevention on Grant No. RO4/CCR008515* (Tech. Report No. 96-06). Seattle: University of Washington, Fetal Alcohol and Drug Unit.

Streissguth, A.P., Clarren, S.K., & Jones, K.L. (1985). Natural history of the fetal alcohol syndrome: A ten-year follow-up of eleven patients. *Lancet, 2,* 85–91.

Streissguth, A.P., LaDue, R.A., & Randels, S.P. (1988). *A manual on adolescents and adults with fetal alcohol syndrome with special reference to American Indians* (2nd ed.). (Available from the National Clearinghouse for Alcohol and Drug Information, P.O. Box 2345, Rockville, MD 20847, Inventory # IHS002.)

Streissguth, A.P., Landesman-Dwyer, S., Martin, J.C., & Smith, D.W. (1980). Teratogenic effects of alcohol in humans and laboratory animals. *Science, 209,* 353–361.

Sullivan, W.C. (1899). A note on the influence of maternal inebriety on the offspring. *Journal of Mental Science, 45,* 489–503.

Surgeon General's Advisory on Alcohol and Pregnancy. (1981). *FDA Drug Bulletin, 11*(2). Rockville, MD: Department of Health and Human Services.

Ulleland, C.N. (1972). The offspring of alcoholic mothers. *Annals of the New York Academy of Sciences, 197,* 167–169.

Ulleland, C.N., Wennberg, R.P., Igo, R.P., & Smith, N.J. (1970). The offspring of alcoholic mothers. *Pediatric Research, 4,* 474.

Warner, R.H., & Rosett, H.L. (1975). The effects of drinking on offspring: An historical survey of the American and British literature. *Journal of Studies on Alcohol, 36*(11), 1395–1420.

Wenner, K. (Executive Producer). (1990, March 30). What's wrong with my child? *20/20.* Seattle, WA: American Broadcasting Co.

West, J.R. (Ed.). (1986). *Alcohol and brain development.* New York: Oxford University Press.

II

The Science of
Fetal Alcohol Syndrome

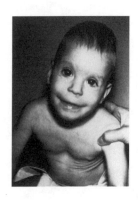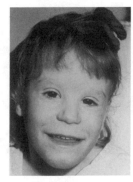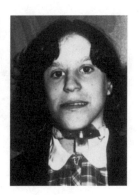

4

Alcohol as
a Teratogen

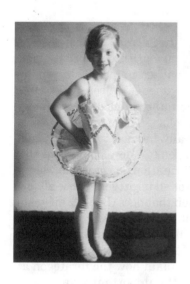

In Washington, D.C., in 1957, Papara-Nicholson and Telford gave alcohol to pregnant guinea pigs several times a week and observed abnormally low birth weights, poor locomotion, incoordination, and feeding and suckling difficulties in their offspring. They published these findings, which may well be the first study of the neurobehavioral effects of alcohol, as an abstract.

In Romania in 1968, Sandor injected chicken eggs with alcohol and observed malformations and growth deficiencies in the baby chicks (Sandor, 1968; Sandor & Elias, 1968). In 1971, Sandor and Amels published similar studies with laboratory rats and warned that the findings provided a serious danger signal of prenatal risk of ethanol intoxication during early pregnancy in humans.

Many questions were raised in 1973 when fetal alcohol syndrome (FAS) was named and identified as a birth defect: Does alcohol damage the fetus or are the other drugs or substances often used by alcoholics really the culprits? Could the symptoms of FAS be attributed to the poor nutrition that many alcoholics manifest? Could one of the by-products of alcohol (e.g., acetaldehyde) be responsible for the prenatal damage? Could the poverty conditions in which many alcoholic women live, or the abuse and neglect with which many of their children live, be the cause of the disabilities associated with FAS? Does alcoholism in fathers affect children prenatally? The world was restless for answers, yet many of the human studies necessary to answer them would involve long, complex, expensive years of research to carry out. Meanwhile, public health questions needed addressing: What about dose and timing of exposure? Should all women or just alcoholics be advised to cut down or stop drinking during pregnancy?

These questions could be addressed in the experimental animal laboratory. Animal studies could easily control whether or not the alcoholic rats smoked cigarettes, had alcoholic husbands, or neglected their children. Soon, a scientific methodology was developed for how best to get alcohol into rats and mice (they aren't as fond of it as humans are), how to maintain equivalent calories in the alcohol and the control dams, and how to cross-foster the offspring (so they wouldn't be raised by their alcoholic mothers). The science that addresses such issues is called teratology.

UNDERSTANDING TERATOLOGY

Teratogens are substances or conditions that disrupt typical development in offspring as a result of gestational exposure and cause birth defects. As a science, teratology was formalized in the 1970s, primarily from research on laboratory animals. James G. Wilson (1973, 1977; Wilson & Fraser, 1977), often called the father of modern teratology, established the basic principles of teratology. These apply to teratogens, in general, and to alcohol, specifically, because it is a teratogen. There are four main things that can happen to a developing fetus that is exposed to a teratogen: death, malformations, growth deficiency, and functional deficits (see Table 4.1). Not all teratogens cause all four outcomes; alcohol, however, is a teratogen that does (Bond & diGuisto, 1977; Brown, Goulding, & Fabro, 1979; Ellis & Pick, 1980; Martin, Martin, Sigman, & Radow, 1977; Randall, 1977, 1987; Randall & Taylor, 1979; Riley & Vorhees, 1986; West, 1986).

The principles of teratology help explain how the teratogen affects the developing offspring. One of the important principles of teratology is the *dose–response relationship:* the greater the dose, the larger the anticipated response (i.e., the effect on the off-

Table 4.1.   Teratogens can cause four distinct
types of outcomes in exposed offspring

Death
Malformations
Growth deficiency
Functional deficits

spring). Another important concept of teratology is that the pattern
and timing of the dose affect the type and severity of the response.
For example, administration of a teratogenic dose during the early
period of embryonic development causes deviations in the physical
structure of the offspring; administration during the final
trimester affects the overall size of the offspring. The brain, however, which develops throughout gestation, is vulnerable during all
trimesters of the pregnancy. The patterning of the exposure is also
an important component. Heavy episodic exposure (e.g., binge
drinking), even if only occasional, affects the offspring differently
from more frequent, light exposure. The principles of teratogenics
and behavioral teratology have been developed to apply to teratogenic agents in general (X-irradiation, heavy metals such as mer-
cury and lead, and drugs such as certain anticonvulsants and alcohol). FAS quickly emerged as the largest and broadest line of
research in behavioral teratology. "FAS represents the largest environmental cause of behavioral teratogenesis yet discovered and,
perhaps, the largest single environmental cause that will ever be
discovered" (Riley & Vorhees, 1986, p. 13).

Another important concept of teratology theory is that genes
and teratogens interact to cause deviant development. In addition
to variations in dose, pattern, and timing of exposure, the genetic
makeup of both the mother and child greatly influence whether a
particular fetus will be adversely affected. For example, some
species are more vulnerable to the teratogenic effects of a given
drug, and not all offspring share the same vulnerability to specific
teratogens. Within a litter of laboratory rats (all, of course, having
the same exposure to alcohol), some of the offspring will be born
with obvious birth defects while others will not. (For further details,
see Chernoff, 1980; Gilliam, Kotch, Dudek, & Riley, 1988; and Goodlett, Gilliam, Nichols, & West, 1989.)

An important aspect of teratogenic study is to determine how
a specific teratogen produces an effect. Once the mechanisms of
action are understood, the evidence that that agent causes the

birth defect is stronger. This is how alcohol causes prenatal brain damage: Alcohol disrupts and impedes prenatal development in several ways. Alcohol has a direct toxic effect on cells and can produce cell death, thereby causing certain areas of the brain to actually contain fewer cells than normal. The brain regions affected by prenatal alcohol exposure in animal models include the hippocampus, cerebellum, corpus callosum, and cortex. Alcohol can impede the transport of amino acids (which are the important building blocks of proteins) and glucose (which is the main energy source for cells). Alcohol can also impair the placental–fetal blood flow, causing hypoxia (oxygen deprivation), or derange the hormone and chemical regulatory systems that control the maturation and migration of nerve cells in the brain (Michaelis & Michaelis, 1994; Randall, Ekblad, & Anton, 1990; Schenker et al., 1990; West, 1986).

Animal Studies of Alcohol Teratogenesis

After the identification of FAS in 1973, research funds were available through the National Institute on Alcohol Abuse and Alcoholism (NIAAA), and experimental animal laboratories across the country began addressing the questions raised by the first clinical reports. Within 2 years the first studies were published. For the next 15 years, these studies addressed six questions of particular interest to humans:

1. Is alcohol teratogenic?
2. Could episodic or a single episode of alcohol exposure produce an effect, or are only chronic alcoholics at risk?
3. What are the mechanisms through which the teratogenic effects of alcohol are produced?
4. Can lower or less chronic doses of alcohol cause brain damage but no physical effects?
5. Is the brain damage caused by alcohol permanent?
6. Are the outcomes produced by prenatal alcohol in animal models comparable to those observed in children and adults with FAS and FAE?

The early studies concentrated on rat mothers who were "chronic alcoholics," heavily exposing their fetuses to alcohol throughout their pregnancies. Physical malformations of limbs, digits, eyes, ears, internal organs, and brain were significantly more frequent in alcohol-exposed offspring than in the pair-fed controls. Growth deficiency (see Figure 4.1), decreased litter size, and increased resorptions (the rodent equivalent of miscarriages) also increased with

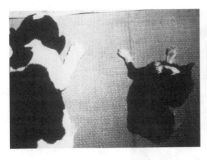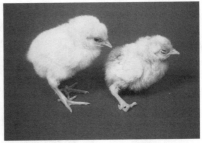

Figure 4.1. Malformations and growth deficiency in pup and chick produced by heavy prenatal alcohol exposure. (From Ellis & Pick, 1980, p. 131; reprinted by permission from Williams & Wilkins; and Streissguth & Little, 1994, p. 10; reprinted by permission. Chick photograph courtesy of Dr. William Shoemaker.)

prenatal alcohol exposure. Explicit brain damage and developmental delays were also observed (Brown et al., 1979; Ellis & Pick, 1980; Randall, 1977, 1987; Randall & Taylor, 1979 [see Figure 4.2]).

In 1981, the work of Sulik, Johnson, and Webb made a significant breakthrough in terms of the morphological effects of episodic exposure by demonstrating, in a mouse model how the face of FAS could be produced by just two heavy doses of ethanol on Day 7 of gestation: "Striking histological [tissue] changes occurred in the developing brain within 24 hours after exposure" (Sulik et al., 1981, p. 936) (see Figure 4.3). Confirming the influence of genetic variance, Sulik and her colleagues also noted that not all exposed fetuses in a litter were affected, and some were much more severely affected than others, although they all received the same dose and timing of alcohol exposure. This study also demonstrated that chronic or regular alcohol use was not necessary to produce changes in brain development.

In 1992, Goodlett and West described a series of studies they and their colleagues had carried out in West's laboratory over the prior 8 years. They investigated a binge-like pattern of drinking in rats and found that drinking during the third trimester equivalent was associated with damage to the hippocampal and cerebellar regions of the brain and that different cell groups had differential sensitivities to alcohol. Massing the alcohol into one daily drink was more likely to produce neuronal damage in the developing brain (particularly the cerebellum) than drinking the same amount of alcohol slowly throughout the day. Obviously a "day" for a rat is more like a "week and a half" for a woman. This binge model in rats is similar to the model used for nonhuman primate studies.

Clarren and colleagues (Clarren, Astley, & Bowden, 1988; Clarren, Astley, Gunderson, & Spellman, 1992) conducted alcohol teratology studies with macaques (i.e., primates) using a "Saturday

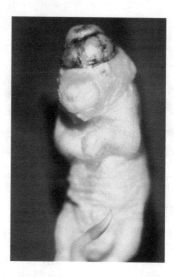

Figure 4.2.   Exencephaly in mouse produced by heavy prenatal alcohol exposure; note extruded brain tissue. (Photograph courtesy of Dr. Carrie Randall.)

night binge" model of exposure. This model replicates the drinking habits of those women who do not drink every day but binge once a week. Although none of the macaque mothers had alcohol more than once a week while pregnant, some were given a large amount of alcohol at this time, whereas others had the equivalent of only a couple of drinks. Their offspring were examined on cognitive tasks similar to the Wisconsin General Test Apparatus (WGTA) (Harlow, 1959), which measures the ability to generalize from one visual stimulus to a series of stimuli with similar characteristics. Almost all of the offspring of the heaviest binge-drinking mothers had learning difficulties, although not all failed on any one task, and no offspring were deficient on all tasks. Dose-dependent neuronal deficits in the brain were also demonstrated, specifically in the number of Purkinje cells in the cerebellum (Bonthius et al., 1996). This important nonhuman primate study, carried out over many years by Clarren and colleagues, demonstrated that alcohol-induced neurochemical abnormalities, neuronal depletion, and cognitive and motor deficits and delays can occur in individuals who have normal head circumference, typical appearance (i.e., no FAS faces), and normal brain images.

Goodlett and West (1992) note that neuronal depletion (cell loss) may be one of the most extreme effects of alcohol exposure during development. In studying the effects of low blood alcohol concentrations (BACs) and low-level alcohol exposure, acute astrogliosis in the deep layers of the cortex (Goodlett et al., 1989; Goodlett & West, 1992) and

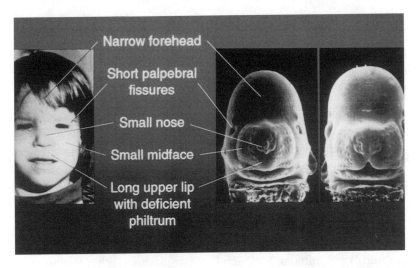

Figure 4.3. How prenatal alcohol produces the face of FAS in boy and mouse. (From Sulik et al., 1981, p. 937; reprinted by permission.)

permanent reductions in zinc density in the mossy fibers of the hippocampus (Savage, Montano, Paxton, & Kasarskis, 1989; Savage et al., 1991) have been demonstrated at peak BACs, beginning at around 50 milligrams per deciliter, which is less than two drinks (J. West, personal communication, May 23, 1993). Mossy fiber zinc reduction in different parts of the hippocampus ranged from 20% to 36%. Goodlett and West (1992) concluded: "With regard to the controversial issue of what degree of alcohol consumption constitutes a risk to the developing CNS, these studies suggest that identifiable, presumably deleterious effects on CNS structure can result from even moderate levels of exposure. Other studies using a prenatal exposure paradigm via a liquid diet producing low maternal BACs (peak BACs of 30–40 milligrams per deciliter) indicate that neurochemical and neurophysiological alterations are very sensitive markers of long-lasting neurological effects of gestational alcohol exposure. The only prudent conclusion is that alcohol can affect the developing brain even at low exposure levels. Abstinence during pregnancy is the only way to avoid such effects." (Goodlett & West, 1992, pp. 64–65).

NEUROBEHAVIORAL TERATOLOGY OF ALCOHOL

Because alcohol produces CNS damage, it is classified as a *neurobehavioral teratogen,* which is a special group of teratogens that cause brain damage and modify behavior (see Riley & Vorhees, 1986). Because it takes a larger dose of a neurobehavioral teratogen to produce physical malformations than it does to cause CNS damage, the neurobehavioral effects of a teratogenic agent such as alcohol can be observed at levels of exposure that produce no physical abnormalities whatsoever.

Pennington and colleagues conducted a classic neurobehavioral teratology study by injecting alcohol into the airspace of chicks' eggs. Although their dosing levels were not high enough to impair physical growth or produce malformations, they were associated with delayed cell division in the brain and slower brain growth. During early development, these alcohol-injected chicks were slower to learn a detour learning task that rewarded them with food (see Figure 4.4). In fact, some of them never learned how to get to the food, even after being shown every day for 4 days. Virtually none of the control chicks (who had received a water injection) had this much difficulty learning the detour (Means, Burnette, & Pennington, 1988; Means, McDaniel, & Pennington, 1989; Pennington, Boyd, Kalmus, & Wilson, 1983).

Hyperactivity was one of the first behaviors to be investigated in the animal studies on the behavioral teratology of alcohol. Increased activity in these early animal models was measured with activity wheels or open-field paradigms. In the late 1970s, researchers from four separate laboratories demonstrated that prena-

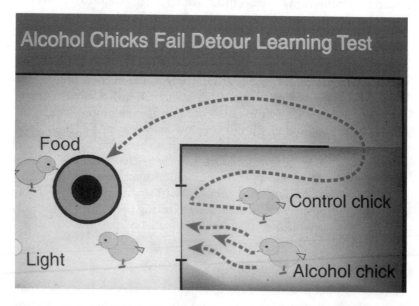

Figure 4.4.   Alcohol chick fails detour learning test. (Data from Means et al., 1988, 1989. Diagram from Streissguth & Little, 1994; reprinted by permission.)

tal alcohol exposure caused young rats to be hyperactive (Bond & diGuisto, 1977; Caul, Osborne, Fernandez, & Henderson, 1979; Martin, Martin, Sigman, & Radow, 1978; Shaywitz, Griffieth, & Warshaw, 1979).

Problems with *response inhibition* were also reported from several studies of young rats prenatally exposed to alcohol. These studies examined how quickly an animal learns to avoid a negative reinforcement (usually an electric shock). Martin et al. (1977) found that alcohol-exposed rat pups did not learn as quickly as those who had not been exposed when the negative reinforcement paradigm was used and were significantly poorer at discriminating contingencies (i.e., they continued to press the wrong bar at the wrong time, even though they got shocked for doing it). This suggested that perhaps alcohol-exposed animals do not cope with stress as well as nonexposed animals.

In 1979, Riley and colleagues (Riley, Lochry, & Shapiro, 1979; Riley, Lochry, Shapiro, & Baldwin, 1979) found response-inhibition impairments in rats prenatally exposed to alcohol using two types of maze conditions. Again, the alcohol-exposed rat pups were slower than those not exposed in learning not to run into a compartment in which they got shocked. They also showed an increase in perseverative behavior by returning to the arm of the maze where the food *used* to be, long after the reinforcement had been changed to the other arm of the maze (Riley, Barron, & Hannigan, 1986). This work was particularly interesting because poor response inhibition is a behavioral impairment often associated with hippocampal lesions—the part of the brain that Goodlett and West (1992) had demonstrated to be damaged by prenatal alcohol exposure.

Although most of the early behavioral teratology studies dealt with younger animals, several followed the animals into adulthood. Phillips and Stainbrook (1976) found that the adult offspring of mother rats given wine during pregnancy and while nursing made significantly fewer correct responses (i.e., they generalized more poorly from their previous experience) on the WGTA, thereby demonstrating that the developmental delays produced by alcohol may be lifelong impairments.

Riley (1990) summarized the research literature on the effects of prenatal alcohol exposure on adolescent and adult animals. The neurobehavioral effects of alcohol do not diminish with age, but as Goodlett and West (1992) noted, it may be necessary to use more sophisticated learning tasks to measure this effect as the animals mature. Riley also observed unusual behavior patterns in adult rats that were prenatally exposed to alcohol. For example, although the alcohol-exposed animals could successfully navigate the easier T-maze as they aged, they reverted to perseverative behaviors when confronted with the more complex 10-arm radial maze. Here, they repeatedly entered arms that were once baited but from which they had already eaten the food and also repeatedly entered arms in which they had never found food. In support of Riley (1980), Dumas and Rabe (1994) have shown long-term memory impairments in aging mice produced by a single heavy dose of alcohol during early embryonic development.

Few animal studies have investigated social interaction problems in prenatally exposed offspring, although one early study from Czechoslovakia reported increased aggressive behavior among alcohol-exposed mouse pups in a social situation (Elis & Krsiak, 1976). Two studies have shown longer latency for alcohol-exposed male rats to achieve appropriate sexually specific behaviors (mounting and copulation) (Barron, Tieman, & Riley, 1988; Parker, Udani, Gavaler, & Van Thiel, 1984). Two studies have shown marked impairments in appropriate maternal behaviors in fetal alcohol-exposed adult females (Barron & Riley, 1985; Hård et al., 1985).

Hård and colleagues (1985) studied the interactions of fetal-alcohol–exposed rat mothers with their 4-day-old pups that had been removed from the nest. Compared with control mothers, the prenatally exposed mothers built nests of inferior quality and took, on average, twice as long to retrieve the first pup to the nest. After 30 minutes, half of the fetal-alcohol mothers had not retrieved their litters. The offspring themselves (that had not been alcohol exposed) did not show any disturbances of physical or behavioral development (e.g., the emission of disturbed vocalizations), which might have triggered a differential response from the mothers. Although the brain weights of the mothers prenatally exposed to alcohol were not significantly different from the control mothers, they did have decreased serotonin synthesis in the brain, which has been associated with disturbed maternal behavior in rats. The retrieval behavior of the fetal-alcohol rat mothers was disoriented, unmotivated, and disorganized. They sometimes carried a pup halfway to the nest and then dropped it to pick up another pup, or they spent much time grooming themselves and eating and drinking and ignored their pups. In contrast, the control mothers retrieved all the pups in rapid succession and then licked them and crouched over them protectively.

Hård and colleagues (1985) suggested that the disorganized behaviors of the fetal-alcohol mother rats may reflect damage to the hippocampal region of the brain, which, when damaged, can produce this type of spatial disorganization. Similar results have been reported by Barron and Riley (1985).

Alcohol and Pregnancy: The Relevance of the Animal Findings for Humans

By the 1990s, animal studies were using dosing paradigms that were well within the equivalent range of those used by women (e.g., Goodlett & West, 1992; Savage et al., 1992). And Driscoll, Streissguth, and Riley (1990) demonstrated the remarkable similarity in the animal behavioral teratology literature and the human epidemiological and clinical studies of children who were prenatally exposed to alcohol. Response inhibition impairments, learning difficulties, gait disturbances, suckling and balance problems, and many other limitations have been demonstrated in both children and animals affected by prenatal alcohol exposure (see Table 4.2). From the clinical and public health perspective, there are six main implications to be drawn from research on the teratogenic effects of alcohol:

Table 4.2.   Behavioral effects following prenatal alcohol exposure in humans and animals

Humans	Animals
Hyperactivity	Increased activity, exploration, and reactivity
Attention deficits, distractibility	Decreased attention
Lack of inhibition	Inhibition deficits
Mental retardation, learning disabilities	Impaired associative learning
Reduced habituation	Impaired habituation
Perseveration	Perseveration
Feeding difficulties	Feeding difficulties
Gait abnormalities	Altered gait
Poor fine and gross motor skills	Poor coordination
Developmental delays (motor, social, language)	Developmental delay
Hearing abnormalities	Altered auditory evoked potentials
Poor state regulation	Poor state regulation

Reprinted by permission of the publisher from Driscoll, C.D., Streissguth, A.P., & Riley, E.P. (1990). Prenatal alcohol exposure: Comparability of effects in human and animal models. *Neurobehavioral Toxicology and Teratology, 12,* 232; copyright ©1990 by Elsevier Science, Inc.

1. **Alcohol is a teratogenic drug.** Two decades of animal research (the 1970s and 1980s) have demonstrated that alcohol can damage and disrupt the developing embryo and fetus.

   Implications: To prevent FAS/FAE, the Surgeon General's warning against drinking during pregnancy or when planning a pregnancy should be followed (Surgeon General's Advisory on Alcohol and Pregnancy, 1981). Also, clinical services should be targeted at the heaviest-drinking women.

2. **Dose, timing, and pattern of exposure modify the prenatal effects of alcohol.** Animal research has demonstrated that the teratogenic effects of alcohol are not limited to heavy chronic exposure. Moderate alcohol and episodic exposure also produce deleterious effects on offspring, as do exposure both early and late in gestation.

   Implications: Not only are children of mothers who are chronic alcoholics at risk. Women who drink before they know they are pregnant or have an occasional heavy dose of alcohol (binge) may also cause damage to their children.

3. **Individual differences in the mother and the child modify the effect of prenatal exposure in the individual animal, in terms of both the severity and the type of offspring effect.** Alcohol causes a wide variety of CNS effects in offspring that are manifest at various ages. Alcohol causes the damage; genes modify the effect. This is demonstrated by studies of human twins born to alcoholic mothers. Both twins are exposed to the same amount of alcohol, yet when the twins are dizygotic (2-egg) twins, they are more likely to be differentially affected by the alcohol than when they are monozygotic (1-egg) twins (Streissguth & Dehaene, 1993).

   Implications: The fact that some offspring appear unaffected by prenatal alcohol at any point in time does *not* mean that alcohol is not teratogenic or that an individual who is free of alcohol-caused disabilities at one age will necessarily be free of them at another.

4. **Brain damage from prenatal alcohol can occur without accompanying physical manifestations and from lower doses and frequency of exposure.**

   Implications: Children with FAS are not the only ones damaged by prenatal alcohol. Those with FAE and ARND can have brain damage just as surely caused by alcohol as those with FAS, and it can occur at lower exposure levels.

5. **Brain–behavior relationships have been well established in animal studies.** Disrupted brain development caused by prenatal alcohol can cause aberrant behavior in the offspring. But in

the living organism, the actual brain damage is more difficult to assess than the disrupted behavior. Specifically, prenatal alcohol can cause hyperactivity, difficulty withholding a response (impulsivity), difficulty learning from experience, and perseverative problem-solving approaches.

Implications: Many of the puzzling and bizarre behaviors that people with FAS engage in may be caused by their brain damage. This has major implications for their daily living and their social interactions—FAS is not just a learning problem in the classroom.

Mother of a girl with FAS: She just doesn't seem to learn the same way that other children do. She doesn't learn from experience. Punishment or logic has no effect on her. She just keeps doing the same dumb things time after time, although they never lead to a satisfactory solution.

Father of a son with FAS: My adolescent son just keeps doing things over and over again. I can't understand it. He never seems to learn. Even when it makes the other kids turn away from him, he stands too close to them, touches them too much, and says all the wrong things. He's not stupid—he just doesn't get it.

6. **The effects of prenatal alcohol exposure last into adulthood.** Aberrant behaviors resulting from prenatal alcohol exposure are still observable in adult animals. They are observed in animals raised in standard rearing environments that otherwise produce healthy adults.

Implications: Aberrant behaviors in children, adolescents, and adults can be caused by prenatal damage. Understanding this can be useful in responding constructively to the aberrant behaviors. A diagnosis of FAS/FAE can be an important link.

Mother of a son with FAS: We raised Pierre just like our other children, but he responded totally differently—we couldn't figure it out. It was as though all the typical ways of teaching our other children about how to behave had no effect on Pierre. It wasn't until we read about FAS, went back and got more information from the adoption agency, and found out that his mother was an alcoholic that we finally figured out what the problem was.

REFERENCES

Barron, S., & Riley, E.P. (1985). Pup-induced maternal behavior in adult and juvenile rats exposed to alcohol prenatally. *Alcoholism: Clinical and Experimental Research, 9*(4), 360–365.

Barron, S., Tieman, S.B., & Riley, E.P. (1988). Effects of prenatal alcohol exposure on the sexually dimorphic nucleus of the preoptic area of the hypothalamus in male and female rats. *Alcoholism: Clinical and Experimental Research, 12*(1), 59–64.

Bond, N.W., & diGuisto, E.L. (1977). Effects of prenatal alcohol consumption on shock avoidance learning in rats. *Psychological Reports, 41,* 1269–1270.

Bonthius, D.J., Bonthius, N.E., Napper, R.E., Astley, S.J., Clarren, S.K., & West, J.R. (1996). Purkinje cell deficits in nonhuman primates following weekly exposure to ethanol during gestation. *Teratology, 53,* 230–236.

Brown, N.A., Goulding, E.H., & Fabro, S. (1979). Ethanol embryotoxicity: Direct effects on mammalian embryos *in vitro. Science, 206,* 573–575.

Caul, W.F., Osborne, G.L., Fernandez, K., & Henderson, G.I. (1979). Open-field and avoidance performance of rats as a function of prenatal ethanol treatment. *Addictive Behaviors, 4*(4), 311–322.

Chernoff, G.F. (1980). The fetal alcohol syndrome in mice: Maternal variables. *Teratology, 22,* 71–75.

Clarren, S.K., Astley, S.J., & Bowden, D.M. (1988). Physical anomalies and developmental delays in nonhuman primate infants exposed to weekly doses of ethanol during gestation. *Teratology, 37*(6), 561–569.

Clarren, S.K., Astley, S.J., Gunderson, V.M., & Spellman, D. (1992). Cognitive and behavioral deficits in nonhuman primates associated with very early embryonic binge exposures to ethanol. *Journal of Pediatrics, 121,* 789–796.

Driscoll, C.D., Streissguth, A.P., & Riley, E.P. (1990). Prenatal alcohol exposure: Comparability of effects in humans and animal models. *Neurotoxicology and Teratology, 12,* 231–237.

Dumas, R.M., & Rabe, A. (1994). Augmented memory loss in aging mice after one embryonic exposure to alcohol. *Neurotoxicology and Teratology, 16,* 605–612.

Elis, J., & Krsiak, M. (1976). Proceedings: Effect of alcohol administration during pregnancy on social behavior of offspring of mice. *Activitas Nervosa Superior, 17,* 281–282.

Ellis, F.W., & Pick, J.R. (1980). An animal model of the fetal alcohol syndrome in beagles. *Alcoholism: Clinical and Experimental Research, 4,* 123–134.

Gilliam, D.M., Kotch, L.E., Dudek, B.C., & Riley, E.P. (1988). Ethanol teratogenesis in mice selected for differences in alcohol sensitivity. *Alcohol, 5*(6), 513–519.

Goodlett, C.R., Gilliam, D.M., Nichols, J.M., & West, J.R. (1989). Genetic influences on brain growth restriction induced by developmental exposure to alcohol. *Neurotoxicology, 10*(3), 321–334.

Goodlett, C.R., & West, J.R. (1992). Fetal alcohol effects: Rat model of alcohol exposure during the brain growth spurt. In I.S. Zagon & T.A. Slotkin (Eds.), *Maternal substance abuse and the developing nervous system* (pp. 45–75). San Diego: Academic Press.

Hård, E., Musi, B., Dahlgren, I.L., Engel, J., Larsson, K., Liljequist, S., & Lindh, A.S. (1985). Impaired maternal behaviour and altered central serotonergic activity in the adult offspring of chronically ethanol treated dams. *Acta Pharmacologica et Toxicologica, 56,* 347–353.

Harlow, H.F. (1959). The development of learning in the rhesus monkey. *American Scientist, 47*(4), 459–479.

Martin, J.C., Martin, D.C., Sigman, G., & Radow, B. (1977). Offspring survival, development, and operant performance following maternal ethanol consumption. *Developmental Psychobiology, 10*(5), 435–446.

Martin, J.C., Martin, D.C., Sigman, G., & Radow, B. (1978). Maternal ethanol consumption and hyperactivity in cross-fostered offspring. *Physiological Psychology, 6,* 362–365.

Means, L.W., Burnette, M.A., & Pennington, S.N. (1988). The effect of embryonic ethanol exposure on detour learning in the chick. *Alcohol, 5*(4), 305–308.

Means, L.W., McDaniel, K., & Pennington, S.N. (1989). Embryonic ethanol exposure impairs detour learning in chicks. *Alcohol, 6*(4), 327–330.

Michaelis, E.K., & Michaelis, M.L. (1994). Cellular and molecular bases of alcohol's teratogenic effects. *Alcohol Health and Research World, 18*(1), 17–21.

Papara-Nicholson, D., & Telford, I.R. (1957). Effects of alcohol on reproduction and fetal development in the guinea pig. *Anatomical Record, 127,* 438–439.

Parker, S., Udani, M., Gavaler, J.S., & Van Thiel, D.H. (1984). Adverse effects of ethanol upon the adult sexual behavior of male rats exposed in utero. *Neurobehavioral Toxicology and Teratology, 6*(4), 289–293.

Pennington, S.N., Boyd, J.W., Kalmus, G.W., & Wilson, R.W. (1983). The molecular mechanism of fetal alcohol syndrome (FAS): I. Ethanol-induced growth suppression. *Neurobehavioral Toxicology and Teratology, 5*(2), 259–262.

Phillips, D.S., & Stainbrook, G.L. (1976). Effects of early alcohol exposure upon adult learning abilities and taste preferences. *Physiological Psychology, 4,* 473–475.

Randall, C.L. (1977). Teratogenic effects of in utero ethanol exposure. In K. Blum, D. Bord, & M. Hamilton (Eds.), *Alcohol and opiates: Neurochemical and behavioral mechanisms* (pp. 91–107). New York: Academic Press.

Randall, C.L. (1987). Alcohol as a teratogen: A decade of research in review. *Alcohol and Alcoholism (Suppl.),* 125–132.

Randall, C.L., Ekblad, J., & Anton, R.F. (1990). Perspectives on the pathophysiology of fetal alcohol syndrome. *Alcoholism: Clinical and Experimental Research, 14,* 807–812.

Randall, C.L., & Taylor, W.J. (1979). Prenatal ethanol exposure in mice: Teratogenic effects. *Teratology, 19,* 305–312.

Riley, E.P. (1990). The long-term behavioral effects of prenatal alcohol exposure in rats. *Alcoholism: Clinical and Experimental Research, 14*(5), 670–673.

Riley, E.P., Barron, S., & Hannigan, J.H. (1986). Response inhibition deficits following prenatal alcohol exposure: A comparison to the effects of hippocampal lesions in rats. In J.R.West (Ed.), *Alcohol and brain development* (pp. 71–102). London : Oxford University Press.

Riley, E.P., Lochry, E.A., & Shapiro, N.R. (1979). Lack of response inhibition in rats prenatally exposed to alcohol. *Psychopharmacology, 62*(1), 47–52.

Riley, E.P., Lochry, E.A., Shapiro, N.R., & Baldwin, J. (1979). Response perseveration in rats exposed to alcohol prenatally. *Pharmacology, Biochemistry, and Behavior, 10*(2), 255–259.

Riley, E.P., & Vorhees, C.V. (Eds.). (1986). *Handbook of behavioral teratology.* New York: Plenum.

Sandor, S., (1968). A new method for *in ovo* time-lapse cinematography of the chick embryo during the first three days of development. *Revue Roumaine d'Embryologie Cytologie Serie d'Embryologie, 5*(1), 77–80.

Sandor, S., & Amels, D. (1971). The action of ethanol on the prenatal development of albino rats. *Revue Roumaine d'Embryologie Cytologie Serie d'Embryologie, 8,* 101–118.

Sandor, S., & Elias, S. (1968). The influence of ethyl-alcohol on the development of the chick embryo. *Revue Roumaine d'Embryologie Cytologie Serie d'Embryologie, 5*(1), 51–76.

Savage, D.D., Montano, C.Y., Paxton, L.L., & Kasarskis, E.J. (1989). Prenatal ethanol exposure decreases hippocampal mossy fiber zinc in 45-day old rats. *Alcohol: Clinical and Experimental Research, 13,* 588–593.

Savage, D.D., Queen, S.A., Paxton, L.L., Goodlett, C.R., Mahoney, J.C., & West, J.R. (1991). Postnatal ethanol exposure decreases hippocampal mossy fiber zinc density in 45-day-old rats. *Alcohol: Clinical and Experimental Research, 15,* 339.

Savage, D.D., Queen, S.A., Sanchez, C.F., Paxton, L.L., Mahoney, J.C., Goodlett, C.R., & West, J.R. (1992). Prenatal ethanol exposure during the last third of gestation in rat reduces hippocampal NMDA agonist binding site density in 45-day-old offspring (RSA abstracts 164). *Alcohol, 9,* 37–41.

Schenker, S., Becker, H.C., Randall, C.L., Phillips, D.K., Baskin, G.S., & Henderson, G.I. (1990). Fetal alcohol syndrome: Current status of pathogenesis. *Alcoholism: Clinical and Experimental Research, 14*(5), 635–647.

Shaywitz, B.A., Griffieth, G.G., & Warshaw, J.B. (1979). Hyperactivity and cognitive deficits in developing rat pups born to alcoholic mothers: An experimental model of the expanded fetal alcohol syndrome (EFAS). *Neurobehavioral Toxicology, 1,* 113–122.

Streissguth, A.P., & Dehaene, P. (1993). Fetal alcohol syndrome in twins of alcoholic mothers: Concordance of diagnosis and IQ. *American Journal of Medical Genetics, 47,* 857–861.

Streissguth, A.P., & Little, R.E. (1994). *Alcohol, pregnancy, and the fetal alcohol syndrome: Unit 5. Biomedical education: Alcohol use and its medical consequences* (slide lecture series, 2nd ed.). Hanover, NH: Dartmouth Medical School, Project Cork. (Available by calling 1-800-432-8433.)

Sulik, K.K., Johnson, M.C., & Webb, M.A. (1981). Fetal alcohol syndrome: Embryogenesis in a mouse model. *Science, 214,* 936–938.

Surgeon General's Advisory on Alcohol and Pregnancy. (1981). *FDA Drug Bulletin, 11*(2). Rockville, MD: U.S. Department of Health and Human Services.

West, J.R. (Ed.). (1986). *Alcohol and brain development.* New York: Oxford University Press.

Wilson, J.G. (1973). *Environment and birth defects.* New York: Academic Press.

Wilson, J.G. (1977). New area of concern in teratology. *Teratology, 16,* 227–228.

Wilson, J.G., & Fraser, F.C. (Eds.). (1977). *Handbook of teratology: Vol. 1. General principles, etiology.* New York: Plenum.

5

Alcohol's Impact on Children

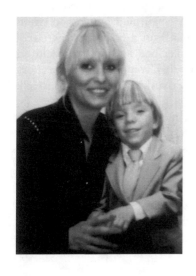

In Russia in 1974, Shurygin published a study in a pediatrics journal comparing 19 children of alcoholic mothers who were born before *their mothers became alcoholic with 23 children born* after *their mothers became alcoholic. Those born prior to the onset of alcoholism began at 9–10 years of age to display symptoms that were primarily vegetative, emotional, and behavioral in nature, and their symptoms tended to diminish with improved social circumstances. Many of the children born after the onset of their mothers' alcoholism, however, had profound central nervous system (CNS) impairments that were manifest in infancy, and 14 of the 23 had mental retardation (Shurygin, 1974).*

I came across this study a couple of years after we'd seen the first children with fetal alcohol syndrome (FAS) in Seattle, Washington. Shurygin, in Russia, must have been doing this work while Lemoine was studying similar children in France. I never knew who Shurygin was, never even knew his— or her—first name or other research. As far as I knew, Shurygin was a solitary figure carrying out a highly original piece of research from what seemed to be personal experience. What was it about the children of those alcoholic mothers who drank during pregnancy that so distinguished them from other children raised in alcoholic families, even from their own siblings?—It was organic brain damage from the toxic effects of alcohol that the children born to alcoholic mothers sustained before they were born. Shurygin's study, combined with the case reports of children with FAS, pointed to the importance of when in the course of her childbearing a mother drank. These studies also pointed to the unique role of the mother in contributing to the etiology of the child's problems.

It is hard to imagine in 1997, with the full impact of 24 years of research on alcohol and pregnancy, how exciting it was in the early 1970s to hear of the work of Lemoine in France, Shurygin in Russia, Sandor in Romania, or Papara-Nicholson and Telford in the United States. I remember vividly my own dismay in 1973, before the days of computer-generated searches, sitting in the University of Washington Health Sciences Library and having my stylus come up empty from the state-of-the-art international alcohol files as I "fished" for reference cards on alcohol and pregnancy using a manual system involving long boxes of 5″ × 7″ cards with holes punched along their edges according to predetermined categories.

I'll begin with a little history to help explain why what we take for granted today was not even imagined in the early 1970s. Surprisingly, the alcoholic family, as depicted and detailed in the scientific literature of the past, had typically referred to those families in which the father was identified as being alcoholic. Because alcohol researchers were used to studying the impact of liquor on the livers of heavy-drinking men, there was some skepticism in those early days that the "small" amounts of liquor consumed by women (relative to men) could have any impact at all on a fetus. In the early 1970s when risks to the fetus were described as being associated with 1–2 ounces of absolute alcohol per day, some male researchers were incredulous. "You'd call *that* heavy drinking?" they used to ask of me in disbelief.

Heavy-drinking fathers often felt the same: They tended to underplay the significance of their wives' drinking. For some, the realization came too late. A father whose son was diagnosed with FAS as a young adult said the following:

Looking back on it, I guess I was just totally unaware of how much my wife was drinking. It never seemed like much compared to what I drank. We always drank together at the officers' club; our social activities revolved around alcohol—it was just our way of life. Wherever we were in the world, the officers' club was always available. I did know that she'd pass out sometimes, and I'd have to help her home; but I know she never drank as much as I did. She tried to stop a couple of times but just couldn't seem to. She finally died of her alcoholism when our son was 13.

With the awareness of FAS in the mid-1970s, alcoholic mothers also became a focus of interest. This finally led to a better understanding of the impact of the mothers' alcoholism on her children and on the mother herself.

During the years between 1973 and 1997, many reports described the children of alcoholic mothers. These studies revealed the range of neurobehavioral difficulties detectable across the life span—not only in children with the physical features of FAS but also in other children without the full FAS who were born to alcoholic mothers. This chapter discusses how alcohol affects the sexes differently, describes the impact of alcoholic families and fathers, and then examines the effects of alcohol at social-drinking levels on children's neurobehavioral development.

CHILDREN OF ALCOHOLIC MOTHERS

Quickly on the heels of the alarming early reports from Nantes, France, and Seattle, Washington, clinicians in several countries began studies of children born to alcoholic mothers. Those studies described here have, for the most part, taken a developmental approach so that the natural history of children with FAS and of other children born to alcoholic mothers can be understood across the life span.

Göteborg, Sweden

In 1974, Marita Aronson, a psychologist in Göteborg, Sweden, began a series of studies on children of alcoholic mothers. In the first round of studies, Aronson and Olegård (1985) evaluated 99 children (with an average age of 14 years) who comprised all living offspring of 33 alcoholic mothers: 15% had low birth weight, and 10% had malformations. Half of the children had borderline or retarded mental development; 49% were classified as neuropsychologically atypical (which, in this study, was defined as having at least three of the following: hyperactivity, impulsiveness, distractibility, temper tantrums, short memory span, concentration difficulties, perseveration, and perceptual disorders). Aronson and Olegård (1985) also found that the rearing environments of the children were not related to their mental abilities or neuropsychological symptoms. Another important finding was that the children had significantly lower mental abilities than their own mothers.

In another study, 21 of the children from the first study were matched to a comparison group. Aronson and Olegård (1987) found that the young children of the alcoholic mothers had an average IQ score of 95, whereas the comparison group children had an average IQ score of 112. Even more important, 76% of the study-group children had delayed visual-perceptual ability, and 62% had attentional difficulties (hyperactivity, distractibility, or short attention span). None of the comparison-group children displayed either of these conditions (Aronson, Kyllerman, Sabel, Sandin, & Olegård, 1985).

More generally, Aronson (1984) found that children of alcoholic mothers have a wide range of mental disabilities and that increased severity of physical malformations is associated with decreased intellectual performance. This parallels the earlier findings of Streissguth, Herman, and Smith (1978a). But even children without any facial anomalies who were born to alcoholic mothers had significantly lower IQ scores than children born to mothers who did not drink while pregnant (Aronson, 1984; Jones, Smith, Streissguth, & Myrianthopoulos, 1974; Streissguth, Little, Woodell, & Herman, 1979). Aronson (1984) stated, "Reduced size and malformations are the most *visible* aspects of the fetal alcohol syndrome, but mental retardation and neuropsychological disturbances seem to be the most *serious* defect" (p. 24; emphasis added).

In fact, 12 years later, Aronson (1996) conducted a third study, examining 24 of the study-group children as young adolescents, and found continuing neuropsychological impairments; more than 60% of the cohort had also developed neuropsychiatric impairments. Three of the 24 children had autistic-type disorders (including two with a dual diagnosis of Asperger syndrome and FAS/FAE), two had attention-deficit/hyperactivity disorder, two had motor perception dysfunction (MPD), and eight had deficits in attention, motor control, and perception (DAMP). (Two reports from Canada had previously described the coexistence of FAS/FAE with autism or autistic behaviors [Harris, MacKay, & Osborn, 1995; Nanson, 1992].) Although two thirds of the study-group children had been placed in foster care and received intervention and support services, they remained difficult to raise. Aronson (1996) concluded that early fostering did not eliminate the harmful effects of exposure to alcohol in utero.

Berlin, Germany

In 1977, Spohr, a pediatrician, and Steinhausen, a child psychiatrist, began the Berlin FAS Study. A number of papers have described the physical, intellectual, and psychiatric problems of 158 children with FAS (Spohr & Steinhausen, 1987; Spohr, Willms, & Steinhausen, 1993; Steinhausen, Gobel, & Nestler, 1984; Steinhausen, Willms, & Spohr, 1993, 1994).

Spohr, Willms, and Steinhausen (1994) presented follow-up data on 44 of these individuals ages 14 and older, describing how, with age, their behavioral functioning became more delayed, their intellectual functioning remained stable, and their physical symptoms of FAS became less prominent. As adolescents, only 10% still had the pronounced and recognizable dysmorphic features of FAS, yet 75% did not function at an age-appropriate level, manifesting distinct mental and social impairments. Spohr et al. (1994) described a trend in their development in which, after an initial stage of age-appropriate performance, they developed increasing problems with abstract reasoning and central cognitive processing. Almost 50% were described as having emotional disorders and stereotypic behavior. Approximately 35% had speech disorders, and 30% had hyperkinesis. Although 30% had attended a general education primary school, none attended general education high schools. About one third were eventually hospitalized in institutions for individuals with mental retardation. Behaviorally, German adolescents with FAS were much like those described in France and Seattle. Spohr et al. (1994) noted, "Sometimes serious intellectual shortcomings were masked by a lively friendliness or a very effective superficial skill in language" (p. 26).

In 1996, Steinhausen traced the prevalence of a group of psychopathologies in these children from preschool to later school age. Altogether, 63% of the children displayed symptoms of one or more psychiatric disorders as they aged. Although some disorders decreased in frequency (e.g., eating disorders, enuresis), others increased (e.g., emotional disorders, habits, stereotypes, speech disorders). A third group of symptoms (characteristic of conduct disorders and hyperkinetic disorders) remained constant. Attentional deficits were the most frequent problem reported by parents and teachers, followed by social relationship problems (Steinhausen, 1996a, b).

Nantes, France

In Nantes, France, Lemoine, who in 1968 published results of the first study of FAS, conducted in his retirement an heroic 30-year

follow-up study (Lemoine & Lemoine, 1992). Among 50 of his former patients with severe FAS, five had died in childhood, primarily
from cardiac or respiratory problems. Among 28 with mild FAS, two
had committed suicide as adults, and five others had attempted suicide. After examining 99 of his patients with FAS, many of whom he
found in state institutions, Lemoine concluded that mental problems constituted the most severe manifestations of FAS in adulthood, including both intellectual mental retardation and behavior
problems (Lemoine & Lemoine, 1992). This extraordinary report
from Lemoine and his physician son is a landmark work that has
not received the worldwide attention it deserves. Published in
French, it has never been officially translated. An English account
of Lemoine's paper is included in Streissguth (1994).

Lemoine also examined 16 former patients who, as children,
had *not* exhibited the physical manifestations of FAS, although they
had been born to alcoholic mothers and had early psychomotor retardation. He found that, as adults, these individuals had significant behavior problems and were unable to stay focused on any activity. Six of these individuals were found in centers for adults with
moderate disabilities. It is also interesting to note that Lemoine
also encountered 10 of the original mothers from his study who had
since been treated for their alcoholism and given birth to normal
children who grew into normal adults.

In the first study to address the prevalence of individuals with
alcohol-related birth defects in institutions treating individuals
with disabilities, Lemoine and Lemoine (1992) made some remarkable observations. In the course of tracing his former patients,
Lemoine examined additional individuals in each of the various institutions who were known to have been born to alcoholic mothers.
He estimated that in five centers serving adults with moderate disabilities, 20% (33 individuals) of the population were born to alcoholic mothers. Of these 33, 25 individuals had severe FAS, and 8 had
FAE and displayed no dysmorphic characteristics. In three institutions serving younger and less severely affected children and adolescents, Lemoine estimated that 14% of the population had been born
to alcoholic mothers (of these 42 individuals, 6 were dysmorphic and
36 were not).

Lemoine and Lemoine (1992) concluded that there are severe
long-term psychological challenges associated with FAS that indicate the need for long-term professional services, even when the individuals lack the characteristic dysmorphic features.

Helsinki, Finland

In 1979, the first child with FAS was reported in the Finnish medical literature. Four years later, in 1983, Finnish researchers began a major campaign to counsel women in antenatal clinics to reduce their drinking during pregnancy. Of 85 women detected to be problem drinkers in Helsinki, Finland, and outlying suburbs, 55 women (65%) reduced their alcohol intake by at least 50% (Halmesmäki, 1988). Nevertheless, 20 infants (24%) were born with full FAS and 22 (26%) were born with FAE.

In a follow-up study of these same infants, Autti-Rämö (1993) found that FAS facial dysmorphology and growth deficiency were most characteristic of offspring of women who drank throughout pregnancy, but that even those who cut down in the second trimester had children with a significantly higher occurrence of delayed psychomotor, cognitive, and speech development by 18–27 months of age. Decreasing alcohol use during the first trimester, which was possible for about one third of the mothers, was the most efficacious for the offspring.

These comprehensive studies, spanning the life span of children with FAS from Göteborg, Berlin, Nantes, and Helsinki, as well as Tübingen (Majewski, 1993) and Münster, Germany (Löser, 1995), complement those from Seattle (as reported in Chapters 2 and 3) (Hanson, Jones, & Smith, 1976; Jones et al., 1974; LaDue, Streissguth, & Randels, 1992; Streissguth, 1976; Streissguth et al., 1991; Streissguth, Clarren, & Jones, 1985; Streissguth, Herman, & Smith, 1978a, b). There is now no doubt that children born to alcoholic mothers who drank during pregnancy are at risk for numerous and varied adverse neurodevelopmental outcomes that do not ameliorate as they mature and that this risk also extends to those without the typical FAS features.

HOW A MOTHER'S ALCOHOLISM
AFFECTS HER CHILDREN AND HER HEALTH

My wife came from a distinguished family with good academic credentials. She herself had an advanced degree and taught at our local college. Her mother had been a professional before her. My wife began drinking heavily when she gave up her job to become a mother. She was already drinking during her pregnancy with our first baby (later identified as having FAE) and was drinking even more during her second pregnancy—more than I ever realized. Staying home with a baby was very difficult for her. Our second child (diagnosed with FAS at 6 years of age) was born a couple of years after our first. My wife was dead of cirrhosis by the time our younger child was 1 year old.

Not all children whose mothers abuse alcohol during pregnancy have FAS, and it is not uncommon for a child with the FAS to have an older sibling with only partial or mild effects. Both mothers and infants differ greatly in their vulnerability to alcohol damage. Chronicity or stage of alcoholism may also be relevant. Yet, many mothers who have produced children with FAS during their alcoholism have produced normal children after being in recovery. Likewise, many mothers who have produced children with FAS during a period of alcohol abuse had previously produced normal children during an alcohol-free period.

Dehaene (1995; Dehaene et al., 1981) examined the reproductive histories of five mothers with chronic alcoholism and found that these mothers gave birth to infants with FAS after a string of children with successively lower birth weights (see Figure 5.1). Clinicians note that children with FAS are often produced at or near the end of an alcoholic mother's reproductive history and that once an alcoholic mother has produced a child with FAS, she is likely to con-

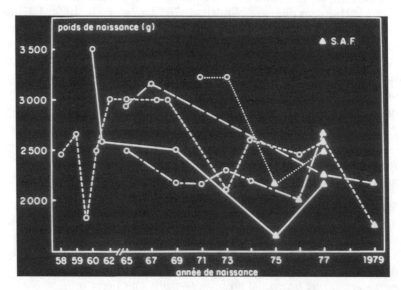

Figure 5.1. Birth weight of successive offspring of five mothers who have chronic alcoholism. (SAF = syndrome d'alcoolisme fœtal = fetal alcohol syndrome.) (From Dehaene et al., 1981, p. 2641; reprinted by permission.)

tinue producing more children with FAS unless she stops drinking or dies (Dehaene et al., 1981; see also Abel, 1988). This early observation has now been confirmed by Spohr (1996) in a study of 76 siblings of 56 children with FAS. Siblings older than the index child by at least 5 years were reported to be normal in terms of schooling and professional education. The closer they were to the index FAS child, the more likely the older siblings were to have FAE; the youngest children were often the most affected.

In the 1970s and 1980s, researchers began to more closely examine the different ways in which alcohol affects both of the sexes. They found that females appear to attain higher peak blood concentrations than males with a given dose of alcohol (Frezza et al., 1990); to be more susceptible to liver damage from alcohol (Norton, Batey, Dwyer, & MacMahon, 1987); to develop alcoholism at younger ages than men and after fewer years of heavy drinking; and to die at an earlier age of alcohol-related diseases (Ashley et al., 1977; Deal & Gavaler, 1994). These studies are important for understanding the biological impact of alcohol on both the mothers themselves and on their fetuses and may help explain the compounding impact that chronic maternal alcoholism appears to have on the offspring. Research also indicates that among alcoholic women, a binge pattern of alcohol consumption is particularly associated with premature death (Smith, Lewis, Kercher, & Spitznagel, 1994). This relates to one of the shocking findings from follow-up studies of children with FAS: A high proportion (69% in one study) of the biological mothers of children with FAS were dead before their children were grown up (Aronson, 1996; May, Hymbaugh, Aase, & Samet, 1983; Streissguth et al., 1991; Streissguth et al., 1985).

Could the deteriorating biological state of the mother as the disease of alcoholism progresses have an impact on the children she produces? In an important early study, researchers from Tübingen, Germany, studied this question by examining the children born to alcoholic mothers who were in different stages of their alcoholism (Majewski, 1981; Seidenberg & Majewski, 1978). Women in the earliest stages of alcoholism had fewer children with FAS, and those they did have were more lightly affected. Women in the most chronic and severe stage of alcoholism had a higher proportion of children with FAS, and these children were much more severely affected, for example, having more major malformations in addition to FAS. Majewski did not find large enough differences in what these women reported drinking to account for the large differences in the outcomes of their children, but obtaining accurate drinking histories from active alcoholics is difficult. Majewski concluded that the stage of the mother's alcoholism is an important factor in the health of the offspring.

We also studied this question in Seattle in the late 1970s by examining the children of alcoholic mothers who were in recovery. We included 50 recovered alcoholic mothers who were drinking during a target pregnancy; 50 recovered alcoholic mothers who were not drinking during a target pregnancy, and 50 nonalcoholic mothers who were not drinking during a target pregnancy. Target infants (matched across groups for age and sex) born to the alcoholic mothers who drank during their pregnancies had significantly lower birth weights than those born to the alcoholic mothers who abstained from alcohol during their pregnancies, yet both groups had significantly lower birth weights than women who had never been alcoholic (Little, Streissguth, Barr, & Herman, 1980.) The average IQ scores of the three groups of offspring followed a similar pattern, with the control children earning the highest scores, followed by the children of the abstinent alcoholics, and the children of the drinking alcoholics earning the lowest scores (Streissguth et al., 1979).

The best estimate from existing data is that between 25% and 45% of women with chronic alcoholism will give birth to children with FAS if they continue to drink heavily during pregnancy (Aronson, 1984; Bingol et al., 1987; Jones et al., 1974; Majewski, 1981; Majewski & Majewski, 1988; May et al., 1983; Olegård et al., 1979; Seidenberg & Majewski, 1978).

Perhaps some of the prenatal effects of alcohol, even those that occur while an alcoholic mother refrains from drinking during pregnancy, can be explained by the damage that alcohol does to the female reproductive system. In the first data ever available on drinking and reproductive dysfunction from a representative national sample of women, Wilsnack, Klassen, and Wilsnack (1984) found that dysmenorrhea, heavy menstrual flow, and premenstrual discomfort increased with drinking level and were particularly strongly associated with six or more drinks per day at least once a week. Mello, Mendelson, and Teoh (1989) also found that female alcohol abuse and alcoholism are associated with a broad spectrum of reproductive system disorders including amenorrhea, anovulation, lateral phase dysfunction, and ovarian pathology. The reproductive consequences can range from infertility and increased risk of spontaneous abortion to impaired fetal growth and development.

Joseph A. Califano, Jr., former Secretary of Health, Education, and Welfare, said the following in a 1996 news release:

> These 2 years of work have uncovered a tremendous void in research on women and substance abuse. . . . The more recent recognition that

women's problems require separate attention has served to underscore how much we do not know. . . . In 1989, the year of the most recent comprehensive survey, less that 14% of all women and 12% of pregnant women who needed treatment received it. (pp. 3, 11–12)

More research on female alcohol abuse is certainly needed, particularly in the treatment arena.

CHILDREN OF ALCOHOLIC FATHERS AND FAMILIES

"Your talk on FAS was very interesting, doctor, but what happens to the baby when the man is drinking the alcohol?" After lecturing on FAS for 23 years, this is absolutely the most frequent question I am asked, and it is almost always asked by women. The many challenges that beset families of alcoholics and their impact on the welfare of the children are widely known. Yet the alcoholic family, as depicted and detailed in the scientific literature of the past, has typically referred to those families in which the identified alcoholic is the father. Nylander's (1960) classic study of children of alcoholic fathers, for example, revealed that these children had more emotional challenges, were more often neglected, and had more somatic and psychiatric symptoms and behavior problems than comparison-group children. A 20-year follow-up of these children revealed that boys of alcoholic fathers had more challenges with psychosocial adaptation than comparison-group boys (Rydelius, 1981). Frequently, researchers find that children of alcoholic fathers have lower IQ scores and more episodes of social and psychiatric disturbances, delinquency, defiance of authority, alcoholism, and hyperactivity than children of fathers who are not alcoholic (Abel & Lee, 1988; Drake & Vaillant, 1988; Earls, Reich, Jung, & Cloninger, 1988; El-Guebaly & Offord, 1977; Ervin, Little, Streissguth, & Beck, 1984; Sher, 1991; von Knorring, 1991). For the most part, these studies have focused on the rearing father, not necessarily the biological father. Since the mid-1980s, more attempts to study the biological effects of paternal alcohol use and abuse have been undertaken.

Reproductive effects associated with male alcoholism have included problems with sperm production, quality, and motility. One study reported small birth weights in offspring of fathers who drank regularly or heavily (Little & Sing, 1986), but another study failed to replicate the results when the fathers used considerably less alcohol (Savitz, Zhang, Schwinge, & John, 1992). A few animal studies have addressed this topic. Abel and Lee (1988), for example, found decreased activity and serum testosterone in rat and mouse pups sired by alcohol-consuming males but no effect on body or organ weights. Rat studies by Cicero (1994) have suggested that a period of moderate alcohol consumption by males during sexual maturation, followed by a drug-free period sufficient to restore normal hormonal status, resulted in atypical offspring development. The results were highly selective, involving decreases in different hormone levels in male versus female offspring and impairments in visual-spatial performance in males only. Another line of studies reported cognitive impairments in nondrinking sons of male alcoholics (e.g., Ozkaragoz & Noble, 1995; Tarter, Jacob, & Bremer, 1989), but, again, these findings have not been consistently reported (e.g., Gillen & Hesselbrock, 1992). In fact, the paternal effects literature is small and inconsistent compared with the vast and systematic base of scientific knowledge developed since the 1970s on FAS and the adverse effects of prenatal alcohol exposure on offspring.

The Children of Kauai

Werner's landmark study of an entire population of children born in 1955 on the island of Kauai, Hawaii, demonstrates the long-term impact of maternal versus paternal alcoholism on children when mothers abused alcohol while pregnant. In a series of books published since the 1970s, Werner painstakingly described this cohort of 700 children from birth to adulthood. In her 1986 paper, Werner described the long-term outcomes of 200 children designated to be at risk of adverse outcome due to a variety of circumstances. Of these 200, 43 had alcoholic fathers, and 11 had alcoholic mothers. Of the 11 with alcoholic mothers, 10 developed serious learning and behavior problems by 18 years of age. These 10 included all 9 children of those alcoholic mothers known to have been drinking during pregnancy. By contrast, only 10 of the 43 children who had an alcohol-abusing father developed serious learning and behavior problems (Werner, 1986). Although much has been written about resiliency in childhood and the environmental factors that promote resiliency even in alcoholic families (e.g., Children of Alcoholics Foundation, Inc., 1992), Werner's research clearly indicates that the children of alcoholic mothers were not resilient, especially when the mothers were drinking during pregnancy.

Outcomes of Children Removed from Alcoholic Homes

Several researchers have explored the issue of whether children with FAS show improved performance when removed from their alcoholic homes. Several studies note that an improved environment does not improve the cognitive or intellectual level of children with FAS (e.g., Aronson, 1984; Spohr et al., 1994), presumably because they reflect the basic CNS effects of in utero alcohol exposure. An improved living situation, however, does seem to improve their psychosocial functioning. Aronson (1984) found that half of the children born to alcoholic mothers in her study exhibited psychosocial symptoms (defined as any three of the following: difficulty relating to others, aggressiveness, poor self-confidence, psychosomatic symptoms, insecurity, anxiety, truancy, juvenile delinquency, or drug abuse). Those in foster or adoptive homes had fewer psychosocial symptoms than those living in their biological homes. In particular, those removed from their biological mothers before 6 months of age had fewer psychosocial symptoms than the others (Aronson, 1984; Aronson & Olegård, 1987). Findings from our secondary disabilities study of 415 people of all ages with FAS/FAE confirmed these findings: Living in a stable and nurturing environment (for at least the median duration for the group) was the most important "universal" protective factor studied. Individuals who lived in such homes were less likely to have disrupted school experiences, inappropriate sexual behaviors, trouble with the law, and alcohol or other drug problems (Streissguth, Barr, Kogan, & Bookstein, 1996).

ALCOHOL AND CHILDREN WHEN MOTHERS DRINK SOCIALLY

Women of childbearing age use alcohol more frequently than cigarettes or any of the illegal drugs (Day & Richardson, 1994) (see Figure 5.2). One of the most serious consequences of alcohol use by women is the intra-uterine impact on their children. Although mothers who are alcoholic or abusing alcohol are at highest risk of having children with FAS, even women who drink socially are at increased risk of poor pregnancy outcomes and of having children with subtle yet long-lasting neurodevelopmental problems.

The National Institute on Alcohol Abuse and Alcoholism (NIAAA) funded several large prospective studies on alcohol and pregnancy to examine the effects of prenatal alcohol exposure. These studies used maternal self-report (usually obtained during pregnancy) to examine the relationship between alcohol dose and offspring outcomes at various ages; they used "blind" assessments and adjusted statistically, or through the study design, for potential confounders. The role of the human social-drinking studies is to determine the breadth and magnitude of the prenatal damage from alcohol in offspring at varying ages as well as the relationship to dose, timing, and pattern of exposure. New analytical techniques

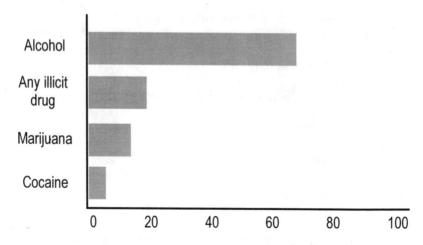

Figure 5.2.   Alcohol and other drug use among women of childbearing age. (From Streissguth & Little, 1994, p. 3; reprinted by permission.)

have permitted examination of multiple outcomes of multiple measures of dose within a single analysis (see Bookstein, Sampson, Streissguth, & Barr, 1996; Streissguth, Bookstein, Sampson, & Barr, 1993).

These studies have revealed many types of adverse pregnancy outcomes associated with varying levels of prenatal alcohol exposure. Findings have included increased frequency of miscarriages and stillbirths; increased frequency of premature babies and babies who were of low birth weight for their gestational ages; and decreased average birth weight, length, and head circumference (see Coles, 1992; Day, 1992; Kaminski & Larroque, 1996; Little & Wendt, 1991; Streissguth, Barr, Sampson, & Bookstein, 1994; and Streissguth et al., 1993, for reviews). Not all studies reported all findings; differences in study design, sample size, presence of other risk factors, level of alcohol use in the sample, number of heavier drinkers in the sample, and methods of measuring exposure may account for the discrepancies. The studies have included populations of inner-city African American mothers, lower-class Caucasian mothers, and middle-class mothers receiving prenatal care through prepaid health plans. Prenatal alcohol exposure cuts a wide swath.

CNS Dysfunction in Neonates

A few studies went beyond the traditional endpoints of epidemiology and conducted detailed examinations of newborns, measuring alcohol-related disruptions in typical sleep/wake cycles (Rosett et al., 1979); atypical electroencephalogram (EEG) patterns, which are particularly associated with maternal binge drinking (Day, 1992; Ioffe & Chernick, 1988); and increased frequency of poor habituation to redundant stimuli, weak suck and longer latency to initiate suckling, and poor reflex development (Streissguth et al., 1994; Streissguth, Bookstein, & Barr, 1996).

Habituation is a basic characteristic with which human infants and most other species are born. It represents the ability of an organism to "tune out" the many stimuli confronting it that are not relevant to its well-being. Brazelton (1973) developed a method of measuring habituation in newborns by repeatedly shining a flashlight beam across their eyelids while they are sleeping lightly. Typically, the baby makes a couple of twitches or squints but then resumes sleeping. Those infants exposed prenatally to alcohol, however, were not as adept at habituation. The more alcohol to which the infant was exposed prenatally, the more his or her sleep was disrupted by the light beam. Habituation to auditory stimuli was similarly measured with a rattle and a bell.

Poor habituation is thought to be one of the earliest signs of CNS dysfunction. It is thought to be analogous to the response inhibition deficits produced by prenatal alcohol exposure with animal models (Driscoll, Streissguth, & Riley, 1990). Indeed, these studies later found that "habituation to light" on day 1 of life turned out to be the outcome most highly related to prenatal alcohol exposure out of the hundreds of outcomes subsequently examined in this longitudinal prospective study during the first 7 years of life (Streissguth et al., 1983, 1993).

These studies are of particular interest because they measured adverse effects of prenatal alcohol in the newborn period even before the later postnatal environment impinged on the child. Thus, these newborn studies provided some of the strongest evidence for the impact of prenatal alcohol exposure on the CNS of exposed human offspring. These findings are not limited to newborns of alcoholics, but rather are generally associated with alcohol exposure in a dose-dependent fashion (i.e., the higher the exposure, the greater the effects).

Infancy Impairments in Information Processing and Mental and Motor Functioning

Longitudinal prospective studies of inner-city African American children in Detroit, Michigan, have demonstrated reaction-time impairments at age 6½ months (Jacobson, Jacobson, & Sokol, 1994) and impairments in information processing associated with prenatal alcohol exposure in 12-month-old infants (Jacobson, Jacobson,

Sokol, Martier, & Ager, 1993). In this latter study, the more alcohol to which the infants had been exposed prenatally, the longer they took to process the information (i.e., to turn their gaze to a novel photograph). These findings are consistent with a study of information-processing difficulties with prenatal alcohol exposure in 4- and 7-year-old children (Streissguth et al., 1994; Streissguth, Bookstein, et al., 1996).

Several longitudinal prospective studies have also found alcohol-related decrements in mental or motor functioning during infancy (Day, 1992; Jacobson, Jacobson, Sokol, Martier, Ager, & Kaplan-Estrin, 1993; Streissguth et al., 1993). O'Connor, Brill, and Sigman (1986) studied well-educated older mothers and found not only that there were dose-related effects on infant mental tests but also that the 12-month-old infants of mothers drinking moderately to heavily (averaging 1 or more ounces of absolute alcohol per day) had IQ scores that were 24 points lower (on average) than their own mothers' IQ scores. Infants of nondrinking or lightly drinking mothers in the comparison group had a discrepancy of only three IQ points on average from their mothers' IQ scores.

Prenatal alcohol effects on infant mental and motor development are often not detected at ages 18–24 months (e.g., Euromac, 1992; Richardson, Day, & Goldschmidt, 1995; Streissguth et al., 1993). Global developmental tests may not be sensitive enough to detect subtle alcohol-related individual differences in infants born to mothers who drink only socially in the late infancy period. In general, the lower the level of exposure to be detected, the more sensitive and specific must be the tests used.

Neurobehavioral Findings in Preschool and Early School–Age Children

During the preschool and early school–age years, prenatal alcohol effects on cognitive, attentional, and motor performance have now been shown in seven different cohorts of children (Brown et al., 1991; Coles et al., 1991; Goldschmidt, Richardson, Stoffer, Geva, & Day, 1996; Landesman-Dwyer, Ragozin, & Little, 1981; Larroque et al., 1995; Russell, 1991; Streissguth et al., 1993). Sensitive neurobehavioral tests detected alcohol-related impairments on attention, spatial memory and integration, verbal memory and integration, flexible problem solving, and perceptual motor function at the end of the first year of school (see Streissguth et al., 1993, 1994; Streissguth, Bookstein, & Barr, 1996; for reviews.) Based on ratings by second-grade teachers, the classroom behaviors most salient for prenatal alcohol were difficulty retaining information; impulsivity/poor cooperation; and poorer comprehension of words, grammar, word recall, and tactfulness. These were important findings, as they indicated that the kinds of dysfunctional behaviors and neurobehavioral impairments measurable in the laboratory were also observed in the second-grade classroom.

Dysfunctional classroom behaviors were still associated with prenatal alcohol exposure when the children were 11 years old, namely problems with distractibility, restlessness, lack of persistence, reluctance to meet challenges, low arithmetic skills, and low overall achievement scores on standardized national achievement tests (Carmichael Olson, Sampson, Barr, Streissguth, & Bookstein, 1992). In both laboratory assessments (at 7 and 14 years of age) and classroom behavior ratings (at 7 and 11 years of age), arithmetic disability and attentional deficits were related to prenatal alcohol exposure (Streissguth, Bookstein, & Barr, 1996).

Longitudinal prospective studies have established that all four of the primary outcomes caused by prenatal alcohol exposure in experimental animals have also been associated with prenatal alcohol exposure in humans, including an increased rate of death (miscarriages and stillbirths), growth deficiency, minor physical anomalies, and CNS dysfunction. In well-nourished humans as in animal models, the growth deficiency may be more transient than the CNS effects (e.g., Sampson, Bookstein, Barr, & Streissguth, 1994), although in lower-class populations both types of effects of prenatal alcohol appear to persist into childhood (Day, Richardson, Geva, & Robles, 1994).

In some studies, because there are a variety of dose scores available, the relative salience of different timings and patterns of exposure can be evaluated. The salience of alcohol for attention, memory, and neurobehavioral outcomes is higher for alcohol exposure during early pregnancy (before a woman knows she is pregnant), and for a "binge" pattern of consumption. These data do not suggest a "safe threshold" of alcohol exposure.

CONCLUSIONS

Research from several types of studies has answered many questions about alcohol and pregnancy since the 1970s. All women are now advised to abstain from alcohol use during pregnancy. Whereas mothers who are alcoholic or abusing alcohol during pregnancy are at highest risk of having children with FAS, even social-drinking women are at risk of having children with subtle yet long-lasting neurodevelopmental problems.

Mothers who are the most chronically alcoholic appear to be at highest risk of producing children with FAS/FAE and of producing the most severely affected children. Children with full FAS are more likely to appear later in the childbearing trajectory of alcoholic women, often following instances of poor pregnancy outcome or of children with only partial or mild features of FAS.

Women who have borne children with FAS during a period of alcohol abuse have borne healthy children in their sobriety. Alcoholic women who are able to stop drinking during a pregnancy, particularly early in pregnancy, are less likely to have children with FAS/FAE and to have improved pregnancy outcomes. It seems fitting to appreciate the work of Shurygin in recognizing that the critical variable in the lives of children of alcoholics is whether they were prenatally exposed to alcohol.

REFERENCES

Abel, E.L. (1988). Fetal alcohol syndrome in families. *Neurotoxicology and Teratology, 10,* 1–2.

Abel, E.L., & Lee, J.A. (1988). Paternal alcohol exposure affects offspring behavior but not body or organ weights in mice. *Alcoholism: Clinical and Experimental Research, 12*(3), 349–355.

Aronson, M. (1984). *Children of alcoholic mothers.* Unpublished doctoral dissertation, University of Göteborg, Departments of Pediatrics and Psychology, Sweden.

Aronson, M. (1996, July 28–30). *Neuropsychological and neuropsychiatric disorders in children exposed to alcohol during pregnancy: A follow-up study of 24 children born to alcoholic mothers in Göteborg, Sweden.* Paper presented at the International Symposium on Neurobehavioral Effects of Prenatal Alcohol Exposure, Missilac, France.

Aronson, M., Kyllerman, M., Sabel, K.G., Sandin, B., & Olegård, R. (1985). Children of alcoholic mothers: Developmental, perceptual and behavioral characteristics as compared to matched controls. *Acta Paediatrica Scandinavica, 74*(1), 27–35.

Aronson, M., & Olegård, R. (1987). Children of alcoholic mothers. *Pediatrician, 14,* 57–61.

Ashley, M.J., Olin, J.S., leRiche, W.H., Kornaczewski, A., Schmidt, W., & Rankin, J.G. (1977). Morbidity in alcoholics: Evidence for accelerated development of physical disease in women. *Archives of Internal Medicine, 137,* 883–887.

Autti-Rämö, I. (1993). *The outcome of children exposed to alcohol in utero: A prospective follow-up study during the first three years.* Helsinki, Finland: University of Helsinki, Department of Child Neurology.

Bingol, N., Schuster, C., Fuchs, M., Iosub, S., Turner, G., Stone, R.K., & Gromisch, D.S. (1987). The influence of socioeconomic factors on the occurrence of fetal alcohol syndrome. *Advances in Alcohol and Substance Abuse, 6*(4), 105–118.

Bookstein, F.L., Sampson, P.D., Streissguth, A.P., & Barr, H.M. (1996). Exploiting redundant measurement of dose and developmental outcome: New methods from the behavioral teratology of alcohol. *Developmental Psychology, 32*(3), 404–415.

Brazelton, T.B. (1973). Neonatal Behavioral Assessment Scale. *Clinics in Developmental Medicine, 50.* London: William Heinemann Medical Books, Ltd.

Brown, R.T., Coles, C.D., Smith, I.E., Platzman, K.A., Erickson, S., & Falek, A. (1991). Effects of prenatal alcohol exposure at school age: II. Attention and behavior. *Neurotoxicology and Teratology, 13*(4), 369–376.

Califano, J.A., Jr. (1996). *Substance abuse and the American woman* (Executive summary and foreword). New York: Columbia University, National Center on Addiction and Substance Abuse.

Carmichael Olson, H., Sampson, P.D., Barr, H.M., Streissguth, A.P., & Bookstein, F.L. (1992). Prenatal exposure to alcohol and school problems in late childhood: A longitudinal prospective study. *Development and Psychopathology, 4,* 341–359.

Children of Alcoholics Foundation, Inc. (1992). *Report of the Forum on Protective Factors, Resiliency, and Vulnerable Children.* New York: Author.

Cicero, T.J. (1994). Effects of paternal exposure to alcohol on offspring development. *Alcohol Health and Research World, 18*(1), 37–41.

Coles, C.D. (1992). Prenatal alcohol exposure and human development. In M.W. Miller (Ed.), *Development of the central nervous system: Effects of alcohol and opiates* (pp. 9–36). New York: John Wiley & Sons.

Coles, C.D., Brown, R.T., Smith, I.E., Platzman, K.A., Erickson, S., & Falek, A. (1991). Effects of prenatal alcohol exposure at school age: I. Physical and cognitive development. *Neurotoxicology and Teratology, 13*(4), 357–367.

Day, N.L. (1992). Effects of prenatal alcohol exposure. In I.S. Zagon & T.A. Slotkin (Eds.), *Maternal substance abuse and the developing nervous system* (pp. 27–43). San Diego: Academic Press.

Day, N.L., & Richardson, G.A. (1994). Comparative teratogenicity of alcohol and other drugs. *Alcohol Health and Research World, 18*(1), 42–48.

Day, N.L., Richardson, G.A., Geva, D., & Robles, N. (1994). Alcohol, marijuana, and tobacco: Effects of prenatal exposure on offspring growth and morphology at age six. *Alcoholism: Clinical and Experimental Research, 18*(4), 786–794.

Deal, S.R., & Gavaler, J.S. (1994). Are women more susceptible than men to alcohol-induced cirrhosis? *Alcohol Health and Research World, 18*(3), 189–191.

Dehaene, P. (1995). La grossesse et l'alcool [Alcohol and pregnancy]. *Que Sais-Je?, 2934.* Paris: Presses Universitaires de France.

Dehaene, P., Crépin, G., Delahousse, G., Querleu, D., Walbaum, R., Titran, M., & Samaille-Villette, C. (1981). Aspects épidémiologiques du syndrome d'alcoolisme fœtal: 45 observations en 3 ans [Epidemiological aspects of fetal alcohol syndrome: 45 observations in 3 years]. *La Nouvelle Presse Médicale, 10,* 2639–2643.

Drake, R.E., & Vaillant, G.E. (1988). Predicting alcoholism and personality disorder in a 33-year longitudinal study of children of alcoholics. *British Journal of Addiction, 83*(7), 799–807.

Driscoll, C.D., Streissguth, A.P., & Riley, E.P. (1990). Prenatal alcohol exposure: Comparability of effects in humans and animal models. *Neurotoxicology and Teratology, 12*, 231–237.

Earls, R., Reich, W., Jung, K.G., & Cloninger, R.C. (1988). Psychopathology in children of alcoholic and antisocial parents. *Alcoholism: Clinical and Experimental Research, 12*(4), 481–487.

El-Guebaly, N., & Offord, D. (1977). Offspring of alcoholics: A critical review. *American Journal of Psychiatry, 134*(4), 357–365.

Ervin, C.S., Little, R.E., Streissguth, A.P., & Beck, D.E. (1984). Alcoholic fathering and its relation to child's intellectual development: A pilot investigation. *Alcoholism: Clinical and Experimental Research, 8*(4), 362–365.

Euromac. (1992). A European concerted action: Maternal alcohol consumption and its relation to the outcome of pregnancy and child development at 18 months. *International Journal of Epidemiology, 21*(4, Suppl.), 1–87.

Frezza, M., di-Padova, C., Pozzato, G., Terpin, M., Baraona, E., & Lieber, C.S. (1990). High blood alcohol levels in women. The role of decreased gastric alcohol dehydrogenase activity and first-pass metabolism. *New England Journal of Medicine, 322*(2), 95–99.

Gillen, R., & Hesselbrock, V. (1992). Cognitive functioning, ASP, and family history of alcoholism in young men at risk for alcoholism. *Alcoholism: Clinical and Experimental Research, 16*(2), 206–214.

Goldschmidt, L., Richardson, G.A., Stoffer, D.S., Geva, D., & Day, N.L. (1996). Prenatal alcohol exposure and acedemic achievement at age six: A nonlinear fit. *Alcoholism: Clinical and Experimental Research, 20*(4), 763–770.

Halmesmäki, E. (1988). Alcohol counselling of 85 pregnant problem drinkers: Effect on drinking and fetal outcome. *British Journal of Obstetrics and Gynaecology, 95*, 243–247.

Hanson, J.W., Jones, K.L., & Smith, D.W. (1976). Fetal alcohol syndrome: Experience with 41 patients. *Journal of the American Medical Association, 235*(14), 1458–1460.

Harris, S.R., MacKay, L.L., & Osborn, J.A. (1995). Autistic behaviors in offspring of mothers abusing alcohol and other drugs: A series of case reports. *Alcoholism: Clinical and Experimental Research, 19*(3), 660–665.

Ioffe, S., & Chernick, V. (1988). Development of the EEG between 30 and 40 weeks' gestation in normal and alcohol-exposed infants. *Developmental Medicine and Child Neurology, 30*(6), 797–807.

Jacobson, S.W., Jacobson, J.L., & Sokol, R.J. (1994). Effects of fetal alcohol exposure on infant reaction time. *Alcoholism: Clinical and Experimental Research, 18*(5), 1125–1132.

Jacobson, S.W., Jacobson, J.L., Sokol, R.J., Martier, S.S., & Ager, J.W. (1993). Prenatal alcohol exposure and infant information processing ability. *Child Development, 64*(6), 1706–1721.

Jacobson, J.L., Jacobson, S.W., Sokol, R.J., Martier, S.S., Ager, J.W., & Kaplan-Estrin, M.G. (1993). Teratogenic effects on alcohol on infant development. *Alcoholism, Clinical and Experimental Research, 17*(1), 174–183.

Jones, K.L., Smith, D.W., Streissguth, A.P., & Myrianthopoulos, N.C. (1974). Outcome in offspring of chronic alcoholic women. *Lancet, 1*(866), 1076–1078.

Kaminski, M., & Larroque, B. (1996). Alcohol use during pregnancy and its effects on developmental outcome. In H-L. Spohr & H-C. Steinhausen (Eds.), *Alcohol, pregnancy, and the developing child* (pp. 41–60). New York: Cambridge University Press.

LaDue, R.A., Streissguth, A.P., & Randels, S.P. (1992). Clinical considerations pertaining to adolescents and adults with fetal alcohol syndrome. In T.B. Sonderegger (Ed.), *Perinatal substance abuse: Research findings and clinical implications* (pp. 104–131). Baltimore: Johns Hopkins University Press.

Landesman-Dwyer, S., Ragozin, A.S., & Little, R.E. (1981). Behavioral correlates of prenatal alcohol exposure: A four-year follow-up study. *Neurobehavioral Toxicology and Teratology, 3*(2), 187–193.

Larroque, B., Kaminski, M., Dehaene, P., Subtil, D., Delfosse, M-J., & Querleu, D. (1995). Moderate prenatal alcohol exposure and psychomotor development at preschool age. *American Journal of Public Health, 85*(12), 1654–1661.

Lemoine, P., & Lemoine, P. (1992). Avenir des enfants de mères alcooliques (Étude de 105 cas retrouvés à l'âge adulte) et quelques constatations d'intérêt prophylactique [Following the infants of alcoholic mothers (Study of 105 cases through adulthood and some notes on prophylaxis)]. *Annales de Pédiatrie (Paris), 39,* 226–235.

Little, R.E., & Sing, C.F. (1986). Association of father's drinking and infant's birth weight. *New England Journal of Medicine, 314,* 1644–1645.

Little, R.E., Streissguth, A.P., Barr, H.M., & Herman, C.S. (1980). Decreased birth weight in infants of alcoholic women who abstained during pregnancy. *Journal of Pediatrics, 96*(6), 974–977.

Little, R.E., & Wendt, J.K. (1991). The effects of maternal drinking in the reproductive period: An epidemiologic review. *Journal of Substance Abuse, 3*(2), 187–204.

Löser, H. (1995). *Alkohol-embryopathie und alkoholeffekte [Alcohol embryopathy and fetal alcohol syndrome].* Stuttgart, Germany: Gustav Fischer Verlag.

Majewski, F. (1981). Alcohol embryopathy: Some facts and speculations about pathogenesis. *Neurobehavioral Toxicology and Teratology, 3*(2), 129–144.

Majewski, F. (1993). Alcohol embryopathy: Experience with 200 patients. *Developmental Brain Dysfunction, 6,* 248–265.

Majewski, F., & Majewski, B. (1988). Alcohol embryopathy: Symptoms and auxological data and frequency among the offspring and pathogenesis. In K. Kuriyama, A. Takada, & H. Ishii (Eds.), *International Conference Series: No. 805. Biomedical and social aspects of alcohol and alcoholism* (pp. 837–844). Amsterdam, NY: Excerpta Medica.

May, P.A., Hymbaugh, K.J., Aase, J.M., & Samet, J.M. (1983). Epidemiology of fetal alcohol syndrome among American Indians of the Southwest. *Social Biology, 30*(4), 374–387.

Mello, N.K., Mendelson, J.H., & Teoh, S.K. (1989). Neuroendocrine consequences of alcohol abuse in women. In D.E. Hutchings (Ed.), *Prenatal abuse of licit and illicit drugs* (pp. 211–240). New York: Annals of the New York Academy of Sciences.

Nanson, J.L. (1992). Autism in fetal alcohol syndrome: A report of six cases. *Alcoholism: Clinical and Experimental Research, 16*(3), 558–565.

Norton, R., Batey, R., Dwyer, T., & MacMahon, S. (1987). Alcohol consumption and the risk of alcohol related cirrhosis in women. *British Medical Journal Clinical Research Edition, 295*(6590), 80–82.

Nylander, I. (1960). Children of alcoholic fathers. *Acta Paediatrica Scandinavica, 49*(121), 1–34.

O'Connor, M.J., Brill, N.J., & Sigman, M. (1986). Alcohol use in primiparous women older than 30 years of age: Relation to infant development. *Pediatrics, 78*(3), 444–450.

Olegård, R., Sabel, K.G., Aronsson, M., Sandin, B., Johansson, P.R., Carlsson, C., Kyllerman, M., Iversen, K., & Hrbek, A. (1979). Effects on the child of alcohol abuse during pregnancy. *Acta Paediatrica Scandinavica, 275*(Supp.), 112–121.

Ozkaragoz, T.Z., & Noble, E.P. (1995). Neuropsychological differences between sons of active alcoholic and non-alcoholic fathers. *Alcohol and Alcoholism, 30*(1), 115–123.

Richardson, G.A., Day, N.L., Goldschmidt, L. (1995). Prenatal alcohol, marijuana, and tobacco use: Infant mental and motor development. *Neurotoxicology and Teratology, 17*(4), 479–487.

Rosett, H.L., Snyder, P., Sander, S., Lee, A., Cook, P., Weiner, L., & Gould, J. (1979). Effects of maternal drinking on neonatal state regulation. *Developmental Medicine and Child Neurology, 21*(4), 464–473.

Russell, M. (1991). Clinical implications of recent research on the fetal alcohol syndrome. *Bulletin of the New York Academy of Medicine, 67*(3), 207–222.

Rydelius, P.A. (1981). Children of alcoholic fathers: Their social adjustment and their health status over 20 years. *Acta Paediatrica Scandinavica, 286*, 1–89.

Sampson, P.D., Bookstein, F.L., Barr, H.M., & Streissguth, A.P. (1994). Prenatal alcohol exposure, birthweight, and measures of child size from birth to age 14 years. *American Journal of Public Health, 84*(9), 1421–1428.

Savitz, D.A., Zhang, J., Schwinge, P., & John, E.M. (1992). Association of paternal alcohol use with gestational age and birth weight. *Teratology, 46*, 465–471.

Seidenberg, J., & Majewski, F. (1978). Zur häeufigkeit der alkoholembryopathie in den Verschjidenen phasen der müettlichen alkoholkrankheit [Frequency of alcohol embryopathy in the different phases of maternal alcoholism]. *Suchtgefahren, 24*, 63–75.

Sher, K.J. (1991). *Children of alcoholics: A critical appraisal of theory and research*. Chicago: University of Chicago Press.

Shurygin, G.I. (1974). Ob osobennostyakh psikhicheskogo razvitiya detei ot materei, stradayushchikh khronicheskim alkogolizmom [Characteristics of the mental development of children of alcoholic mothers]. *Pediatriya Moskva, 11*, 71–73.

Smith, E.M., Lewis, C.E., Kercher, C., & Spitznagel, E. (1994). Predictors of mortality in alcoholic women: A 20-year follow-up study. *Alcoholism: Clinical and Experimental Research, 18*(5), 1177–1186.

Spohr, H-L. (1996). Fetal alcohol syndrome in adolescence: Long-term perspective of children diagnosed in infancy. In H-L. Spohr & H-C. Steinhausen (Eds.), *Alcohol, pregnancy, and the developing child* (pp. 207–226). New York: Cambridge University Press.

Spohr, H-L., & Steinhausen, H-C. (1987). Follow-up studies of children with fetal alcohol syndrome. *Neuropediatrics, 18*(1), 13–17.

Spohr, H-L., Willms, J., & Steinhausen, H-C. (1993). Prenatal alcohol exposure and long-term developmental consequences. *Lancet, 341*(8850), 907–910.

Spohr, H-L., Willms, J., & Steinhausen, H-C. (1994). The fetal alcohol syndrome in adolescence. *Acta Paediatrica, 83*(404), 19–26.

Steinhausen, H-C. (1996a, July 28–30). *Long-term outcome of children with FAS: Psychopathology, behavior, and intelligence.* Paper presented at the International Symposium on Neurobehavioral Effects of Prenatal Alcohol Exposure, Missilac, France.

Steinhausen, H-C. (1996b). Psychopathology and cognitive functioning in children with fetal alcohol syndrome. In H-L. Spohr & H-C. Steinhausen (Eds.), *Alcohol, pregnancy, and the developing child* (pp. 227–246). New York: Cambridge University Press.

Steinhausen, H-C., Gobel, D., & Nestler, V. (1984). Psychopathology in the offspring of alcoholic parents. *Journal of the American Academy of Child Psychiatry, 23*(4) 465–471.

Steinhausen, H-C., Willms, J., & Spohr, H-L. (1993). Long-term psychopathological and cognitive outcome of children with fetal alcohol syndrome. *Journal of the American Academy of Child and Adolescent Psychiatry, 32*(5), 990–994.

Steinhausen, H-C., Willms, J., & Spohr, H-L. (1994). Correlates of psychopathology and intelligence in children with fetal alcohol syndrome. *Journal of Child Psychology and Psychiatry and Allied Disciplines, 35,* 323–331.

Streissguth, A.P. (1976). Psychologic handicaps in children with the fetal alcohol syndrome. In F.A. Seixas & S. Eggleston (Eds.), *Work in progress in alcoholism* (Vol. 273, pp. 140–145). New York: Annals of the New York Academy of Sciences.

Streissguth, A.P. (1994). A long-term perspective of FAS. *Alcohol Health and Research World, 18*(1), 74–81.

Streissguth, A.P., Aase, J.M., Clarren, S.K., Randels, S.P., LaDue, R.A., & Smith, D.F. Fetal alcohol syndrome in adolescents and adults. (1991). *Journal of the American Medical Association, 265*(15), 1961–1967.

Streissguth, A.P., Barr, H.M., Kogan, J., & Bookstein, F.L. (1996). *Understanding the occurrence of secondary disabilities in clients with fetal alcohol syndrome: Final report to the Centers for Disease Control and Prevention on Grant No. RO4/CCR008515* (Tech. Report No. 96-06). Seattle: University of Washington, Fetal Alcohol and Drug Unit.

Streissguth, A.P., Barr, H.M., Sampson, P.D., & Bookstein, F.L. (1994). Prenatal alcohol and offspring development: The first fourteen years. *Drug and Alcohol Dependence, 36,* 89–99.

Streissguth, A.P., Bookstein, F.L., & Barr, H.M. (1996). A dose-response study of the enduring effects of prenatal alcohol exposure: Birth to 14 years. In H-L. Spohr & H-C. Steinhausen (Eds.), *Alcohol, pregnancy and the developing child* (pp. 141–168). New York: Cambridge University Press.

Streissguth, A.P., Bookstein, F.L., Sampson, P.D., & Barr, H.M. (1993). *The enduring effects of prenatal alcohol exposure on child development: Birth through 7 years, a partial least squares solution.* Ann Arbor: University of Michigan Press.

Streissguth, A.P., Clarren, S.K., & Jones, K.L. (1985). Natural history of the fetal alcohol syndrome: A ten-year follow-up of eleven patients. *Lancet, 2,* 85–91.

Streissguth, A.P., Herman, C.S., & Smith, D.W. (1978a). Intelligence, behavior, and dysmorphogenesis in the fetal alcohol syndrome: A report on 20 patients. *Journal of Pediatrics, 92,* 363–367.

Streissguth, A.P., Herman, C.S., & Smith, D.W. (1978b). Stability of intelligence in the fetal alcohol syndrome: A preliminary report. *Alcoholism: Clinical and Experimental Research, 2*(2), 165–170.

Streissguth, A.P., & Little, R.E. (1994). *Alcohol, pregnancy, and the fetal alcohol syndrome: Unit 5. Biomedical education: Alcohol use and its medical consequences* (slide lecture series, 2nd ed.). Hanover, NH: Dartmouth Medical School, Project Cork. (Available by calling 1-800-432-8433.)

Streissguth, A.P., Little, R.E., Woodell, S., & Herman, C.S. (1979). IQ in children of recovered alcoholic mothers compared to matched controls. *Alcoholism: Clinical and Experimental Research, 3*(2), 197.

Tarter, R.E., Jacob, T., & Bremer, D.A. (1989). Cognitive status of sons of alcoholic men. *Alcoholism: Clinical and Experimental Research, 13*(2), 232–235.

von Knorring, A-L. (1991). Annotation: Children of alcoholics. *Journal of Child Psychology and Psychiatry and Allied Disciplines, 32*(3), 411–421.

Werner, E.E. (1986). Resilient offspring of alcoholics: A longitudinal study from birth to age 18. *Journal of Studies on Alcohol, 47*(1), 34–40.

Wilsnack, S.C., Klassen, A.D., & Wilsnack, R.W. (1984). Drinking and reproductive dysfunction among women in a 1981 national survey. *Alcoholism: Clinical and Experimental Research, 8*(5), 451–458.

6

Primary and Secondary Disabilities

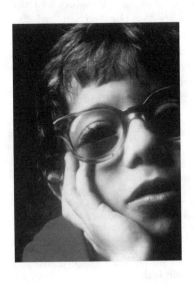

Mrs. Hallowell was a well-educated woman and the wife of a college professor. Dr. and Mrs. Hallowell had two children: The first was born before she became an alcoholic, and the second was born after. Their firstborn son had an extremely high IQ, whereas their second son, Jeremy, scored in the low to normal range when I first examined him as an adult. Although he did not have mental retardation, Jeremy's IQ score of 94 represented a clear cognitive impairment with respect to his genetic potential. Although some children of more typical parents are able to function adequately with an IQ score of 90 or 100, Jeremy's accompanying prenatal brain damage rendered him dysfunctional.

While Jeremy was growing up, however, he was never diagnosed as having FAS or FAE—these terms had not yet been invented. In retrospect, his mother, already in recovery for many years when we first met, described Jeremy as a disorganized, dependent, and forgetful child without much use for learning. He had small horizons and gave up easily. He was disoriented but sweet, and, as an adolescent, more depressed than hyperactive. He never seemed to comprehend social cues.

Individuals with FAS/FAE exhibit two types of disabilities across the life span. Primary disabilities are those that the child is born with. They reflect the CNS dysfunction inherent in the diagnosis. Secondary disabilities are those that an individual is not born with and that could presumably be ameliorated through better understanding and appropriate interventions.

PRIMARY DISABILITIES ARISE FROM ORGANIC BRAIN DAMAGE

Although most people understand brain damage quite well when it occurs after a child is born, children who are born with prenatal brain damage are more of a puzzle. Because there are no pre–post behavior changes to evaluate, people often have difficulty understanding the true disability that accompanies FAS/FAE. In addition, symptoms may be so subtle at birth that they are unrecognizable or indistinguishable from transitory behaviors resulting from a difficult delivery or from medications taken by the mother just prior to delivery. By the time the child manifests dysfunctional behaviors, the temptation is to attribute them to any convenient postnatal event rather than to prenatal trauma.

Children with FAS/FAE experience brain damage because exposure to prenatal alcohol can disrupt the normal proliferation and migration of brain cells, which produces structural deviations in brain development. Prenatal alcohol exposure can also disrupt the electrophysiology and neurochemical balance of the brain, so that messages are not transmitted as efficiently or as accurately as they should be. In some children with FAS/FAE, the "wiring" of the brain's message system is dysfunctional, causing message receptors to be faulty. Prenatal exposure to alcohol does not always cause these primary disabilities any more than encephalitis always causes postnatal brain damage. But when it does, the damage lasts a lifetime. Data from two types of studies are presented.[1]

---

[1] For understanding FAS-associated primary brain damage in humans, I present two types of data: test data from specific individuals with FAS or FAE and averaged data from groups of people with FAS or FAE. These average scores may be presented by themselves or contrasted with some type of comparison group or some normative data available on the tests. Sometimes group data are presented as scores that have standardized the amount of variability that exists among the members of the group (standard deviations). When there is much variability in a group, the average score may be less accurate as a characterization of the typical group member than when there is less variability. In most patient populations and especially among individuals with FAS and FAE, the group variability is unusually high.

The first 11 children identified with FAS had many direct and indirect indicators of prenatal brain damage. Ten had microcephaly (small head circumference, which relates to small brain size) and developmental delays; and nine had fine-motor problems, manifest in early infancy by tremulousness. These functional impairments were thought to result from brain dysfunction. All 11 also had short palpebral fissures that were thought to be a consequence of reduced ocular growth and alcohol-related alterations in early brain development (see Jones, 1986; Sulik, Johnson, & Webb, 1981).

FAS-associated brain damage in humans has been studied via autopsies and brain imaging studies, which reveal structural abnormalities, and electrophysiological studies, functional MRI (magnetic resonance imaging), and PET (positron emission tomography), which reveal functional disruptions. Despite the extensive experimental animal studies on prenatal alcohol and the brain, in 1997 this work in humans is just in its infancy.

Structural Brain Damage

Evaluating Brain Structure in Individuals with FAS Via Autopsies

Jones and Smith (1973) first described the structural brain damage associated with FAS after examining a 5-day-old infant who had died because of complications associated with FAS. "This first necropsy performed on a patient with FAS disclosed serious dysmorphogenesis of the brain that may be responsible for some of the functional abnormalities and the joint malposition seen in this syndrome" (Jones & Smith, 1973, p. 999). The authors described serious disorientation of both neuronal and glial elements as well as incomplete development of the brain that was thought to have started before the 80th day of gestation, based on the absence of the corpus callosum.

In 1978, a paper by Clarren, Alvord, Sumi, Streissguth, and Smith described autopsies on three additional children exposed to alcohol prenatally, each of whom exhibited similar malformations stemming from abnormalities in migration of neuronal and glial elements. Yet, only one had microcephaly; two others had hydrocephalus. From the external criteria, only two of the four were diagnosed as having FAS, which indicates that a small head size or FAS facial characteristics do not always accompany alcohol-related structural damage to the fetal brain. It is also interesting to note that two of the four mothers were not identified as chronic alcoholics during their pregnancies. Both had reported an occasional "binge" of five or more drinks at a time (one mother reported drinking 3–4 times a week, the other 2–3 times a month). Clarren and colleagues (1978) speculated that the observed interference with cerebellar and brain stem development occurred by 45 days' gestation, whereas the cerebral abnormalities were initiated by 85 days' gestation. They concluded that "in some infants, problems of brain structure and/or function may occur as the only apparent abnormality in the wake of intrauterine alcohol exposure" (p. 67). Since 1978, autopsies on a few more individuals with FAS have confirmed and expanded these findings (e.g., Clarren, 1986; Majewski, 1993). Russian researchers studying 44 embryos and 1 fetus discovered brain pathology in the offspring of all 10 mothers who were alcoholic. Among the progeny of the nonalcoholic mothers, researchers found decreasing frequency of brain pathology in proportion to their reported alcohol use (Kovetskii, Konovalov, Orlovskaia, Semke, & Solonskii, 1991).

Evaluating Brain Structure in Individuals with FAS Via MRI Researchers can directly evaluate the brain structure of individuals with FAS with MRI, a technique that produces pictures of "slices" of the brain in living subjects. Studies from San Diego, California (e.g., Mattson & Riley, 1995; Riley et al., 1995), where a special research MRI protocol has been developed, revealed structural brain damage in adolescents with FAS and others prenatally exposed to alcohol. These individuals generally had small brain volume; small cerebellum (involved in posture, balance, coordination, and some aspects of cognition); disproportionately small basal ganglia (associated with memory problems); small diencephalon (an important "relay center" of the brain, involved in transferring messages from one part of the brain to another); and small or absent corpus callosum (which carries bundles of nerve fibers that connect the right and left sides of the brain) (see Figure 6.1). As the controlled research studies with laboratory animals demonstrate (see Chapter 4), brain abnormalities such as these can be explicitly caused by the teratogenic effects

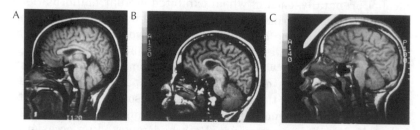

Figure 6.1. MRI showing normal corpus callosum (a) compared with a thin (b) and absent (c) corpus callosum in individuals with FAS, respectively. (From Mattson et al., 1994, p. 276; reprinted by permission.)

of alcohol, as it interferes with the actual brain cells' ability to multiply and divide and migrate to the parts of the brain where they are supposed to be for proper functioning (Becker, Randall, Salo, Saulnier, & Weathersby, 1994; Goodlett & West, 1992; Michaelis & Michaelis, 1994; National Institute on Alcohol Abuse and Alcoholism [NIAAA], 1990, 1993). In a replication of their earlier MRI studies, Mattson et al. (1996) extended their basal ganglia work to a more careful examination of the caudate nucleus, which they report is smaller in six children with FAS compared with seven typically developing children.

The research MRI protocol being utilized in San Diego is based on volumetric assessment, which permits a much more precise reading than that usually available in clinical settings. The usual radiographic analyses that are read clinically often fail to detect structural brain abnormalities in children with FAS, even though these children may have substantial mental impairments and behavior problems (Clarren et al., 1995; Knight et al., 1993).

Functional Brain Damage

Although studies of the architecture of the brain are of great interest, it is unlikely that they will ever be able to reveal all of the types of brain disturbances that affect individuals with FAS. Many of the ways that brain function can go awry are not observable by measuring brain structure—measurements of the brain "at work" are also important for understanding FAS-associated behaviors, but very few such studies have been carried out.

Electroencephalograms (EEGs) In 1977, Havlicek, Childiaeva, and Chernick began studying the functional brain damage associated with FAS by charting EEG abnormalities in groups of children with alcoholic mothers. In 1990, Ioffe and Chernick extended this work to show that these abnormalities can persist until 6 weeks of age in infants exposed to varying amounts of alcohol in utero. These abnormalities were not due to illicit drug use, smoking, or other ingestants and were not restricted to infants with a diagnosis of FAS. Neonates exposed to alcohol in utero, even those without FAS, showed, on average, more EEG activity during REM sleep (rapid eye movement, indicating a state of deep sleep) and quiet sleep, which correlates with poor motor and mental development at 10 months. Ioffe and Chernick (1990) believe that this methodology of computerized EEG analysis, which appears to be a sensitive index of prenatal alcohol effects on the fetal brain, will have clinical usefulness in terms of identifying exposed infants at later risk of alcohol-related neurodevelopmental delays.

Positron Emission Tomography (PET)　PET scans can also be used to examine brain function in individuals with FAS. In 1993, Loock, Conry, and Clark, using a PET scan technique, described a 16-year-old female with FAS who had marked metabolic disregulation but whose brain looked normal according to a clinically read MRI. In a larger study of 19 adolescents and adults with FAS and an average IQ score of 80, PET scans also revealed a higher proportion of functional abnormalities than a structural (non-volumetric) analysis of clinical MRI readings (Cambell, Loock, Conry, & Conry, 1996). In 1997, however, studies using PET scans are just commencing. As research methodology improves, important findings will likely emerge to shed further light on the genesis of alcohol-related CNS dysfunctions.

BRAIN–BEHAVIOR RELATIONSHIPS
THAT CONTRIBUTE TO PRIMARY DISABILITIES

Studies correlating behavior problems with either structural or functional brain damage caused by prenatal alcohol exposure are beginning to emerge in the experimental animal literature. For example, the following correlations have been found: hippocampal dendritic impairments with learning impairments (Abel, Jacobson, & Sherwin, 1983); decreased volumes of the olfactory bulb with impaired odor-associative learning (Barron & Riley, 1992); optic nerve hypoplasia with impaired vision (Strömland & Pinazo-Durán, 1994); reduction in cerebellar size with impaired motor development and ability (Meyer, Kotch, & Riley, 1990a,b); decreased serotonin synthesis with impairments in instinctive maternal behaviors (Hård et al., 1985); and decreased callosal size with hyperactivity (Zimmerberg & Mickus, 1990). (For a review of some of these studies, see Goodlett, Bonthius, Wasserman, & West, 1992.)

These animal behaviors show a marked similarity to the behaviors of children prenatally exposed to alcohol (see Table 4.2). There is also comparability between the doses required for these effects in these populations, after adjustments for differences in alcohol metabolism (Driscoll, Streissguth, & Riley, 1990). Studies such as these provide the scientific background for appreciating the organic basis of the primary disabilities in individuals with both FAS and FAE.

Neuropsychological Impairments

Documentation of specific neuropsychological impairments in individuals with FAS should eventually help explain the magnitude of their difficulties with adaptive living. By understanding which parts of the brain are impaired, professionals should be better able to utilize effective interventions developed for similar types of brain injury. Although the magnitude of the impairments measured behaviorally will depend, to some extent, on the degree of mental retardation in the individuals studied and on the sensitivity of the tests, findings suggest the following types of cognitive and neuropsychological impairments.

Auditory memory impairments for verbal recall, particularly for the manipulation of verbal material, have been found. Auditory recall appears to be impaired (compared with the norms) even in those with FAS/FAE who have IQ scores in the normal range. This impairment manifests itself in several conditions: in the face of distraction, when mental calculations must be performed on the remembered material, or after a delay. In one study, adolescents and adults with FAS often had unusual difficulty recalling lists of words even after five presentations (Kerns, Don, Mateer, & Streissguth, 1997). They also averaged numerous "intrusive errors," an unusual phenomenon in which individuals add in words that were not on the original list. Mattson and colleagues (1994) compared individuals with FAS with those with Huntington disease, a degenerative disease that affects the basal ganglia and produces subcortical dementia. Both groups of individuals made repetitive or perseverative errors, and both were better at recognizing words they had heard before than at recalling them when given no cues. Mattson and colleagues (1996) reviewed a number of studies linking basal ganglia and especially caudate damage, with behavioral impairments documented with prenatal alcohol exposure. These include impairments in spatial learning, evidence of kinetic tremor, attentional disorders, perseverative behaviors, and response inhibition. Impairments in response inhibition are thought to be at the root of the impulsive and hyperactive behaviors often noted in individuals with FAS/FAE. Mattson and colleagues speculate that these behavioral impairments in these individuals arise from abnormalities of the basal ganglia and in particular the caudate nucleus. Church, Eldis, Blakley, and Bowle (in press) describe a high prevalence of sensorineural, conductive, and central hearing impairments in individuals with FAS.

Uecker and Nadel (1996) demonstrated spatial memory impairments in children with FAS. On average, the children had difficulty with delayed recall of objects previously observed and represented the original visual displays in a distorted fashion, which are thought to be consistent with an interpretation of hippocampal dysfunction. Many of the children with FAS performed in a fashion similar to that of individuals with right temporal lobectomies and a large excision from the hippocampus. Uecker and Nadel (1996) speculated that children with FAS do not adequately form internal representations of spatial relations in the environment and thus have a disrupted "cognitive map." On a design copying task, children with FAS, on average, copied fewer designs correctly and more frequently made qualitative errors in copying corners and in distorting the basic shape of the design than those in a comparison group. They also had difficulty drawing a clock from memory and in drawing the hands for a specified time. This so-called constructional apraxia has been associated with parietal lobe damage, according to Uecker and Nadel, who describe another small FAS study that showed abnormal parietal lobe activity on magnetoencephalographic (MEG) imaging. They noted, "Gestational alcohol exposure can have a wide range of neural effects, not only on single brain structures, but also on neural networks of information processing. Typically cooperative brain functions are probably awry in FAS individuals" (Uecker & Nadel, 1996, p. 217).

Other studies have suggested that many individuals with FAS/FAE have impairments in "executive function" tasks, involving forming, planning, and carrying out goal-directed behaviors, which are often attributed to frontal lobe function. Decreased verbal and nonverbal fluency are also found in individuals with FAS as are impairments in cognitive estimation (see Carmichael Olson, Feldman, & Streissguth, 1992; Kerns et al., 1997; Kodituwakku, Handmaker, Cutler, Weathersby, & Handmaker, 1995; and Kopera-Frye, Dehaene, & Streissguth, 1996, for further details).

As of 1997, these studies are only beginning. Although it is clear that there is an organic basis for FAS-associated behavior problems, much more research is necessary to make this information clinically useful in helping individuals.

MEASURING PRIMARY DISABILITIES IN GROUPS OF INDIVIDUALS WITH FAS/FAE

Because it has not been possible to precisely measure the structural and functional workings of the brain in large numbers of people with FAS/FAE, psychological test scores have been used as surrogate measures of their primary disabilities, including data from intelligence tests, achievement tests, tests of adaptive behavioral functioning, and behavioral observations. The largest group of individuals with FAS/FAE to have received standardized IQ evaluations are the 473 individuals in our FAS follow-up study (Streissguth, Barr, Kogan, & Bookstein, 1996). Primarily ascertained by clinical referrals for FAS diagnostic examinations at the University of Washington Medical School over a 23-year period, all were diagnosed by dysmorphologists familiar with FAS. Figure 6.2 depicts the distribution of IQ scores for those with FAS and those with FAE. The 178 individuals diagnosed with FAS had IQ scores ranging from 20 (indicating severe mental retardation) to 120 (indicating above average intelligence). The mean IQ score for those with FAS was 79. The IQ scores of the 295 individuals with FAE, PFAE, or ARND ranged from 49 to 142; the mean IQ score was 90 (Streissguth, Barr, Kogan, et al., 1996).

Mental retardation has never been a defining characteristic of FAS. In earlier small sample studies, however, more children with mental retardation were described. (For example, Clarren & Smith, 1978, noted that 80% of the children with FAS described in the literature up to that time were mentally retarded.) Ascertainment of a broader spectrum of individuals with FAS has occurred since these early reports. As Figure 6.2 shows, mental retardation (IQ score less than 70) is now not the norm for a large sample of people with FAS/FAE. The practical consequence of this new finding is the realization that only 25% of individuals with the full FAS and less than 10% of those with FAE would readily qualify for special educational and vocational services that use mental retardation as their qualifying criterion. Besides IQ impairments, individuals with FAS manifest CNS dysfunction in numerous primary disabilities (see Table 6.1).

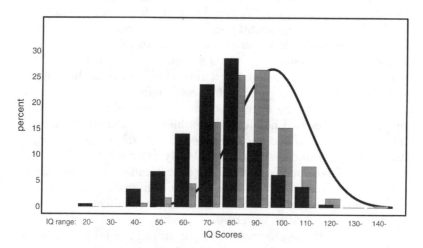

Figure 6.2.   IQ distributions for FAS ■ and FAE ■ compared with the normal curve (*N* = 473). (*Source:* Streissguth, Barr, et al., 1996.)

Table 6.1. Maladaptive behaviors and symptoms in people with FAS/FAE that indicate or suggest possible organic etiology

Behavior	Percentage
Attention deficits (SCL)	80
Memory problems (SCL)	73
Hyperactivity (SCL)	72
Expresses thoughts that are not sensible (VABS)	38
Rocks back and forth, sitting or standing (VABS)	33
Is unaware of what is happening in immediate surroundings (VABS)	27
Extremely peculiar mannerisms or habits (VABS)	20
Exhibits tic (VABS)	15
Excessive preoccupation with objects or activities (VABS)	15
Self-injurious behavior (VABS)	15
Seizure disorders (SCL)	10

Note: SCL = Symptom checklist from LaDue, Streissguth, and Randels, 1992; VABS = Vineland Adaptive Behavior Scale (Sparrow, Balla, & Cicchetti, 1984). Data from LaDue et al., 1992; *N* = 62–74, depending on the SCL item; *N* = 54 for VABS items.

MEASURING SECONDARY DISABILITIES
IN GROUPS OF INDIVIDUALS WITH FAS/FAE

Since 1985, our Fetal Alcohol and Drug Unit, with funding from the Indian Health Service, has published three longitudinal studies of children with FAS. Although our focus was on primary disabilities, these studies offered the first glimpse of what we now term secondary disabilities. In the first (Streissguth, Clarren, & Jones, 1985), we carried out a 10-year follow-up with 8 of the first 11 children diagnosed with FAS. We found that the four with IQ scores below 70 had more appropriate school placements and were more likely to be in stable living environments than the four with higher IQ scores. The latter four with IQ scores above 70 were not recognized by their schools as having a developmental disability and, as a result, were not receiving much special help or encouragement at school. These four who were *not* officially "mentally retarded" were the ones who seemed headed for trouble. Subsequent events confirmed this. One of the boys dropped out of school for his entire fifth-grade year and resumed school only after moving to another state. One girl dropped out of middle school and had a baby soon afterward. Another reportedly dropped out of high school, became an unmarried teenage mother, and had a transient lifestyle. Only one of the four continued on in school.

Based on these observations, our next FAS follow-up study (LaDue, Streissguth, & Randels, 1992; Streissguth, Aase, et al., 1991; Streissguth, Randels, & Smith, 1991) focused exclusively on individuals older than 12 years—the age at which children with FAS seemed to encounter trouble both at school and at home. This study involved psychological examinations of 61 adolescents and adults, ranging from 12 to 40 years old (with an average age of 17 years), diagnosed with FAS/FAE. As a group, they had academic impairments as would be expected. Although some read and spelled at a fifth-grade level or even beyond, their average level of academic functioning was at a second- to fourth-grade level. Their pattern of academic disabilities (with arithmetic skills worse than reading and spelling) resembled that noted in studies of children of social drinkers (see Chapter 5); however, the magnitude of their impairments was much greater.

In an effort to document and quantify clinically noted adaptive living impairments, we administered the Vineland Adaptive Behavior Scales (VABS) (Sparrow, Balla, & Cicchetti, 1984) to caregivers of these 61 individuals and found that these individuals (with an average age of 17 years) operated, on average, at a 7-year-old level (Streissguth, Aase, et al., 1991). Of the three domains measured by the VABS (daily living skills, socialization, and community skills), the individuals with FAS/FAE performed best on daily living skills (at an average 9-year-old level) and most poorly on socialization skills (at an average 6-year-old level). Although a few individuals had age-appropriate daily living skills, none were age appropriate in terms of socialization or communication. Even those who did not have mental retardation were frequently identified by such VABS items as failing to consider consequences of their actions, lacking appropriate initiative, being unresponsive to subtle social cues, and lacking reciprocal friendships.

In 1992, we published an expanded sample of 92 adolescents and adults with FAS and FAE using the VABS Maladaptive Behavior Scale and found that 58% of the individuals scored in the "significantly maladaptive" range (LaDue et al., 1992). This is a much higher proportion of individuals with severe behavior problems than is found, for example, in individuals with Down syndrome.

In 1992, our unit utilized the construct of secondary disabilities to encompass the measurable difficulties that people with FAS/FAE face as they mature and launched a major research effort funded by the Centers for Disease Control and Prevention to study this topic. Some of the common secondary disabilities we measured included disrupted school experiences, problems with alcohol and other drug abuse, irresponsible parenting, joblessness, homelessness, mental health problems, victimization, trouble with the law, and premature death.

The stories of these individuals' lives were sad and shocking, and it quickly became clear that these were not youth with mild disabilities who were fitting neatly into existing services for those with disabilities. Table 6.2 briefly conceptualizes the relationship between the apparent CNS dysfunctions characteristic of individuals with FAS/FAE and their maladaptive behaviors in the community (see also Chapter 8). This table represents my conceptualization of the relationship among some of the types of cognitive impairments that people with FAS/FAE have and the day-to-day difficulties they encounter. Imagine these disabilities in a person who generally looks and acts retarded; such behaviors would not be surprising and would probably generate sympathy, nurturance, and the desire to help. If, however, you imagine these behaviors in a person who seems to be quite "normal" in speech and affect and does not have mental retardation, either to the casual observer or according to IQ tests, then it is much more difficult to view these as reasonable behaviors. Some common reactions include "He doesn't learn well? He must not be trying." "She can't balance her checkbook? Her parents must not have taught her properly." Faced with the discrepancy between *how* people behave and how we *expect* them to behave, we derive our own hypotheses. If someone has recently been in an automobile accident, we might link the unexpected behavior to some brain trauma. In the absence of a meaningful "causal event," it is unlikely that the "brain damage" hypothesis will be brought into play by the observer. The diagnosis or knowledge of significant prenatal alcohol exposure might be enough for the observer to generate the correct hypothesis, but only if the observer actually understands the meaning of FAS/FAE or of significant prenatal alcohol exposure. It is out of this discrepancy between what we expect of people with FAS/FAE and what we perceive them actually doing that the climate for secondary disabilities is created. Other secondary disabilities may arise more directly from the things that

Table 6.2.   Clinical implications of characteristic FAS/FAE cognitive impairments

Poor judgment	easily victimized
Attention deficits	unfocused/distractible
Arithmetic disability	difficulty handling money
Memory impairment	difficulty learning from experience
Difficulty abstracting	difficulty understanding consequences
Disorientations in time and space	difficulty perceiving social cues
Impulsivity	poor frustration tolerance

Note: Constructed from clinical experience.

happen to children in their lives—because of the environments in which they live, because of being less able to protect themselves, and so forth. Theoretically, if we understood the primary disabilities of FAS/FAE better, some secondary disabilities might be prevented.

We thought Diane was a success story. Diagnosed with FAS as a baby, she was raised by a relative during much of her life and had an IQ score in the 80s. Her caregiver gave a glowing account of her progress when Diane was 10 years old. When we contacted her caregiver several years later, we were astonished to learn that Diane had dropped out of school, run away, lived on the streets, and had a baby she wasn't able to care for. What had gone wrong?

One problem was the fact that Diane was diagnosed with FAS in 1973, before professionals really comprehended the effects of the diagnosis across the life span, particularly in a child who obviously did not have mental retardation. Because there were no definable effects, such as mental retardation, Diane's caregivers and teachers assumed that she was a typically developing child and did not offer her any special services, considerations, or advocacy. I can still remember how Diane's sensible caregiver had bristled in recounting how a psychologist in another state had attempted to convince her that Diane must have mental retardation if she had FAS. In this indignation to assert her normality, her caregivers neglected to consider the hidden but very real disabilities that are associated with FAS, which, when left untreated, can easily develop into secondary disabilities.

I was truly stunned by the difficulties that Diane, and so many like her, faced as they entered adolescence. Although learning difficulties were expected in these children, the overwhelming problems with daily living and even socialization were not. Diane's poor judgment seemed to intensify and control her approach to each of life's challenges as she entered her teenage years. Diane— like so many individuals with FAS—simply made terrible decisions when left to her own devices. The older she got, and the more opportunity for making bad choices she confronted, the worse her problems became.

Our 4-year study on secondary disabilities (Streissguth, Barr, et al., 1996) involved 415 individuals (6–51 years old) with FAS (33%) or FAE (67%). Two data collection instruments were developed; both were administered to caregivers. The Fetal Alcohol Behavior Scale (FABS) reflects the behavioral phenotype of typical fetal alcohol behaviors (Streissguth, Bookstein, Barr, & Press, 1996; see Chapter 7). The life history interview (LHI) is a 70-minute, 37-page comprehensive structured interview designed to obtain information from a primary caregiver about an individual's secondary disabilities across the life span. It also compiles information on possible risk and protective factors characteristic of either the individual or his or her environment.

Six secondary disabilities were measured by the LHI. Mental health problems were defined by having had problems with treatment for any one of a long list of problems including attention-deficit/hyperactivity disorder (ADHD), depression, suicide threats or attempts, panic attacks, psychosis (hearing voices, seeing visions), behavior or conduct disorders (aggressive or assertive behaviors), sexual acting out, and so forth. Disrupted school experiences were defined as ever being suspended or expelled or dropping out of school. Trouble with the law was defined as ever being charged, convicted, or in trouble with authorities for any one of a list of criminal behaviors. Confinement was defined as having been incarcerated for a crime or having received inpatient treatment for mental health problems or for alcohol and other drug problems. Inappropriate sexual behavior was defined as having "repeatedly" had one or more problems with inappropriate sexual advances, sexual touching, promiscuity, exposure, compulsion, voyeurism, masturbation in public places, incest and so forth, or having been sentenced to a sexual offender's treatment program. Alcohol and drug problems were defined as having had alcohol abuse problems, drug abuse problems, and/or inpatient or outpatient treatment for such problems. Figure 6.3 presents data on the frequency of these six secondary disabilities in these 415 patients with FAS/FAE. Those who were 6–11 years of age can be compared with those 12 and older.

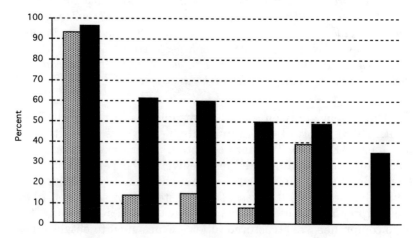

Figure 6.3. Secondary disabilities in FAS/FAE. (Key: ▨ = 6–11 years; ■ = 12 years and older; N = 415; columns, left to right, represent mental health problems, disrupted school experiences, trouble with the law, confinement, inappropriate sexual behaviors, and alcohol and drug problems.) (*Source:* Streissguth, Barr, et al., 1996.)

Mental Health Problems

More than 90% of the individuals in our study had mental health problems, and more than 80% had had treatment for mental health problems. There was no difference in the prevalence of mental health problems for children versus adolescents and adults, but the children and adolescents were more likely to have attentional deficits (61%), whereas depression (more than 50%) was the most prevalent mental health problem among adults.

Disrupted School Experiences

More than 60% of the adolescents and adults had had a disrupted school experience and, surprisingly, so had 14% of the children. Suspensions were the most frequent disrupted school experience among individuals of all ages, but the drop-out rate among adults was almost as high (almost 40%). Students with disrupted school experiences had twice as many learning and behavior problems as those without disrupted school experiences. The most frequent learning problems for all ages were problems with attention (70%) and repeatedly incomplete school work (55%–60%). The most frequent behavior problems were getting along with peers (about 60%) and repeatedly being disruptive in class (55%–60%).

Trouble with the Law

Sixty percent of the adolescents and adults and even 14% of the children had trouble with the law. Shoplifting/theft was the most frequent crime. Among individuals older than 12 years of age who had had trouble with the law, the most prevalent types of sentencing were juvenile justice (more than 60%) and juvenile detention (more than 40%). The most prevalent sentencing alternatives were probation (46%) and community service (39%). Trouble with the law is usually strongly related to disrupted school experiences. Individuals who didn't have disrupted school experiences were only 40% as likely to be in trouble with the law.

Confinement

Fifty percent of the adolescents and adults but less than 10% of the children had been confined. Adolescents and adults were more likely to have been incarcerated (32% and 42%, respectively) than to have been in either inpatient mental health programs (20%–28%) or inpatient alcohol and other drug treatment programs (12%–20%).

Inappropriate Sexual Behavior

Forty-nine percent of adolescents and adults and 39% of children had displayed inappropriate sexual behavior, making this category the next most common secondary disability for children. The most frequent inappropriate sexual behaviors were sexual advances, sexual touching, and promiscuity at 18%, 16%, and 16%, respectively.

Alcohol and Other Drug Problems

Problems with alcohol and other drugs were reported for 35% of adolescents and adults but were not reported as a problem for children. Many patients did not drink at all. The most popular reasons for abstinence according to caregivers' reports were "no access to alcohol" and "against the patient's beliefs" (both at about 35%).

In summary, people with FAS/FAE have a shocking level of secondary disabilities that severely impair their quality of life and is extremely costly to society. The low level of societal protection and support given to people with FAS/FAE and their families is unacceptable and further compromises their lives. In order to receive more appropriate levels of protection and support, their primary disabilities must be better understood by families, service providers, and society at large. The permanent, organic brain damage of people with FAS/FAE is often "hidden" because it does not conform to current system guidelines for providing services, such as a low IQ score, a debilitating physical disability, serious mental illness, or even a characteristic FAS face. By understanding the devastating secondary disabilities that characterize most individuals with FAS/FAE and by understanding the intrinsic and extrinsic risk and protective factors that exacerbate or ameliorate these disabilities, we should be able to improve the quality of life for people with FAS/FAE and their families and reduce the costs to society.

It is not enough to just document the presence or absence of secondary disabilities in people with FAS/FAE. Secondary disabilities should not be viewed as unavoidable; they have arisen out of the responses of the environment to those innate brain dysfunctions with which people with alcohol-related birth defects are born. As with any medical condition, understanding and providing appropriate interventions are the tools of change.

RISK AND PROTECTIVE FACTORS
ASSOCIATED WITH SECONDARY DISABILITIES

To facilitate understanding, our secondary disabilities study also examined risk and protective factors associated with secondary disabilities. Risk factors are those that are associated with elevated rates of secondary disabilities. Protective factors are associated with lower rates of secondary disabilities. Our analyses revealed eight factors that were almost universally protective in terms of the secondary disabilities evaluated. There were five environmental factors: 1) living in a stable and nurturing home of good quality, 2) not having frequent changes of household, 3) not being a victim of violence, 4) having received developmental disabilities services, and 5) having been diagnosed before 6 years of age. These protective factors give clear indication to families, service providers, policy planners, and communities about necessary actions to take to prevent and overcome these devastating secondary disabilities. There were also several intrinsic factors (characterizing the individuals themselves) that were risk factors for secondary disabilities. In general, higher rates of secondary disabilities were observed for people who had FAE rather than FAS; higher FABS scores rather than lower; and an IQ score above rather than below 70.

These risk factors give clear indication of who among the population of people with FAS/FAE that we studied were most at risk for secondary disabilities. They are those who are less disabled by conventional standards (i.e., do not have the full FAS and do not have mental retardation) but still possess obvious fetal-alcohol behaviors that get them into trouble.

Together, evaluation of risk and protective factors point to specific community interventions. Some, such as protecting children from physical and sexual abuse, are obvious. Others, such as assuming that children throughout the country have easy access to early and appropriate diagnostic evaluations for alcohol-related birth defects, are far from a reality anywhere. From the life-span perspective, an early diagnosis was related to more independent living and fewer employment problems as an adult. Knowing the diagnosis and understanding the cause and nature of the disability helps families and communities obtain the services they need for people with FAS/FAE early enough in life to prevent secondary disabilities and achieve a better lifetime outcome. Two models for providing community FAS/FAE diagnostic services have already been developed (Clarren & Astley, 1997; May & Hymbaugh, 1982). Making an early diagnosis a reality is an urgent priority.

CONCLUSIONS

Among 415 individuals of all ages with FAS/FAE, secondary disabilities were abundant: 94% had mental health problems, 45% had inappropriate sexual behaviors, 43% had disrupted school experiences, and 42% had trouble with the law. This level of serious secondary disabilities is unacceptable but not inevitable in people born with birth defects. Distressing as these new data are, it is important not to overgeneralize these findings. They are, after all, only a glimpse at what has happened to 415 people born with alcohol-related birth defects in the Pacific Northwest between 1973 and 1993. Only 11% of the 253 who were 12 years and older had actually been diagnosed with FAS/FAE by age 6. Many of them grew up in communities and even in families that had no knowledge of what it meant to have FAS/FAE. The term ARND hadn't even been invented when they were growing up.

This is not a hopeless, frightening problem that has no solution. On the contrary, these data present the blueprints for solutions that can be achieved in every community. The following eight chapters of this book (see also Streissguth & Kanter, 1997) help set the stage for ensuring that there will be fewer available participants for a future study of FAS/FAE and that earlier identification and greater understanding of their needs will result in an improved quality of life for all individuals involved.

REFERENCES

Abel, E.L., Jacobson, S., & Sherwin, B.T. (1983). In utero alcohol exposure: Functional and structural brain damage. *Neurobehavioral Toxicology and Teratology, 5,* 363–366.

Barron, S., & Riley, E.P. (1992). The effects of prenatal alcohol exposure on behavioral and neuroanatomical components of olfaction. *Neurobehavioral Toxicology and Teratology, 14*(4), 291–297.

Becker, H.C., Randall, C.L., Salo, A.L., Saulnier, J.L., & Weathersby, R.T. (1994). Animal research: Charting the course for FAS. *Alcohol Health and Research World, 18*(1), 10–16.

Cambell, C., Loock, C., Conry, J., & Conry, R. (1996). Functional metabolic integrity of the brain in FAS. *Alcoholism: Clinical and Experimental Research, 20*(2), 32A.

Carmichael Olson, H., Feldman, J., & Streissguth, A.P. (1992). Neuropsychological deficits and life adjustment in adolescents and adults with fetal alcohol syndrome. *Alcoholism: Clinical and Experimental Research, 16*(2), 380.

Church, M.W., Eldis, F., Blakley, B.W., & Bowle, E.V. (in press). Hearing, language, speech, vestibular and dentofacial disorders in the fetal alcohol syndrome (FAS). *Alcoholism: Clinical and Experimental Research.*

Clarren, S.B., Clarren, S.K., Astley, S.J., Shurtleff, H., Unis, A., & Weinberger, E. (1995). *A neurodevelopmental psychoeducational profile of children with fetal alcohol syndrome.* Unpublished manuscript.

Clarren, S.K. (1986). Neuropathy in fetal alcohol syndrome. In J.R. West (Ed.), *Alcohol and brain development* (pp.158–166). New York: Oxford University Press.

Clarren, S.K., Alvord, E.C., Jr., Sumi, S.M., Streissguth, A.P., & Smith, D.W. (1978). Brain malformations related to prenatal exposure to ethanol. *Journal of Pediatrics, 92*(1), 64–67.

Clarren, S.K., & Astley, S. (1997). The development of the FAS diagnostic and prevention network in Washington State. In A. Streissguth & J. Kanter (Eds.), *The challenge of fetal alcohol syndrome: Overcoming secondary disabilities* (pp. 38–49). Seattle: University of Washington Press.

Clarren, S.K., & Smith, D.W. (1978). The fetal alcohol syndrome. *New England Journal of Medicine, 298*(19), 1063–1067.

Driscoll, C.D., Streissguth, A.P., & Riley, E.P. (1990). Prenatal alcohol exposure: Comparability of effects in humans and animal models. *Neurobehavioral Toxicology and Teratology, 12,* 231–237.

Goodlett, C.R., Bonthius, D.J., Wasserman, E.A., & West, J.R. (1992). An animal model of CNS dysfunction associated with fetal alcohol exposure: Behavioral and neuroanatomical correlates. In I. Gormezano & E.A. Wasserman (Eds.), *Learning and memory: The behavioral and biological substrates* (pp. 183–208). Mahwah, NJ: Lawrence Erlbaum Associates.

Goodlett, C.R., & West, J.R. (1992). Fetal alcohol effects: Rat model of alcohol exposure during the brain growth spurt. In I.S. Zagon & T.A. Slotkin (Eds.), *Maternal substance abuse and the developing nervous system* (pp. 45–75). San Diego: Academic Press.

Hård, E., Musi, B., Dahlgren, I.L., Engel, J., Larsson, K., Liljequist, S., & Lindh, A.S. (1985). Impaired maternal behavior and altered central serotonergic activity in the adult offspring of chronically ethanol treated dams. *Acta Pharmacologica et Toxicologica, 56,* 347–353.

Havlicek, V., Childiaeva, R., & Chernick, V. (1977). EEG frequency spectrum characteristics of sleep states in infants of alcoholic mothers. *Neuropädiatrie, 8,* 360–373.

Ioffe, S., & Chernick, V. (1990). Prediction of subsequent motor and mental retardation in newborn infants exposed to alcohol in utero by computerized EEG analysis. *Neuropediatrics, 21*(1), 11–17.

Jones, K.L. (1986). Fetal alcohol syndrome. *Pediatrics in Review, 8,* 122–126.

Jones, K.L., & Smith, D.W. (1973). Recognition of the fetal alcohol syndrome in early infancy. *Lancet, 2*(836), 999–1001.

Kerns, K.A., Don, A., Mateer, C.A., & Streissguth, A.P. (1997). Cognitive deficits in non-retarded adults with fetal alcohol syndrome. *Journal of Learning Disabilities, 30*(6).

Knight, J.E., Kodituwakku, P.W., Orrison, W.W., Jr., Lewine, J.D., Maclin, E.L., Weathersby, E.K., Cutler, S.K., McClain, C.H., Handmaker, N.S., & Handmaker, S.D. (1993). Magnetic resonance imaging in high-functioning children with fetal alcohol syndrome who exhibit specific neuropsychological deficits. *Alcoholism: Clinical and Experimental Research, 17*(2), 485.

Kodituwakku, P.W., Handmaker, N.S., Cutler, S.K., Weathersby, E.K., & Handmaker, S.D. (1995). Specific impairments in self-regulation in children exposed to alcohol prenatally. *Alcoholism: Clinical and Experimental Research, 19*(6), 1558–1564.

Kopera-Frye, K., Dehaene, S., & Streissguth, A.P. (1996). Impairments of number processing induced by prenatal alcohol exposure. *Neuropsychologia, 34*(12), 1187–1196.

Kovetskii, N.S., Konovalov, G.V., Orlovskaia, D.D., Semke, V.I., & Solonskii, A.V. (1991). Dizontogenez golovnogo mozga potomstva materey, uptreblyavshikh alkogol' v period beremennosti [Deviations of the brain of offspring of mothers who used alcohol during pregnancy]. *Zhurnal Nevropatologii I Psikhiatrii Imeni S S Korsakova, 91*(10), 57–63.

LaDue, R.A., Streissguth, A.P., & Randels, S.P. (1992). Clinical considerations pertaining to adolescents and adults with fetal alcohol syndrome. In T.B. Sonderegger (Ed.), *Perinatal substance abuse: Research findings and clinical implications* (pp. 104–131). Baltimore: John Hopkins University Press.

Loock, C.A., Conry, J.L., & Clark, C.M. (1993). Disregulation of caudate/cortical metabolism in FAS: A case study. *Alcoholism: Clinical and Experimental Research, 17*(2), 485.

Majewski, F. (1993). Alcohol embryopathy: Experience in 200 patients. *Developmental Brain Dysfunction, 6,* 248–265.

Mattson, S.N., & Riley, E.P. (1995). Prenatal exposure to alcohol: What the images reveal. *Alcohol Health and World Research, 19*(4), 273–278.

Mattson, S.N., Riley, E.P., Jernigan, T.L., Garcia, A., Kaneko, W.M., Enlers, C.L., & Jones, K.L. (1994). A decrease in the size of the basal ganglia following prenatal alcohol exposure: A preliminary report. *Neurobehavioral Toxicology and Teratology, 16*(3), 283–289.

Mattson, S.N., Riley, T.P., Sowell, E.R., Jernigan, T.L.,Sobel, D.F., & Jones, K.L. (1996). A decrease in the size of the basal ganglia in children with fetal alcohol syndrome. *Alcoholism: Clinical and Experimental Research, 20*(6), 1088–1093.

May, P.A., & Hymbaugh, K.J. (1982). A pilot project on fetal alcohol syndrome among American Indians. *Alcohol Health and Research World, 7,* 3–9.

Meyer, L.S., Kotch, L.E., & Riley, E.P. (1990a). Alterations in gait following ethanol exposure during the brain growth spurt in rats. *Alcoholism: Clinical and Experimental Research, 14*(1), 23–27.

Meyer, L.S., Kotch, L.E., & Riley, E.P. (1990b). Neonatal ethanol exposure: functional alterations associated with cerebellar growth retardation. *Neurobehavioral Toxicology and Teratology, 12*(1), 15–22.

Michaelis, E.K., & Michaelis, M.L. (1994). Cellular and molecular bases of alcohol's teratogenic effects. *Alcohol Health and Research World, 18*(1), 17–21.

National Institute on Alcohol Abuse and Alcoholism (NIAAA). (1990). *Alcohol and health: Seventh special report to the U.S. Congress from the Secretary of Health and Human Services* (DHHS Publication No. [ADM] 90–1656). Washington, DC: U.S. Government Printing Office.

National Institute on Alcohol Abuse and Alcoholism (NIAAA). (1993). *Alcohol and health: Eighth special report to the US Congress from the Secretary of Health and Human Services.* Washington, DC: U.S. Department of Health and Human Services, National Institute of Health, Public Health Service. (Available free from National Clearing House for Alcohol and Drug Information [BK 51.8], P.O. Box 2345, Rockville, MD 20852, 1-800-729-6686.)

Riley, E.P., Mattson, S.N., Sowell, E.R., Jernigan, T.L., Sobel, D.F., & Jones, K.L. (1995). Abnormalities of the corpus callosum in children prenatally exposed to alcohol. *Alcoholism: Clinical and Experimental Research, 19*(5), 1198–1202.

Sparrow, S., Balla, D., & Cicchetti, D. (1984). *Vineland Adaptive Behavior Scales (VABS)*. Circle Pines, MN: American Guidance Services.

Streissguth, A.P., Aase, J.M., Clarren, S.K., Randels, S.P., LaDue, R.A., & Smith, D.F. (1991). Fetal alcohol syndrome in adolescents and adults. *Journal of the American Medical Association, 265*(15), 1961–1967.

Streissguth, A.P., Bookstein, F.L., Barr, H.M., & Press, S. (1996). *Fetal Alcohol Behavior Scale* (Tech. Report No. 96-09). Seattle: University of Washington, Fetal Alcohol and Drug Unit.

Streissguth, A.P., Barr, H.M., Kogan, J., & Bookstein, F.L. (1996). *Understanding the occurrence of secondary disabilities in clients with fetal alcohol syndrome (FAS) and fetal alcohol effects (FAE): Final report to the Centers for Disease Control and Prevention on Grant No. RO4/CCR008515* (Tech. Report No. 96-06). Seattle: University of Washington, Fetal Alcohol and Drug Unit.

Streissguth, A.P., Clarren, S.K., & Jones, K.L. (1985). Natural history of the fetal alcohol syndrome: A ten-year follow-up of eleven patients. *Lancet, 2*, 85–91.

Streissguth, A., & Kanter, J. (Eds.). (1997). *The challenge of fetal alcohol syndrome: Overcoming secondary disabilities*. Seattle: University of Washington Press.

Streissguth, A.P., Randels, S.P., & Smith, D.F. (1991). A test-retest study of intelligence in patients with the fetal alcohol syndrome: Implications for care. *Journal of the American Academy of Child and Adolescent Psychiatry, 30*(4), 584–587.

Strömland, K., & Pinazo-Durán, M.D. (1994). Optic nerve hypoplasia: Comparative effects in children and rats exposed to alcohol during pregnancy. *Teratology, 50,* 100–111.

Sulik, K.K., Johnson, M.C., & Webb, M.A. (1981). Fetal alcohol syndrome: Embryogenesis in a mouse model. *Science, 214,* 936–938.

Uecker, A., & Nadel, L. (1996). Spatial locations gone awry: Object and spatial memory deficits in children with fetal alcohol syndrome. *Neuropsychologia, 34*(3), 209–223.

Zimmerberg, B., & Mickus, L.A. (1990). Sex differences in corpus callosum: influence of prenatal alcohol exposure and maternal undernutrition. *Brain Research, 537*(1-2), 115–122.

III

A Life-Span
Approach to
Fetal Alcohol Syndrome

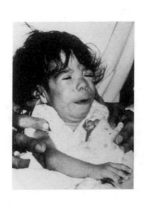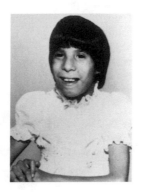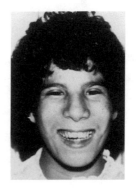

7

Living with Fetal Alcohol Syndrome

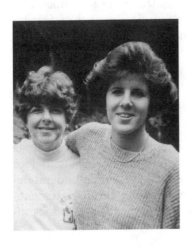

Several years ago, I gave a public lecture to about 70 people. Afterward, three spontaneously came up to tell me their stories. Although the diagnostic speculations of these three adults were never confirmed, they illustrate the diverse faces of alcohol embryopathy that professionals see regularly in clinics serving individuals with FAS/FAE. They also demonstrate the relevance of the research on FAS to the individuals and families coping with related complications. The life stories that were shared with me in that empty auditorium are retold as the opening vignettes for each of the chapters in Part III. The first woman told me the following:

"My younger sister has FAS—I can tell from your pictures. She also has mental retardation. I don't have FAS. I don't look like those pictures, and I don't have mental retardation. But I must have FAE. I've never been able to think like other kids, and school was always very hard. My adoptive family had lots of testing done and sent me to psychiatrists, but they never figured out what was wrong with me. I just found out that my birth mother was an alcoholic. Now I'm 21, working on my GED, living on public assistance with my baby daughter, and I still can't fig-

119

ure things out. I don't even know how to care for my daughter. Can you help me?" (From Streissguth, 1994; reprinted by permission.)

These haunting words have remained with me over the years—yes, I can help; we all can help. Everyone can help individuals with fetal alcohol syndrome (FAS) and fetal alcohol effects (FAE) through understanding, advocacy, and appropriate services. Yet only when communities adopt a life-span approach to understanding and preventing alcohol-related birth defects, extending help to both alcohol-abusing mothers and their children and then to the children as they become parents, can the condition really be ameliorated. With a life-span approach, different services and people can help at many points along the way; any help, whenever it comes, is better than no help at all. This chapter describes the important developmental and familial issues associated with FAS/FAE at key stages throughout the life span.

This section assumes a more personal perspective than the other four, depicting FAS-related brain damage from the standpoint of affected individuals and their families. Everything I know about the personal consequences of FAS I have learned from individuals and families. I've learned by observing, listening, asking questions, and being part of their lives on an ongoing basis. I've learned by being a friend, by being accessible in times of need, and by advocating for them when the system failed them. Initially, each family generalizes about FAS/FAE from its own experiences; but, through networking, sharing, and supporting each other over time, they have learned, as I have, of the rich tapestry of lives and skills that exists under the rubric of FAS/FAE—stories that can't be captured in a single statistic or snapshot. I am in awe of the courage, humor, and good will of these individuals and their families, as they've faced 2 decades of absent services, criticism, and confusion over the nature of their disability.

SEVEN COMMON MISCONCEPTIONS ABOUT FAS/FAE

There are several widespread misconceptions that can be detrimental to understanding the complicated life circumstances of individuals with FAS/FAE and responding appropriately to their needs. Before people can effectively help these individuals, they must understand the true nature of their disability. The following seven statements that are frequently assumed to be true are, in fact, common misconceptions:

1. **MYTH: People with FAS/FAE always have mental retardation.** Although it is true that FAS/FAE is caused by prenatal brain damage and every person with FAS/FAE has specific, individualized cognitive strengths and weaknesses, not all people with FAS/FAE have mental retardation. For example, as one study (Streissguth, Barr, Kogan, & Bookstein, 1996) found, only 25% of 178 individuals with the full FAS were classified as having mental retardation by an IQ score below 70. In fact, it is possible for an individual with FAS/FAE to have an IQ score within the normal range (see Figure 6.2). FAS/FAE diagnostic centers, such as the one at the University of Washington Medical School, see individuals with broad spectrum of IQ scores (Clarren & Astley, 1997). Only the most severely affected children—those with clear microcephaly and other physical malformations—are easily detected at birth (see Darby, Streissguth, & Smith, 1981).

2. **MYTH: The behavior problems associated with FAS/FAE are the result of poor parenting or a bad environment.** Because people with FAS/FAE are born with some brain damage, they do not process information in the same way as most people and do not always behave in a manner that others expect them to. This brain damage, in fact, can permeate even the best environments to cause behavior problems and present parenting challenges. Parents and caregivers need help and support, not criticism. Of course, a loving and understanding environment helps a child with FAS/FAE. But its absence isn't the primary cause of the disability.

3. **MYTH: Admitting that children with FAS/FAE have brain damage means that society has given up on them.** Some people believe that acknowledging the brain damage that accompanies FAS/FAE will depict these individuals as hopeless and devoid of treatment options. Yet, society spends millions of dollars developing treatment procedures for children born with more obvious birth defects and for people sustaining brain damage in more noticeable ways (e.g., auto accidents). As of 1997, the research to understand and ameliorate the specific neuropsychological and cognitive impairments associated with FAS/FAE has not yet been conducted. These individuals are in no way hopeless, but their needs have been sadly overlooked in the allocation of societal resources.

4. **MYTH: Children eventually outgrow FAS/FAE.** FAS/FAE lasts a lifetime, although its manifestations and associated complications vary with age. Children with brain damage (including those with FAS/FAE) usually require a longer period of shel-

tered living, and many need a stronger than usual support system to achieve their best level of adaptive living. Understanding this can help families plan effectively for structured transitions between school and work and can help them spare their children with FAS/FAE the expectation that they should be or must be independent at age 18 or that it is shameful to ask for help.

5. **MYTH: Diagnosing children with FAS/FAE will thwart their development.** Diagnosing is the art or act of recognizing a disease from its symptoms. At a practical level, it is a method of grouping people with some common characteristics together so others like them can be identified, the cause can be identified, and treatments can be provided. The problem is not the diagnosis but the current lack of scientific knowledge about how to treat the disease. An accurate diagnosis does not thwart development in any way whatsoever; it simply alters unrealistic expectations. Most individuals who are diagnosed, and their families, actually feel a sense of relief.

6. **MYTH: It is useless to diagnose FAS/FAE because there is no "real" treatment approach.** This attitude isn't taken toward any other incurable diseases (e.g., childhood autism). Why should it be invoked for FAS/FAE? Any family is in a better position to raise a child once members know the child's diagnosis. Once an individual is diagnosed with FAS/FAE, family members and social services workers can customize developmental approaches and goals to ensure that the individual reaches his or her personal potential. A diagnosis helps everyone understand behaviors that would otherwise be incomprehensible and helps families explain these behaviors to others and to respond more appropriately themselves. A diagnosis helps families build networks of support with others experienced with FAS/FAE. Parents and the individuals themselves need diagnostic information in order to behave rationally and respond realistically. In addition, when no treatment is known, then the acknowledgment of people with this diagnosis motivates the development of appropriate treatments and remediations. Diagnosis provides visibility, and visibility prompts solutions.

7. **MYTH: People with FAS/FAE are unmotivated and uncaring, always missing appointments or acting in ways that society considers irresponsible or inappropriate.** People with FAS/FAE usually care tremendously about pleasing others and want desperately to be accepted, but their basic organic problems with memory, distractibility, processing information, and being overwhelmed by stimulation all work against

their desires. They simply have difficulty understanding the meaning and interrelationships of a complex world that complicate their daily lives. In addition, the repeated experience of failing to meet expectations can generate a general reluctance to meet challenges, even in someone with the best intentions. Some people with FAS/FAE are now learning strategies and techniques for working around these problems.

PROBLEMS, CONCERNS, AND RECOMMENDATIONS

Understanding the realistic problems and concerns of FAS/FAE that individuals, families, and communities face across the life span can help focus action on appropriate solutions. The next two sections describe progress made over a decade (1986–1996) in understanding the lifelong consequences and behavioral manifestations of FAS/FAE.

By 1986, LaDue, Randels, and I had completed a follow-up study of 57 adolescents and adults previously diagnosed by Clarren, Aase, Jones, and Smith. Most had FAS; a few had FAE or possible fetal alcohol effects (PFAE). The document describing this study provided the first systematic account of what happens to young children with FAS/FAE as they mature and gave recommendations for home and community interventions (Streissguth, LaDue, & Randels, 1988). Based on these data and other clinical work, LaDue (1989) formulated a chart of psychosocial problems and concerns associated with FAS/FAE across the life span, with general recommendations (see Table 7.1). This outline, revised in 1992, has been the core of hundreds of lectures and workshops on FAS/FAE since 1989.

Although this chart summarizes some of the clinical problems encountered at each age and provides some comfort to parents experiencing similar problems with their children, it is only a descriptive outline of what was observed from examining the first wave of people identified with FAS/FAE. Most of these individuals were not identified as infants, and most were not raised at a time when there was any general understanding, either among parents or professionals, regarding the long-range impact of this disease.

Since 1990, work has commenced to understand the brain dysfunction associated with FAS/FAE, which may eventually explain the continuity of some of the dysfunctional behaviors. Even now, by understanding the behavioral phenotype of FAS/FAE, parents and caregivers can provide more relevant and helpful interventions throughout the life span.

Table 7.1. Psychosocial needs associated with FAS and FAE

Age	Problems and concerns	Recommendations
Infancy and early childhood: Ages birth–5 years	Poor habituation Sleep disturbances, poor sleep/wake cycles Weak suckle Failure to thrive Delays in walking, talking, and toilet training Distractibility/hyperactivity Difficulty following directions Difficulty adapting to change Irritability, temper tantrums, and disobedience	Early identification Intervention with birth or foster parents Education of parents regarding physical/psychosocial needs of infant or child with FAS/FAE Careful monitoring of physical development and health Safe, stable, structured home Assignment of a case manager to coordinate services and support to parents Placement of the child in preschool Respite care for caregivers Adapt environment to child with moderate stimulation; simple concrete directions; consistent, limited rules
Latency period: Ages 6–11 years	Easily influenced and difficulty predicting and/or understanding consequences Appearance of capability without actual abilities Inappropriate sexual behavior Difficulty separating fact from fantasy Temper tantrums, lying, stealing, disobedience, and defiance of authority Delayed physical and cognitive development Hyperactivity, memory deficits, and impulsivity Poor comprehension of social rules and expectations	Safe, stable, structured home or residential placement Careful, continued monitoring of health issues and existing problems Appropriate educational/daily living skills placement Help caregivers establish realistic expectations and goals Caregivers' support groups and respite care Psychological, educational, adaptive behavior evaluations Use of clear, concrete, predictable, and immediate consequences Case manager role expands to include liaison between parents, schools, health care providers, and social services agencies Mental health care as needed Structuring of leisure time
Adolescence: Ages 12–17 years	Lying, stealing, vandalism, trouble with the law Faulty logic, decompensation Egocentricity; difficulty comprehending and/or responding appropriately to others' feelings, needs, and desires Impulsivity, aggressive, unpredictable behavior Low self-esteem and motivation	Education regarding sexual development, birth control options, and protection from sexually transmitted diseases Implement planning for adult residential placement, financial needs, and vocational/technical training Appropriate mental health interventions if needed Respite care; caregivers' support group Safe, stable, structured homes or other residential placement

	Academic ceiling: lower reading, spelling, and especially arithmetic scores than expected for IQ Depression and suicidal ideation Alcohol and other drug abuse Inappropriate sexual behavior Pregnancy or fathering a child Loss of residential placement	Shifting of focus from academic to daily living and vocational skills Continued monitoring and structuring of leisure time and activities Facilitation of healthy choices and increased responsibility, as appropriate. Case manager role expands to acting as a liaison between individual, family, school, vocational programs, health care providers, residential programs, and court services if needed
Adulthood: Ages 18+ years	Poor comprehension of social expectations Economic support and protection Job training and placement Depression and suicidal ideation and attempts Pregnancy or fathering a child Social, sexual, or financial exploitation and inappropriate behavior Increased expectations of the person by others Increased dissatisfaction toward the person Withdrawal and social isolation Unpredictable and impulsive behavior	Guardianship for funds Subsidized residential placements, financial help for families In-home support services for those able to live independently Case manager support Specialized vocational training and job placements Medical coupons and care Acceptance of the person's "world" Acknowledgment of the person's skills and strengths Encouragement of self-advocacy

From LaDue, 1989; reprinted by permission.

IDENTIFYING THE BEHAVIORAL PHENOTYPE OF FAS/FAE

A phenotype represents the visible characteristics common to a group, as distinguished from their hereditary characteristics (or genotype). The FAS face serves as a physical phenotype for FAS—revealing that prenatal alcohol supersedes familial influences on certain facial features, at least in the young child.

The idea of a behavioral phenotype for FAS occurred to me in the mid-1970s as I listened to so many parents describe their alcohol-affected children with similar phrases. Their descriptions of their children's behavior seemed as unique and specific to these children as the FAS face. Furthermore, it seemed likely that this behavioral phenotype resulted from the central nervous system (CNS) effects of prenatal alcohol exposure. My students and I have gathered data on 78 of these behavioral characteristics over many years from hundreds of parents and caregivers of people of all ages with FAS/FAE. Barr and Bookstein helped carry out analyses to winnow the 78 items down to 36 that clustered together, so that a person characterized by one would be likely to also be characterized by the others. The resulting scale is called the Fetal Alcohol Behavior Scale (FABS) (Streissguth, Barr, & Press, 1996). Our research to date indicates that the average person with FAS/FAE is characterized by three times as many of the 36 FABS items as the average person without known fetal alcohol damage. This "behavioral phenotype" characterizes people with FAS/FAE from childhood to adulthood, but not all items apply to every person. Ongoing research will evaluate the utility of the FABS as a screening tool for FAS/FAE; it is not meant to replace a diagnostic examination.

Some of the more common of the 36 items in the behavioral phenotype follow. Understanding them can be useful in devising interventions for people with FAS/FAE across the life span. They cluster under two general headings: difficulty modulating incoming stimuli and poor cause-and-effect reasoning.

Difficulty Modulating Incoming Stimuli: Poor Habituation

1. Gets overstimulated in social situations, as in a crowded room, or among strangers
2. Overreacts to situations with surprisingly strong emotional reactions
3. Displays rapid mood swings set off by seemingly small events
4. Possesses poor attention spans
5. Has trouble completing tasks
6. Tends to misplace things

Poor Cause-and-Effect Reasoning, Especially in Social Situations

1. Seems unaware of the consequences of his or her behavior, especially the social consequences
2. Shows poor judgment in whom to trust
3. Interrupts with poor timing
4. Cannot take a hint; needs strong, clear commands
5. Loves to be the center of attention; draws attention to self

FOCUSING ON THE INDIVIDUAL

Describing a "behavioral phenotype," a general categorization based on the distinguishing behavioral characteristics of individuals with FAS/FAE, is useful for better understanding the qualitative aspects of the disease, but should never replace or underestimate the value of responding to individuals on the basis of their own particular needs, strengths, and weaknesses. Although people with FAS/FAE exhibit some common characteristics, largely as a result of the brain damage they sustained before they were born, it is important to recognize their individuality, their uniqueness, and their own tempos and temperaments as well. For any life-span approach to be successful, it must focus not only on the life-long effects of the disease but also on the individual manifestations throughout the life span. A life-span approach embraces the concept of emotional well-being and the basic humanity of the individual and should not be preoccupied with only academic yardsticks or conventional markers of success.

My daughter would say to you: I am not a statistic. I am not like you, but my brain works. I am not an FAS case, I am a person with FAS. I have a disability, but my spirit is whole. (Lutke, 1996)

UNDERSTANDING PEOPLE WITH FAS/FAE THROUGHOUT THE LIFE SPAN

A life-span focus helps elucidate the enduring nature of FAS/FAE and suggests how an understanding of the basic disabilities inherent in this disorder enables the implementation of effective interventions at various ages. Understanding the behavioral phenotype of FAS/FAE helps us listen to and interpret the behaviors we observe. Fortunately, articulate adults with FAS/FAE can help explain what it feels like to live with this disease. Their insights can help guide the interventions of parents, caregivers, and professionals.

Kyle: When I go into the supermarket, I feel assaulted with the smells, the sights, and the sounds. . . . Some other times, when a lot is happening at once, I feel just overwhelmed by stimulation—like I can't listen to another thing or take in another word. At these times, my cup is full—at its maximum level. I cannot handle one drop more of input. At this point, I become bristly—bristly like a porcupine, I call it—even abrupt and rude if anyone keeps talking to me. I can't afford to let my cup run over. The best way to communicate with me when I get like this is with a Post-It note. Leave it on the table in front of me, and I'll respond when my cup is not full.

Kyle's insights explain a basic FAS/FAE disability in modulating incoming stimuli that is apparent across the life span. Understanding this from the mouth of an adult can help us sympathize with the baby with FAS who scrunches up his eyes and turns away when someone overwhelms him by being too demanding of his attention. Understanding this in the baby can help explain the behavior of a teenager who dashes to his room and slams the door to be alone when everyone is talking at him at once. Learning to listen to the needs of the individual with FAS/FAE at one age can help explain the seemingly inexplicable behaviors at another. This effective strategy is based on the awareness that there are basic cognitive disabilities in FAS/FAE that are reflected in the behavioral phenotype and that these endure across the life span. Capturing this concept allows the parent or caregiver to become an expert in the care and management of the individual with FAS/FAE, by listening, learning to read the cues, and responding with insight.

Infancy

Infancy is a time for identification and protection: identifying children at risk of FAS/FAE and ensuring that they are in physically safe environments with caregivers in tune with their needs as infants. Infancy is also a time for identifying mothers who are at personal risk because of their alcohol abuse and providing them with the support and advocacy they need for coping with their lives, their alcoholism, and family planning (see Chapter 14). Infancy is a period for helping the mother and safeguarding the child. In this chapter, the needs of the child are paramount.

When an infant is identified as having FAS/FAE, there are often special health complications to consider and monitor. Infants with FAS/FAE have an array of physical complications that are associated with their disease but not necessarily diagnostic of FAS/FAE. These include heart defects; organ and skeletal malformations, particularly cleft lips and palates; hip displacement and scoliosis; seizures; hyper- and hypotonicity; hearing and vision problems; otitis media; and pneumonia. These problems should be routinely detected at delivery or in the course of good medical care and treated by conventional methods.

Conditions associated with FAS/FAE that are of particular interest to caregivers in the infancy period include: tremulousness, irritability, hyperacusis, disrupted sleep/wake cycles, weak suckle, and failure to thrive. These can be signs of an immature or compromised CNS. Recognition of any of these complications can trigger caregiving activities that will benefit both the child and the parent.

Abandoned by his alcoholic mother at birth, Kenny was the first newborn baby in the world diagnosed with FAS (Jones & Smith, 1973). I used to go down to the newborn nursery to play with him and study his behavior. I noticed that the nurses, although they all liked him a lot, complained about how much time it took to feed him. Whenever I stopped by, someone had him in the rocking chair, trying to get him to finish his bottle. I also noticed that when I stimulated him from a light sleep—with a gentle shake of a rattle or bell repeated at brief intervals—he got increasingly aroused and excited, waking up jittery and hyperaroused. He just couldn't seem to habituate.

Habituation is a basic CNS function that protects the newborn from having to respond to the many stimuli in its new environment that have little to do with immediate survival. An infant with habituation problems becomes overwhelmed by stimuli. Research has now shown that poor habituation is one of the earliest and strongest manifestations of the CNS dysfunction associated with prenatal alcohol exposure (Streissguth, Bookstein, Sampson, & Barr, 1993), although alcohol is not the only cause of poor habituation. Infants who habituate poorly are at risk of other types of disorders, either directly or indirectly in terms of caregiver and environmental interactions. This CNS dysfunction makes infants vulnerable to highly stimulating environments because they have difficulty tuning out redundant stimuli.

Caregiver interactions that involve respect for the infant's fragile CNS are helpful in protecting these infants from being overwhelmed by stimulation. When overwhelmed, such infants may startle, shudder, cry, or become agitated. They may avert their gazes; turn their heads away to escape; scrunch their eyes tightly together; frown; and, if the stimulation continues, become increasingly agitated. Learning to read the infant's cues permits the caregiver to avoid overstimulating the infant and to program stimulation into the infant's sleep/wake cycle when the infant will be most responsive. The reciprocity of this interaction, which is especially important to fragile infants, has been likened to a dance.

> Our present view of the mother–infant interaction system is that it should be seen as a dialogue—a mutually adaptive 'dance' between partners. . . . For this dance to proceed smoothly, and for the infant to receive the quantity and quality of stimulation needed for optimum development, both the partners and the dialogue must have certain features. (Barnard et al., 1989, p. 41; see also Sumner & Spietz, 1994).

Caregivers who understand their infants' needs can respond more appropriately.

Much progress was made toward understanding the special needs of fragile infants during the 1970s and 1980s. Some of it stemmed from work with premature infants, other progress came from the special interest in infant behavior generated by the development of the Neonatal Behavioral Assessment Scale by Brazelton (1973) and the observations of other early infant researchers such as Sander (1977) and Wolff (1987). A variety of techniques for enhancing parent sensitivity have been studied, including infant massage (tactile/kinesthetic stimulation), demonstrating the baby's capabilities to parents with the Brazelton scale, and coaching of parents' interactions with the infant (parents are taught specific techniques for slowing down and modulating their responses to correspond to the infant's tempo) (Field, 1993; see also Poulsen, 1995; Villareal, McKinney, & Quackenbush, 1992). Barnard (1990) and colleagues at the Parent–Child Nursing Department at the University of Washington School of Nursing have spent 20 years developing methods for helping nurses help parents be more responsive to the needs of their infants. *Keys to Caregiving* is a self-instructional video series designed to ensure that all caregivers know about the marvelous capacities that newborns bring and in turn to see the capacities of the newborn to enrich the relationship between caregiver and infant (Barnard, 1990). In this spirit, then, the caregiver learns the beauty of timing, of reading the baby's cues for engagement and disengagement, of comforting by touch and swaddling, of stimulating without overwhelming, and, most of all, of the interactive nature of caregiving. Perhaps in a smaller, kinder world, we learned all this from our mothers and grandmothers. Now it is comforting to know that these techniques can be taught through modern technology and are available to a broad audience.

Feeding difficulties during infancy are also associated with prenatal alcohol exposure and can present complications for caregivers of children with FAS/FAE. The Barnard model (1990), which focuses on the interactive elements of feeding, is useful for responding to a weak suckle and avoiding competing stimulation during the feeding process. More active interventions may be needed for infants with FAS/FAE with more severe feeding problems (Randels & Streissguth, 1992; Van Dyke, Mackay, & Ziaylek, 1982). Because some infants with FAS/FAE fail to thrive even when brought into a controlled hospital environment, two cautions are in order: 1) Failure to thrive is not necessarily an indication of child neglect, but rather a signal for careful examination of both prenatal and postnatal factors that could be contributing; 2) all infants being worked up for failure to thrive should be routinely examined for possible fetal alcohol effects and a prenatal alcohol exposure history should be obtained. Postnatal failure to thrive can be triggered by prenatal as well as postnatal events.

Although caregivers may be tempted to surround the infant with a multitude of stimulating sights and sounds in order to enhance development and "increase the IQ score," it is more useful to provide a calm, modulated environment for infants suspected of having FAS/FAE. This environment should be predictable and soothing, not overwhelming—an environment that is interactive with the baby's own responses, respectful of her needs, and oriented toward helping the immature nervous system develop better regulatory control. As mothers of infants affected by fetal alcohol may not have had such caregiving experiences themselves or may not understand the special needs of infants with FAS/FAE, the provision of in-home support and modeling can be especially important during this period.

Finally, infants with FAS/FAE who have not been diagnosed may not be caught by the community safety nets that identify infants at risk of developmental delay primarily on the basis of infant developmental tests like the Bayley Scales of Infant Development (Bayley, 1993). Infant mental and motor development scores do a good job of identifying children with traditional developmental delays at various points in their development; they do less well at clinically detecting children who have specific CNS dysfunction that may result in uneven development in various areas. Children with FAS/FAE who will clearly have mental retardation (e.g., those who will have an IQ score below 70 when they get older) will generally be detected as delayed on mental and motor development as infants. Those with FAS/FAE who will later function in the borderline and normal ranges of intelligence, however, are likely to be missed by this screening. Because people with FAS/FAE with IQ scores in ἐ average range are at greater risk for later secondary disabilities, one could reasonably argue that they might benefit the most from early intervention. Thus, early detection is important. In the absence of better predictors in the infant and young child, the presence of significant prenatal alcohol exposure would appear to be a better selection criterion for early remediation of children at risk of FAS/FAE rather than low scores on infant developmental tests.

Toddler and Preschool Years

The toddler and preschool years are the golden years of FAS/FAE. During these years, many children with FAS/FAE are so petite, elf-like, socially engaging, bright-eyed, and full of promise that it is tempting to think they'll be fine when they finally grow up. Others who have arrived at good homes after early abuse and neglect often make good developmental strides as they respond to nurturing, enrichment, love, and security, leading parents to suspect that they are on the road to recovery. These gains are to be celebrated, as are all signs of emotional well-being and positive personal interactions. The only caution would be to continue listening to the child's own behaviors for guidelines for interventions and planning.

Some children with FAS/FAE are already out of control as preschoolers. For these, professional consultations are urged, along with an early evaluation for FAS/FAE. Violent behavior directed toward self or others, fire-setting, marked hyperactivity, and incorrigibility are all signs for seeking professional treatment. Language delays, motor impairments, significant developmental delays, and unusual sexual behaviors are also indicators for professional intervention. However, no parent seeking professional treatment for such problems should be content with an evaluation that does not involve a careful questioning for prenatal exposure history and a referral for a FAS/FAE diagnostic evaluation when significant exposure is suspected. Local school districts and health departments, mental health centers, university-based child development centers, and state medical genetics programs are all resources for professional consultation and referral.

Early enrichment programs, therapeutic day care, and local Head Start programs may all be appropriate, depending on the needs of the individual child. Preschool programs that encourage organizational "learning-to-learn" skills, positive social interactions, good personal habits, and calm, modulated, predictable environments, such as Montessori Schools or Waldorf Schools, are excellent (see Appendix; see also Hinde, 1993; Tanner-Halverson, 1993).

Although rote learning of preacademic skills often becomes the focus of preschool intervention programs for children with developmental disabilities, for those with FAS/FAE a broader curriculum is desirable, for both home-based and school-based preschool education. Emotional and social development and communication skills are important foci for this age as well (see Nowicki & Duke, 1992).

It is also just as important to attend to the child's nonverbal communications after he or she acquires language as it was in infancy. Parents and teachers who can decode the nonverbal or seemingly inexplicable verbal behaviors of young children with FAS/FAE can help them learn more appropriate and successful interactions. Keeping in mind the behavioral phenotype of prenatal alcohol is useful at each age. Thinking of behavioral disruptions in terms of a basic difficulty with modulating incoming stimuli and poor cause-and-effect reasoning can facilitate understanding of the child's misguided communicative attempts and direct meaningful interventions.

"Kicking me is a strange way to say good morning," Burgess, one of my colleagues who taught in the Special Education Program at the University of Washington College of Education, used to say to one of her students with FAS, demonstrating how to verbalize the appropriate communication for an inappropriate social interaction. Vigilant adults can be particularly effective during the preschool years by keeping situations from getting out of control and communicating these activities to the child, for example, "Let's put away the blocks before playing with the crayons so things don't get all mixed up" or "Let's put the pencils right here so we can find them when we want them."

Teaching children with FAS/FAE to ask for help is yet another useful communicative intervention. Although self-sufficiency is an obvious enduring goal of childhood, the concept of asking for help when needed is an extremely useful technique for situations across the life span. Part of the equation in learning to ask for help is learning to recognize when the task is too hard to achieve alone; the other part is knowing that help is available when you ask for it. Imagine how useful this skill would be to a first-grade child with FAS/FAE who doesn't understand what the teacher expects of her.

Likewise, setting the stage for success is relatively simple in the preschool period if one keeps the child's own developmental skills in mind during play. For example, a child whose motor skills permit only a three-block tower experiences lots of success when there are only three blocks to play with; he experiences some challenge when there are 4 blocks and lots of frustration when there are 10 blocks. Experiencing success is a natural reward that occurs when realistic goals have been set; the adult manipulates the success experience by helping set appropriate goals.

Problems with attention, distraction, and memory can interfere with children's successful compliance with adult requests, no matter how hard the children want to please (see also Lutke, 1997). Following through on picking up toys and cleaning the room are tasks that can be difficult for children with FAS/FAE. Having an adult participate in the task with the child is an easy way to ensure success and a likely strategy for a parent who has already observed that an individual child can't follow more than one or two simultaneous commands. For other tasks, systems involving frequent reminders, a longer-than-anticipated training period, and various systems of sequencing and organizing can be useful. Thus, there are many useful skills, attitudes, and strategies that children with FAS/FAE can be taught by astute adults that will serve them well in the years ahead. In particular, they involve experiencing success, developing strategies to maintain emotional control, learning to recognize and communicate their needs, and becoming aware of cause and effect through daily activities in life. In the young child, these are best taught by programming for success, simple verbalizations, repetition, and an atmosphere of tender support and respect.

The School-Age Years

The bright-eyed manner that belies their cognitive impairments makes children with FAS/FAE especially vulnerable to the vicissitudes of life at school. Parents of children with FAS/FAE should ensure that their child has a sympathetic teacher and should help to educate that teacher so that he or she understands FAS/FAE. The adult who understands the cognitive impairments likely to be experienced by the child with FAS/FAE will remember to keep instructions calm, clear, and short; to set the stage for success, not failure; to teach with both verbal and visual modalities; to break tasks into steps; to keep the situation from getting out of control; to encourage verbalization of needs; to avoid the kind of questioning that makes people without the answers feel as if they are "on the spot;" and to provide support and help rather than employing shame and guilt for failure (see also Rathbun, 1993).

Educated teachers will also listen to the nonverbal communications of the child with FAS/FAE in order to help defuse situations that might become overwhelming for that child, before he or she loses control. Repeated failure, peer pressure and baiting, inability to understand the demands of the task, and insufficient time to complete the task can all contribute to a vulnerable child's loss of control. Yelling, throwing something, stomping out of the room, and slamming the door can all be manifestations of loss of behavioral control. Even after control is lost, the discerning adult can save the situation by helping the child regain control (often achieved by permitting the child to seek a solitary refuge), identifying the triggering events, and using this information in the future to program for success by modifying expectations, providing help and support as needed, reducing the level of environmental stimulation, and sometimes reflecting later on the event by a brief verbal reconstruction. "With kids with FAS and FAE, you've got to know when to talk to them and when not to talk to them," stated one experienced father of several such children. Many parents have said of their children with FAS/FAE, "Each day starts anew without the advantages of what was learned the day before."

The chain of events resulting from the mismatch between the child's needs and abilities and the demands of the day can play out like this: The basic cognitive, attention, and memory problems of children, adolescents, and adults with FAS/FAE set the stage for behavior problems in the classroom and at home because of repeated failure to meet expectations. Basic communication problems and difficulty with self-reflection make verbal communication of needs difficult (e.g., asking for help). Children and even adolescents and adults with FAS/FAE are often overwhelmed by stimulation and unable to either respond appropriately or protect themselves from the overstimulation of competing and ambiguous demands. When they lose control, they are likely to be punished for their unacceptable behavior while the basic problem underlying their lack of compliance is ignored.

Children and adolescents with FAS/FAE often cannot describe clearly what is happening to them, but their responses reveal their lack of comprehension. Thus, they are more dependent than other children on the caring adults in their environments to protect them from overstimulation; to give clear, concise instructions; and gradually, with kindness, to help them learn to monitor and modulate their own responses. Learning to listen to the needs of the child and adolescent with FAS/FAE in relationship to his or her own unique skills and disabilities is an important key to success.

For children without significant hyperactivity, the first three grades of school may be unremarkable. Some of our patients with FAS/FAE are actually overachievers at this age in terms of their ability to read (defined here as decoding words, not necessarily comprehension). Third grade is usually difficult because of underlying problems with number processing; and by fifth grade, with the increased emphasis on abstract thinking, the child with FAS/FAE may be floundering. Although academics may be the most noticeable problem at this age, coping with the increased organizational demands of multiple teachers and multiple classrooms can also be stressful for the child with FAS/FAE and may require special help and understanding. For many, the changing peer social scene with adolescence approaching can be the most stressful part of life at this age.

Adolescence

The adolescent years can be the most difficult for children with FAS/FAE and for their families, especially for those children who have never been diagnosed. During these years, families are faced with the jarring recognition that their child is not fitting the expected pattern of development and is not "catching up." Parental panic and confusion, professional uncertainty in the absence of clear diagnostic information, peer group pressures for independence, decreased interest in school as success diminishes, and normally developing adolescent sexuality all conspire to destabilize whatever equilibrium was developed during childhood.

Problems that families face during this period involve many complex decisions: balancing dependence versus independence, maintaining control, setting expectations, differentiating what behaviors are attributable to normal adolescence and what are caused by the FAS/FAE, and maintaining their own sanity. Problems that teenagers with FAS/FAE face during this period are increased failure and less satisfaction in academic classes, more social isolation as peer interactions are dominated by cliques, uncertainty or unrealistic expectations about what it means to grow up, and a looming sense of low self-esteem and depression. When adolescents have FAS/FAE yet have never been diagnosed, they can't figure out what's wrong. Furthermore, with their poor communication skills, they are, in fact, still dependent on a nurturing family who can listen to their nonverbal communications.

Families who can maintain focus, excitement, and satisfaction at home will be less threatened by the effects of peer pressure. Families who can allow some appropriate sense of autonomy, growth, and increased responsibility within the family context and can provide a supportive and predictable haven of understanding for the teenager will have a greater chance of monitoring and guiding his or her behavior without massive power struggles. Families of adolescents with FAS/FAE need to search creatively for alternate paths to maturity other than total freedom, full independence, and complete lack of supervision. Premature relinquishment of parental control only opens the door for less responsible authorities to assume leadership.

For many children approaching adolescence, tight peer-group bonds are considered the hallmark of the teenage years; but for adolescents with FAS/FAE, the "peer group" they attract on their own can be unpredictable and is often a source of problem behaviors. The use of alcohol and other drugs, out-of-control sexual activity, violence and vandalism, and peers who fail to respect others' needs and take advantage of the most vulnerable in the group are not experiences conducive to a healthy adolescence for people with FAS/FAE. A young teenager with FAS is useful to smart gang members who are quick to exploit his blind loyalty. Even without adverse peer-group interactions, however, some youth with FAS/FAE will have periods of decompensation and regression requiring periodic short-term intensive interventions that cannot be achieved safely or effectively at home.

Parent advocates will demand and work to achieve appropriate school and community resources for helping adolescents with FAS/FAE learn appropriate job skills, engage in appropriate recreation activities, and experience the necessary supervision and appropriate feedback to make these experiences successful at the individual level. They will also work to ensure that there are community resources that are suitable for people with FAS/FAE when their behavior gets out of control (see Hess & Nieman, 1997; see Chapter 10).

During adolescence, it is not uncommon for individuals with FAS/FAE to engage in inappropriate sexual advances that leave them open to victimization, rejection, and, in some instances, prosecution. Close supervision, clear guidance, and the development of rules for appropriate behaviors can help; but if the inappropriate behaviors persist, professional help should be sought (see Chapter 10; Hornby, 1993). Sexual education and birth control issues must, of course, be addressed explicitly by families. In one study of 30 women with FAS/FAE who had had children, 54% did not care for all of their children and 36% had been removed from their care by children's protective services; and 40% were drinking during at least one pregnancy (Grant, Ernst, Streissguth, & Porter, 1997).

Not to be neglected are help and advice on how to appropriately make friends, be a friend, and avoid types of interactions and activities that go against one's personal rules of behavior. Adolescents with FAS/FAE often develop their own rules in order to protect themselves as they face peer influences. Parents who can remain confidantes can continue to help with supportive guidance in the adolescent years.

Many parents derive considerable strength and support from FAS parent support groups in which common concerns and relevant issues are discussed so that the group learns from the personal experiences of others (see Appendix). Mental health professionals, particularly those experienced in FAS/FAE, can also be a source of great comfort for individuals and families dealing with FAS/FAE. Because the family is usually an important source of support and help across the life span of people with FAS/FAE, effective solutions generally focus on adolescent development that doesn't sever family ties. Parents who are knowledgeable about FAS can be on guard against bad advice from less knowledgeable friends and therapists. For example, "kicking Johnny out of the home" makes it harder to monitor and guide his behavior. (Get help before it reaches this stage.) Likewise, therapists who say, "I don't want to talk to your parents, Johnny, because you're an adolescent [adult] now" are really only listening with one ear. Therapists and case managers need input from people with FAS/FAE *and* from their families, even when the individual with FAS/FAE is living apart from his or her family.

Adulthood

Many of the challenges faced by adolescents with FAS/FAE and their families will continue into adulthood. In general, a longer adolescent relationship with the family will more effectively set the stage for adulthood. Topics of continuing relevance during adulthood are money management, medical care, productive work, safe shelter, and a sense of community (see Chapter 10).

Money management is almost always a major problem for people with FAS/FAE. Obviously something that the informed family should begin working on long before adolescence, this is a topic that needs revisiting throughout life. People with FAS/FAE who grow up understanding that this is an arena in which they will continue to need help are less likely to resist the efforts of family to help them.

Johnny went through a $2,000 inheritance in a weekend—he gave it away to his friends. When Sally got her back payments for Supplemental Security Income, a man she'd met at the shelter was waiting for her at the door. He took her to a motel, where he lived with her until her money was all gone.

Protective payees, parents, siblings, spouses, friends, and lawyers have all assumed responsibility for helping people with FAS/FAE live within their means and avoid the victimization generated by available cash. Obtaining appropriate medical care and mental health services are also activities with which adults with FAS/FAE often continue to need help.

Perhaps the most important concept in working toward optimal adult development in people with FAS/FAE is to recognize the life-span nature of the neurobehavioral disabilities discussed earlier. Memory and attentional impairments, difficulty with being overwhelmed by stimulation, and acting impulsively and without consideration of the consequences are characteristics to be considered in developing life plans for adults with FAS/FAE.

Jack was thrilled to get his first paying job as a young adult. He was willing and eager to do a good job. He'd done volunteer work in an office and had responded well to the experience. Therefore, his subsequent work as a busboy at a busy restaurant seemed to be well within his capabilities as a person with FAE and an IQ score within the normal range. To his chagrin, he had great difficulty knowing which tables he was supposed to clear. At this restaurant, the tables to be cleared by the busboys were identified by the waitresses' names: "Jane's table needs clearing." Not only did Jack have difficulty recalling the waitresses' names from day to day, but even when he learned that Jane was the one with braids, he didn't recognize her on a day when she didn't braid her hair. Jack got increasingly discouraged and gradually just stopped showing up for work.

Kyle, older and more experienced than Jack, also knows the sensation of having to process the same information again on each new day, because of a "failure to detail information typically from day to day." At age 45 and after a lifetime of trying, Kyle has learned external techniques for controlling and modulating his sensory input in order to protect himself from overstimulation.

Adults with FAS/FAE, many of whom lack the modulating capacities that most people take for granted to prevent becoming drowned in stimulation, often remain extra-sensitive to sensory stimulation throughout their lifetimes. Bright lights may dazzle these adults, and loud or unexpected noises may startle them. Excessive social stimulation or incomprehensible demands may also be similarly overwhelming. These difficulties are compounded by their difficulty in explaining what is happening to them. It is important to remember that a person on the brink of losing control is not a likely candidate for discussions about why his or her behavior is unacceptable.

Adolescents and adults with FAS/FAE may violate personal space conventions (e.g., stand too close, touch too much) and use inappropriate and ineffectual methods of trying to establish relationships (e.g., "Will you sleep with me?" [teenage girl with FAE to boys at school]; "Will you marry me?" [adult man with FAE and average intelligence to a stranger on a park bench]). They also may misperceive the intentions of others and, therefore, are easily victimized: "He wasn't a stranger, Dr. Ann, I met him at the bus stop" (said an adult with FAS, after a stranger he let sleep over at his apartment stole his money and radio).

Some adults with FAS/FAE reach some self-awareness of these complications. They have helped me understand the pain of having this disease—the pain of being not as smart or as capable as others, yet always wanting desperately to succeed; the pain of not feeling as loved or as wanted as others; the "pain of social banishment," as one adult with FAE described it. Therefore, it is not surprising that depression is the most typical mental health problem, characterizing more than 50% of adolescents and more than 40% of adults with FAS/FAE. Approximately 40% of adults and adolescents with FAS/FAE have made suicide threats, and almost 25% of adults with FAS/FAE have made suicide attempts (Streissguth, Barr, Kogan, et al., 1996). People with FAS/FAE remain especially vulnerable to the vagaries of the environment and the implications of their disease across the life span, which necessitates effective advocacy and better understanding of the syndrome and its accompanying complications.

FOUR WISHES

For everyone affected by prenatal alcohol exposure, I have four wishes:

1. That they receive an appropriate diagnosis early in life
2. That they are raised in a loving, stable, structured family that will use their knowledge about the diagnosis to create a safety net of support in the community
3. That the responses and expectations of his or her family are based on an understanding of that person's own unique needs at each developmental stage
4. That all people with FAS/FAE be given the tools to develop to the best of their abilities into productive adults, living with whatever degree of support is appropriate for them

Accomplishing these four goals will take the concerted efforts of families, professionals, communities, and the individuals themselves—a life-span approach to FAS/FAE.

REFERENCES

Barnard, K.E. (1990). *Keys to caregiving: Self-instructional video series.* (Available from NCAST Publications, University of Washington, Center for Human Development and Disabilities, Seattle, Washington 98195-7920.)

Barnard, K.E., Hammond, M.A., Booth, C.L., Bee, H.L., Mitchell, S.K., & Spieker, S.J. (1989). Measurement and meaning of parent–child interaction. In F.J. Morrison, C.E. Lord, & D.P. Keating (Eds.), *Applied developmental psychology* (Vol. 3). New York: Academic Press.

Bayley, N. (1993). *Bayley Scales of Infant Development–Second edition manual.* San Antonio, TX: The Psychological Corporation.

Brazelton, T.B. (1973). *Neonatal Behavioral Assessment Scale. Clinics in Developmental Medicine, 50.* London: William Heinemann Medical Books.

Clarren, S.K., & Astley, S. (1997). The development of FAS diagnostic and prevention network in Washington State. In A. Streissguth & J. Kanter (Eds.), *The challenge of fetal alcohol syndrome: Overcoming secondary disabilities* (pp. 38–49). Seattle: University of Washington Press.

Darby, B.L., Streissguth, A.P., & Smith, D.W. (1981). A preliminary follow-up of 8 children diagnosed with fetal alcohol syndrome in infancy. *Neurobehavioral Toxicology and Teratology, 3*, 157–159.

Field, T. (1993). Enhancing parent sensitivity. In N.J. Anastasiow & S. Harel (Eds.), *At-risk infants: Interventions, families, and research* (pp. 81–90). Baltimore: Paul H. Brookes Publishing Co.

Grant, T., Ernst, C., Streissguth, A., & Porter, J. (1997). An advocacy program for mothers with FAS/FAE. In A. Streissguth & J. Kanter (Eds.), *The challenge of fetal alcohol syndrome: Overcoming secondary disabilities* (pp. 97–106). Seattle: University of Washington Press.

Hess, J., & Nieman, G. (1997). Residential programs for persons with FAS: Programming and economics. In A. Streissguth & J. Kanter (Eds.), *The challenge of fetal alcohol syndrome: Overcoming secondary disabilities* (pp. 185–193). Seattle: University of Washington Press.

Hinde, J. (1993). Early intervention for alcohol-affected children. In J. Kleinfeld & S. Wescott (Eds.), *Fantastic Antone succeeds! Experiences in educating children with fetal alcohol syndrome* (pp. 131–147). Fairbanks: University of Alaska Press.

Hornby, R. (1993). Helping families and their alcohol affected children. In J. Kleinfeld & S. Wescott (Eds.), *Fantastic Antone succeeds! Experiences in educating children with fetal alcohol syndrome* (pp. 273–294). Fairbanks: University of Alaska Press.

Jones, K.L., & Smith, D.W. (1973). Recognition of the fetal alcohol syndrome in early infancy. *Lancet, 2*(836), 999–1001.

LaDue, R.A. (1989). *Psychosocial problems and concerns* (Tech. Report 89-05). Seattle: University of Washington, Fetal Alcohol and Drug Unit.

Lutke, J. (1996, September). *Hope for children with FAS through understanding.* Lecture presented at the FAS/FAE Secondary Disabilities Conference, Seattle, WA.

Lutke, J. (1997). Spider web walking: Hope for children with FAS through understanding. In A. Streissguth & J. Kanter (Eds.), *The challenge of fetal alcohol syndrome: Overcoming secondary disabilities* (pp. 177–184). Seattle: University of Washington Press.

Nowicki, S., Jr., & Duke, M.P. (1992). *Helping the child who doesn't fit in.* Atlanta: Peachtree.

Poulsen, M.K. (1995). Building resilience in infants and toddlers at risk. In G.H. Smith, C.D. Coles, M.K. Poulsen, & C.K. Cole (Eds.), *Children, families, and substance abuse: Challenges for changing educational and social outcomes* (pp. 95–120). Baltimore: Paul H. Brookes Publishing Co.

Randels, S.P., & Streissguth, A.P. (1992). Fetal alcohol syndrome and nutrition issues. *Nutrition Focus, 7*(3), 1–6.

Rathbun, A. (1993). Overcoming the cycle of failure and frustration. In J. Kleinfeld & S. Wescott (Eds.), *Fantastic Antone succeeds! Experiences in educating children with fetal alcohol syndrome* (pp. 295–313). Fairbanks: University of Alaska Press.

Sander, L. (1977). The regulation of exchange in the infant caregiver systems. In M. Levins & L. Rosenblum (Eds.), *Interaction and conversation and the development of language* (pp. 133–156). New York: John Wiley & Sons.

Streissguth, A.P. (1994). A long-term perspective of FAS. *Alcohol Health and Research World, 18*(1), 74–81.

Streissguth, A.P., Barr, H.M., Kogan, J., & Bookstein, F.L. (1996). *Understanding the occurrence of secondary disabilities in clients with fetal alcohol syndrome (FAS) and fetal alcohol effects (FAE): Final report to the Centers for Disease Control and Prevention (CDC) on Grant No. RO4/CCR008515* (Tech. Report No. 96-06). Seattle: University of Washington, Fetal Alcohol and Drug Unit.

Streissguth, A.P., Barr, H.M., & Press, S. (1996). A Fetal Alcohol Behavior Scale (FABS) for describing children and adults affected by prenatal alcohol exposure. *Alcoholism: Clinical and Experimental Research, 20*(Supp. 2), 73a.

Streissguth, A.P., Bookstein, F.L., Sampson, P.D., & Barr, H.M. (1993). *The enduring effects of prenatal alcohol exposure: Birth through 7 years: A partial least squares solution.* Ann Arbor: University of Michigan Press.

Streissguth, A.P., LaDue, R.A., & Randals, S.P. (1988). *A manual on adolescents and adults with fetal alcohol syndrome with special reference to American Indians* (2nd ed.). National Clearinghouse for Alcohol and Drug Information. (Available from P.O. Box 2345, Rockville, MD 20847, 1-800-729-6686.)

Sumner, G.A., & Spietz, A. (1994). *The NCAST caregiver/parent interaction feeding manual and the NCAST caregiver/parent interaction teaching manual.* Seattle: University of Washington. (Available from NCAST Publications, Box 357920, Seattle, WA 98195-7920; 206-543-8528.)

Tanner-Halverson, P. (1993). Snagging the kite string. In J. Kleinfeld & S. Wescott (Eds.), *Fantastic Antone succeeds! Experiences in educating children with fetal alcohol syndrome* (pp. 201–222). Fairbanks: University of Alaska Press.

Van Dyke, D.C., Mackay, L., & Ziaylek, E.N. (1982). Management of severe feeding dysfunction in children with fetal alcohol syndrome. *Clinical Pediatrics, 21*(6), 336–339.

Villarreal, S.F., McKinney, L.E., & Quackenbush, M. (1992). *Handle with care: Helping children prenatally exposed to drugs and alcohol.* Santa Cruz, CA: ETR Associates.

Wolff, P. (1987). *The development of behavioral states and the expression of emotion in early infancy: New proposals for investigation.* Chicago: University of Chicago Press.

8

The Advocacy Model

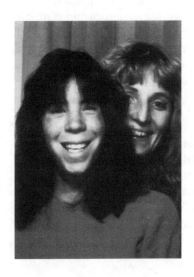

After one of my public lectures on FAS in a distant city, I was approached by a man who said his brother-in-law had FAE. He explained that his wife was the protective payee for her brother, who simply couldn't manage his own affairs. Although the brother attended school to become a chef, he works as a kitchen aide, a job he is comfortable with because of its predictability and repetitive nature. He is surviving marginally in the community except when he drinks; then, he tends to get into trouble. Their mother, who had a graduate degree and worked as a professional in the community, had a serious drinking problem during her pregnancy with this young man but not during the pregnancy with her daughter. Now, as adults, the daughter helps to care for the son.

Although people with fetal alcohol syndrome (FAS) may speak easily—and even colorfully—they often have difficulty speaking effectively for themselves, understanding and expressing their real needs, and applying good judgment to life situations. Naive and trusting, they are vulnerable as both children and adults. Therefore, individuals with FAS (and fetal alcohol effects [FAE]) need advocates, spokes-

145

people who not only have their best interests in mind but also understand the nature of their disability and how best to help them lead healthy, productive lives.

Although many people with developmental disabilities need someone to take care of the activities of life that they can't manage themselves, the situation is somewhat different for people with FAS/FAE. This disease implies some degree of CNS dysfunction, which impairs the ability to clearly visualize one's own problems and to communicate one's needs to others. In addition, the meaning of the FAS diagnosis and the methods of coping with the symptoms are not well known.

Individuals with FAS/FAE are born with organic brain dysfunction, which constitutes their primary disability. Although the manifestations may change as the child matures, the brain damage remains a part of their endowment across the life span. Because of the complexities and unevenness of the brain damage, people with FAS/FAE may be good at some things and disabled at others. They may have normal overall performance on an IQ test but nevertheless have significant disabilities with abstract thinking, learning, and generalizing from their past experiences. They may read well but have difficulty comprehending the subtle social cues of interpersonal relationships. They may talk a lot but lack insight into their own behavior. They may feel distress but be unable to articulate their needs to others. They may have difficulty modulating incoming stimuli and be in danger of being overwhelmed by stimulation and of behaving in an impulsive and maladaptive fashion. They may lack the ability to evaluate their own performance, set realistic goals, and organize their behavior to work toward these goals.

These characteristics, so well known to everyone who lives and works with people with FAS/FAE, are signs of brain dysfunction. They are, in a sense, "hidden disabilities" because they are not necessarily measured by the tests that we have come to rely on to allocate our special services and remedial help. When a child can't see, we get him glasses; when he can't hear, we get him a hearing aid. If he still has trouble, we sit him in the front of the class and make a special effort to be sure the other students understand that he has these disabilities so they can be of help. When a child gets a low score on an IQ test, we call him "mentally retarded," provide special services, and modify our expectations. When a child is "learning disabled," we measure that by a discrepancy between his measured intelligence and his measured academic performance and provide special instruction and remedial help. We call the primary disabilities of people with FAS/FAE hidden because they are not so easily detected by our institutionalized markers, yet they impair learning, adaptive behavior, and independent living nevertheless. The more hidden the disability, the more likely that unrealistic and unattainable expectations will have been established, thus setting up the person with FAS/FAE for frustration, failure, and despair. Whether the despair becomes overt through explosive angry outbursts or through depression and thoughts of suicide, the tendency of society will be to react to the symptoms and not to the cause. This is where the advocate steps in.

The advocate, by understanding the individual's brain damage and evaluating the gulf between expectations and capabilities and between ambitions and success, can individualize responses, help the person with FAS/FAE develop more effective coping strategies, and work within the environmental context to bring expectations in line with capabilities. People with FAS/FAE need advocates to help them in their day-to-day struggles to maintain organization, to avoid being overwhelmed by stimulation, to remain in control of their behavior, and to keep focused on realistic goals. The role of the advocates across the life span is to provide the neurobehavioral infrastructure in which individuals with FAS/FAE may be deficient.

WHAT IS AN ADVOCATE?

An advocate is an active mediator between the person with FAS/FAE and the environment. An advocate helps interpret the child to the world and the child to herself. The advocate is a key figure in preventing or ameliorating the secondary disabilities that can truly change the life trajectory of individuals with FAS/FAE.

If you are a person with FAS/FAE, an advocate is a person who can make things happen on your behalf. An advocate understands your specialized needs and the problems you face in finding solutions. An advocate tries to understand what you are experiencing when you act the way you do. An advocate paces and times her interventions based on your needs at that moment in time and her overall knowledge of FAS/FAE. An advocate helps you strive for reachable goals and plan for successful experiences. She is a sounding board, listening to your pipe dreams but not trying to implement them. An advocate buffers the rebuffs and, as you get older, helps stave off despair. She gently leads you toward your maturity without losing track of who you are. An advocate cherishes your spirit.

People with FAS/FAE need advocates because there is little understanding of how the organic brain damage associated with

FAS/FAE affects the daily lives of people with this disorder. There are no specialized curricula for teaching children with FAS/FAE, and mental health professionals have little experience with this disability per se. Understanding the nature of the primary impairments is the key to success. By understanding the behavioral manifestations of FAS/FAE, the successful advocate keeps the person with FAS/FAE working toward realistic goals and successful solutions.

WHO CAN BE AN ADVOCATE?

Parents are natural advocates, although with biological mothers, their sobriety is a major factor in the degree to which they can reasonably attend to the advocacy needs of their children. Advocacy for alcohol-abusing mothers is an important aspect of advocacy for the child in their care (see Chapter 13). Both foster and adoptive parents can be successful advocates; but without the critical information about the child's prenatal alcohol exposure, their advocacy efforts cannot be targeted to the specific needs of the alcohol-affected child.

Other family members can also be strong advocates. In some instances, fathers are very effective advocates for children whose mothers have succumbed to alcoholism. In other instances, grandparents—both grandmothers and grandfathers—have assumed an advocacy role for grandchildren for whom their children are unable to care. Siblings, particularly in adulthood, can become advocates, as can spouses when they are well informed about FAS/FAE (see Chapter 9).

You don't have to be a relative to be an advocate. Many professionals in the community take on an advocacy role for children and adults with FAS/FAE, although there are no professional qualifications for being an advocate. Teachers and other school personnel can be important advocates (see Chapter 11), working most effectively in conjunction with parent advocates to ensure that the child's best interests are represented at school. Some of the most dedicated advocates for people with FAS/FAE are associated with the criminal justice system. These are professionals from various disciplines who realize that they have people with FAS/FAE in their care and that the institutional or service delivery system is not effectively serving them. Such advocates provide a haven of comfort, understanding, and hope in a situation that might otherwise be bleak.

Hope and a good grasp of reality are two important characteristics of good advocates: hope that a way can be found to promote growth and good sense about which alternatives to try and how to respond creatively to each new challenge. Advocates should never doubt their abilities to find creative solutions and promote individual growth but should approach each challenge with alternatives that are realistic, appropriate, and feasible.

Because the needs of people with FAS/FAE are complex and multidimensional, they can seldom be met by a single advocate or service provider. Advocates must work within the community and with other services providers to orchestrate an appropriate network of services and are often called upon to coordinate between two primary institutions, such as the school and the home or the workplace and the home.

An advocate can be anyone, from a next-door neighbor, to a community religious leader, to a hired caregiver—the necessary and sufficient conditions for effective advocacy are understanding FAS/FAE, a genuine affection for the individual in question, a knack for creative problem solving, and dogged determination.

WHAT MAKES AN ADVOCATE SUCCESSFUL?

There are several basic facts about FAS/FAE that advocates need to know. Every advocate will be more successful once he or she has an understanding of the following points:

1. FAS/FAE is a birth defect that a person is born with, even though the full ramifications may not be visible for many years.
2. The prenatal brain damage from alcohol is manifested behaviorally and cognitively and affects an individual throughout his or her life span, although the manifestations may change from year to year.
3. The range and severity of prenatal alcohol effects are very broad in terms of intellectual and cognitive functioning; within this spectrum every child is unique.
4. Goals and decisions about the individual with FAS/FAE need to be based on a realistic assessment of that individual's own strengths and weaknesses.
5. Alcohol-related brain damage affects both perception and cognition, often rendering the child oblivious to his or her own limitations with memory, attention, cognitive ability, neurobehavioral functioning, and emotional control.

Advocates Help Individuals to Manage the Behavioral Manifestations of Their Brain Damage

"Don't tell me what I can't do. Help me find a way to do it!" (Lutke, 1997, quoting her daughter with FAS)

It is useful for advocates to understand the relationship among prenatal brain damage, the dysfunctional behaviors caused by this damage, the consequences of these dysfunctional behaviors, and some of the likely emotional reactions to these consequences. Understanding these linkages can help advocates make sense out of surprising behaviors caused by these emotions. Advocates seeing these linkages can begin to visualize the kinds of environmental manipulations and interventions necessary to prevent negative outcomes for the person with FAS/FAE. They can also encourage utilization of specific remedial techniques for the problem at hand (see Table 8.1 for a listing of problems, consequences, and solutions).

Mother of a 9-year-old son with FAS: What drives me wild is that one moment he is sweet and charming, the next moment totally out of control. The littlest things seem to set him off. He's like a time bomb—we never know when he'll go off. He becomes completely irrational at a moment's notice.

Many individuals with FAS/FAE fluctuate between states of extreme pleasure and displeasure. This is evident through their erratic and sometimes drastic mood swings. Attaching labels like "willful, spiteful, purposeful" to these overflow behaviors is usually not helpful. Advocates can help to buffer these remarks for individuals with FAS/FAE and mediate adversarial relationships. When confronted with these seemingly "irrational" behaviors, advocates know to first look intently for possible triggers or reinforcers.

Advocates Learn to Infer the Needs of a Person with FAS/FAE from Their Behaviors

People with FAS/FAE are not very self-reflective, especially with regard to their limitations. Unlike people sustaining brain damage in an auto accident or a traumatic illness, people with FAS/FAE have always been as they are. They have no recollection of a more functional time. Thus, it often seems difficult for them to evaluate when they need help or to ask for assistance. Because children and adolescents with FAS/FAE often cannot accurately explain their feelings or their behaviors, advocates learn to infer the nature of the problem from their behaviors and act accordingly. For example, sudden changes in attitudes about school, an upsurge in complaints about a teacher, a sudden change in affect upon returning home from school are subtle cues that an advocate will interpret as signs of frustration and trouble at school. Advocates learn to disentangle the acts of frustration from the incidents that provoke them. Although the inclination is to focus on punishing or extinguishing the act of frustration itself (e.g., slamming the desk top down, throwing the book to the floor, stomping out of the room), the effective advocate needs to understand the setting in which the undesirable behavior occurred. Three important questions are useful in evaluating such situations: 1) Was the setting too distracting or over-stimulating? 2) Was the task too demanding or complex? and 3) Was someone making the person with FAS/FAE feel inadequate, put on the spot, or trapped?

A typical brain can avoid responding to incoming stimuli deemed to be irrelevant to the situation at hand. This ability (called habituation), which most of us take for granted, permits focused attention on the primary task at hand. People with brain damage, however, have difficulty habituating. They tend to become more and more stimulated in complex, multisensory environments, thus becoming overwhelmed with stimulation. In the classroom or in other complex social situations, children with FAS can become hyperstimulated and overaroused to the point of losing emotional control.

Advocates Help Individuals Maintain Emotional Control

Most children with FAS/FAE need more help in maintaining emotional control because of their problems with impulsivity and response inhibition. They benefit from calm, structured settings in which expectations are clear and appropriate responses are reinforced. It is easier to help these individuals refrain from getting out of control than to help them regain control once it is lost. Structure and supervision prevent the situation from getting out of hand. Alert advocates provide enough supervision to be able to intervene as necessary through appropriate redirection of activities. Restructuring activities into shorter periods can avoid the consequences of boredom and repetitive behaviors that often result in explosive tempers and strained nerves. For example, providing only a limited number of toys in a curtailed space can avoid the frustration and confusion that hyperactive children feel in a large roomful of toys. A fenced play area can protect a child who has not yet learned to internalize rules for staying out of the street. Because these individuals frequently do not learn as easily as others do from their own experiences and have more difficulty predicting the consequences of their behaviors, keeping the situation from getting out of hand in the first place is a better strategy than relying on punishment afterward.

Successful advocate strategies to avoid confrontations range from specific interventions for the cognitive impairments and overload to coping with the emotions generated. Avoiding hyperstimulating activities and helping children maintain control over their behaviors by subtle warnings is often necessary. Some parent advo-

Table 8.1. Behavioral and emotional consequences of fetal alcohol–associated brain damage and advocate strategies

Brain damage →	Dysfunctional behavior →	Consequences →	Emotion →	Advocate strategies
Poor habituation	Drowned in stimulation Emotional overload Shuts down discriminations Behaves erratically	Disappoints people Gets criticized	Defensive	Decrease stimulation Teach techniques to reduce stimulation Teach techniques to inhibit behaviors
Poor self-regulation	Out of control behavior Acts without thinking	Gets into trouble	Confused	Reduce settings that induce out-of-control behavior Teach techniques to stay in control
Impulsivity	Quick to anger	Gets punished	Feels picked on	Teach to think before acting Anger management strategies Reward withholding response
Attention deficits	Unfocused/distractible	Incomplete goals	Disappointment Frustration	Reduce distractions Reward paying attention
Slow CNS processing speed	Fails to grasp meaning and meet deadlines	Object of derision Lack of success	Feels dumb Low self-esteem	Give more time Lower expectations Reward success
Arithmetic disability	Cannot handle money	Bungles finances Assigned a payee	Resentful	Develop fail-safe systems Encourage rigid adherence to rules
Difficulty abstracting	Does not understand consequences Does not generalize learning to new situations	Tries hard but fails	Disappointment Frustration	Provide increased structure Modify goals Provide alternative satisfactions

Perseveration	Does same things over and over	Misses the rewards	Confusion Frustration	Teach goal-oriented behaviors with concrete examples Find other behaviors to reward
Memory problems	Does not learn from experience	Makes same mistakes repeatedly	Confusion Frustration	Teach/develop memory aids Develop rigid routines
Disorientation in time and space	Misses appointments Misperceives social cues	Disappoints people Unpredictable	Feels unliked Lonely	Develop coping strategies Have friends be a part of the solution
Poor judgment	Trusts anybody Behaves irrationally	Easily victimized Easily scapegoated	Confused, hurt Low self-esteem	Develop coping strategies Reduce expectations Develop other sources of self-esteem
Difficulty with self-reflection	Cannot express needs	Does not get help Fails to have needs met	Feels a failure Feels dissatisfied	Provide verbal feedback for expressed feelings Reward clear need expression

cates use a gentle, inconspicuous touch to communicate a soothing warning to children before they lose control. Some teacher advocates use a secret message system to communicate impending trouble to children, thus helping them to "save face." In such situations, advocates assess the level of environmental stimulation impinging on the child and adjust the situation before the child gets out of control. Two strategies are useful when the warning systems fail: 1) The advocate can reduce the environmental stimulation (i.e., stop the raucous activity, the peer pressure, the scapegoating, the on-the-spot or demeaning behavior); or 2) the advocate can permit the person with FAS/FAE a graceful exit, physically or verbally, as the situation permits. Environmental manipulations that decrease both stimulation and the distracting influences can greatly improve outcomes and help children maintain emotional control. Preventing outbursts can also help the individual to be more socially acceptable.

Concomitant with environmental manipulation, advocates teach individuals with FAS/FAE techniques to attain better emotional control, including organizational skills to avoid stressful situations and methods of communicating cognitive overload. Advocates plan ahead for transitions, discussing events long before they occur to enable the individual time to ponder, question, and get used to the idea. Individuals with FAS/FAE respond poorly to being rushed. When they are provided plenty of time to accomplish tasks, outcomes can be improved. It is also helpful for advocates to regulate their interactions with the person with FAS/FAE to reduce stress and cognitive overload. Advocates give instructions in a clear, simple, repetitive manner. If the advocate does not demand an explanation when an individual is overloaded but returns to the topic when emotions have calmed down, the situation will be more successfully avoided in the future. In addition, advocates should not demand explanations from children developmentally unable to give them; an effective advocate is skilled at gleaning this knowledge from the child's behavior.

Advocates Help Define an Individual's Limitations and Identify His or Her Strengths

The discrepancy between what individuals with FAS/FAE expect of themselves and their own level of performance can create constant frustration for people of all ages with FAS/FAE. Thus, they often overrespond to insignificant remarks or appear hypersensitive to criticism or teasing. As a result of their FAS-related brain dysfunction that can impair perceptions, these individuals often misinterpret social cues, which fosters frustration and disappointment.

These children, who so often have growth deficiency, have been known to get in trouble for slugging the playground bully, much like adults with FAS/FAE lose their jobs after overreacting to perceived slights from fellow employees. Because people with FAS/FAE at all ages are usually so eager to please and want so much to be competent and liked, they can be devastated by snide remarks, snickers, and the mimicking faces of peers, who are quick to ostracize the nonconforming and provoke the desperate. The poor judgment and difficulty with self-reflection that usually accompany FAS/FAE can also have a profound impact on interpersonal relationships. As a result, many of these individuals are victimized and made into scapegoats. When this happens, advocates can provide protection, support, and understanding.

But not all failures are social in nature. People with FAS/FAE also experience specific cognitive disabilities and slow or uneven central nervous system (CNS) processing. These can result in arithmetic disability, difficulty abstracting, perseveration, memory problems, and disorientation in time and space, which lead to problems with everything from schoolwork to activities of daily living. Repeated failure understandably leads to frustration, disappointment, low self-esteem, and resentment. These individuals are typically motivated and, not realizing their limitations, desperately strive to succeed. Therefore, they are often frustrated when they are unable to perform a task well enough, fast enough, and at the right moment.

Advocates can help to counteract the negativity and low self-esteem that accumulate from day after day of failing to meet expectations and often result in erratic or irrational behavior by teaching better problem-solving skills and finding alternative successes and rewards. When an individual balks at a certain household task, a good advocate can reevaluate the situation and let the person select a chore he'd really like to do and then reward that appropriately. Advocates understand that rewarding a student with FAS/FAE only for receiving a score of 100% on a set of homework problems is not an appropriate response. Instead, advocates examine the general level of problems relative to the child's abilities and attention span. By restructuring the number of steps required, the number of distractions present, and the general level of interest, and by involving the individual in the decision-making process, advocates prompt successful outcomes. However, some people who work with individuals with FAS/FAE maintain the value of positive reinforcement without considering whether they have set the contingencies so high that the reward is seldom, if ever, achieved. In these cases, advocates must educate others to the realities of dealing with FAS/FAE. Advocates also help individuals have more realistic expectations. Often, an advocate protects an adult with FAS/FAE from his own erratic behavior—for example, so that he does not fire his protective payee, quit his job because someone looked at him in the wrong way, or forget to pay his rent and lose his apartment. An advocate is not afraid to tell a person with FAS/FAE when he is doing something really stupid but is clever enough and tactful enough to say it in a way that it can be tolerated.

Advocates Help Individuals Set Realistic Expectations

Often, advocates have no problem setting limits and providing for successes until children with FAS reach adolescence. At that time, when expectations for independence crystallize, the danger is to encourage growth without taking into consideration the individual's inherent limitations. Yet, unless an advocate sets expectations that are relevant and useful, the individual will likely be destined for disappointment and failure.

Janey had FAS, but she did well in her schoolwork and got good grades. As Janey reached adolescence, she wanted to hang out at the mall with the other kids. I strongly advised against this, although it seemed to violate her burgeoning independence. I explained to Janey's parents that kids with all kinds of disabilities have certain restrictions on their behavior, their lives, and their expectations. For example, kids with juvenile diabetes have to learn to manage their medications, and kids with hemophilia can never play contact sports. That's just the way life is. Although these solutions seem more straightforward than limitations to prevent the behavioral challenges posed by FAS/FAE, Janey was able to understand that her FAS is simply a different kind of medical problem. I explained to both Janey and her parents that shopping malls, with their unstructured, unpredictable activities, simply contain too many choices, too many temptations, and too much risk for children and adolescents with FAS/FAE. Although some parents judge their teenager's success by their acceptance among their peers, this family learned that Janey's success must be measured by alternative means. For Janey, success lay in understanding her own limitations, not getting into situations that she couldn't handle, and finding satisfaction in having increased autonomy within a safe setting. Once the family understood the problem, they had no trouble coping with the solution. Janey's parents became effective advocates for her when they realized that her medical diagnosis meant she had special needs and that treating her like a "typical teenager," with all the freedom and risks that that entails, would not be in her best interest. Of course, she had growing to do as an adolescent, but part of her parents' successful advocacy was to find arenas for choice and success within an overall perimeter of protection. The next time I saw the family, Janey was enjoying singing in a choir and special outings with her dad. Her sister, who did not have FAS, was enjoying life at the mall. Advocacy involves keeping each individual moving toward goals and expectations that are appropriate for him or her. Part of this process involves understanding the specific strengths and limitations of each person and how his or her needs and expectations change as he or she matures.

Advocates Teach Individuals with FAS Methods of Compensating for Their Limitations

"When I go into a supermarket, I feel overwhelmed with the sights, the sounds, and the smells. . . ." Kyle is a man with FAS who scores well into the normal range on IQ tests and leads a fairly normal life. Although his limitations are not obvious during casual conversation, he has a problem with stimulus over-load and a memory problem that he must compensate for on a daily basis: "I color code everything. I make my shopping list on a small notepad and write each item on a separate page. That way I only have to attend to one item at a time—when that item has been found, I tear off that page and go to the next item I see. Otherwise, the market is just too overwhelming."

Jack also has FAS and is often disoriented in time and space. He compensates for this limitation by using a cellular phone for getting step-by-step directions for every destination. He also makes it a point to always leave extremely early for appointments so that if he becomes disoriented along the way, he has time to regroup without missing his appointments. He has learned to leave extra early to avoid being late. Although not a fail-safe solution, it gives him the feeling of being in control.

Advocates can help to instill this self-reliance in individuals with FAS by modeling effective interventions and coping techniques. For example, encouraging parents to keep an uncluttered home with objects in the same place every day is helpful, as are meals that are at a predictable time and rituals and traditions that help demarcate the day into a predictable sequence and the months and years into familiar segments.

Advocates will learn the specific needs of a particular individual by listening, watching, trying to help, evaluating success, and trying again. I think often about the first two adults with FAS that I ever knew. Both, at the time I first knew them, were free of the kind of secondary disabilities described in Chapter 6.

Despite markedly different genetic backgrounds and rearing environments, two of the first young men with FAS I ever encountered had not only the facial fea-

tures, growth deficiency, and intellectual impairments characteristic of FAS but also many personality traits in common. Here are their stories:

Jesse was raised since infancy in a state institution for those with mental retardation after he had been abandoned by his alcoholic mother. Sonny, however, was the son of a high-ranking military officer and his alcoholic wife. He had been taken to many famous medical centers for evaluation, starting at age 2, because of his extreme hyperactivity. No one had ever taken a family drinking history or inquired about parental alcoholism. Diagnosed as "hyperactive, unknown etiology," he was given years of psychotherapy. He was raised in an upper-class milieu, with country-club manners.

Both young men were outgoing and friendly, chatty and gracious. At the institution, Jesse would come right up and start talking and laughing with you, like you were old friends. He was like a grown-up child with FAS: no stranger anxiety, curious about everything, and friends with everyone. My first encounter with Sonny was much the same; he came up to me with interest, shook my hand, engaged me in conversation, smiled affably, and radiated openness and trust. Both men had IQ scores in the mentally retarded range: 67 and 57, respectively. Both had a superficial aura of social competency that suggested more normal intellectual functioning than their test scores demonstrated.

When I saw them again 10 years later, the impact of their "advocates" on their lives was clear. Sonny's advocate, his father, was able to take the FAS diagnostic information received when Sonny was about 20 years old and translate it into a protective network of services for Sonny that would, on the one hand, provide the safety and structure he needed but, on the other hand, allow Sonny to grow to the best of his ability. Jesse had no advocate. His case manager might have been an advocate, but no one really knew enough about FAS in those days to know how best to proceed.

Sonny continued to live at home with his widowed father; Jesse lived alone in an apartment under a state disability program called "rent subsidy" in which adults with disabilities are given their own apartments in the community and a case worker visits every few days to help them shop, clean their apartments, cook their meals, and help out as needed. One might think that Jesse had made the better adjustment in terms of independence, yet he has been very lonely since his deinstitutionalization. Not knowing how to obtain companionship, he hung out on the street corner where the action was and got into various predicaments: His few possessions were repeatedly stolen by "friends" he invited to his apartment. One time he let a friend live with him, but his caseworker ousted the friend because she thought they had a homosexual relationship. He dresses as nattily as he can, sometimes has his hair permed, and usually, when we see him, talks of yet another girl with whom he is infatuated but is having trouble attracting or yet another job for which he is hoping that seems just within his reach but always slips away. In the beginning, his case worker described him as lazy and uninterested in working. "He can't really be *that interested in working," she said. "He misses all the appointments I set up for him." We had to intercede for him with his case worker. She wasn't hostile, she just didn't understand FAS and his type of cognitive disabilities, so she wasn't able to be a good advocate. She had unrealistic expectations for him, so she assumed that his lack of compliance was motivational rather than cognitive.*

Sonny, however, lived under his father's supervision. He was not allowed to roam around town on his own, but had a community of people with mild disabilities with whom he associated regularly. He played the trombone in the band at the disability center ("I like it a lot," he said, although he couldn't remember the name of any pieces they played). He did volunteer work at the center and also was involved in job training. His father was an excellent advocate. He sought out activities and gradually, with kindness, taught him the skills he thought Sonny needed, from mastering the bus system to masturbating in the bathroom.

For the next 10 years, Jesse's life continued to be plagued by loneliness and inaction. He had nothing to fill his days. He had seemingly adapted to his life of isolation but by age 40 was getting into trouble in the community for various types of minor inappropriate sexual behaviors. Sonny, however—still in his productive, well-ordered, and protective living arrangement—had finally been able to qualify for a real supervised work experience, real wages, real benefits, and real job satisfaction. It was with great pride that his father told me he is now paying taxes (see Chapter 10).

Both of these men had adequate environments during their early years, even though they were never appropriately diagnosed: Sonny with his retinue of therapists and helpers, Jesse with the clear and unyielding rules of the institution. Although the institution protected Jesse from challenges he could not meet and gave him guidelines for structuring his life by living with simple rules that were within his grasp, society let Jesse down. By expecting him to live alone as an adult without any job skills or ways to structure his own day, they left him at high risk for loneliness, victimization, and failure.

PREVENTING SECONDARY DISABILITIES THROUGH ADVOCACY

Advocates can play a major role in preventing some of the secondary disabilities that affect individuals with FAS/FAE (e.g., alcohol and other drug problems, inappropriate sexual behaviors, trouble with the law). Some advocacy will be accomplished at the interpersonal level. Another level of advocacy will be needed to develop the community infrastructure to support services for people with FAS/FAE. Increased public awareness of FAS/FAE is an important part of public advocacy. Only since the early 1990s have the long-term needs of individuals with FAS/FAE been recognized. Only in 1996 have there been specific outcome data on a large-enough group of individuals with this disease to see clearly the public health implications and the community needs.

Research shows that receiving an accurate and early diagnosis greatly improves the outcomes of individuals with FAS/FAE and helps to prevent secondary disabilities (Streissguth, Barr, Kogan, & Bookstein, 1996). Advocates can work together to raise community awareness and lobby for appropriate diagnostic facilities (see Clarren & Astley, 1997). On an individual level, advocates can ensure that individuals of all ages with signs and symptoms of FAS/FAE are appropriately referred for diagnostic evaluations and that FAS diagnostic clinics, linked to appropriate community services are available. Table 8.2 illustrates some specific strategies.

Research has shown that a disproportionate number of children with FAS/FAE experience early neglect and abuse and multiple disruptive foster placements (Streissguth et al., 1996). To prevent these additional environmental insults and to assist the appropriate and early diagnosis of FAS/FAE, all health professionals working with pregnant and postpartum women can serve as advocates by discussing alcohol and other drug problems with them, providing assistance as needed to their families, recording information about prenatal alcohol and other drug exposure in medical and social service records, and making this information available to foster families to facilitate their advocacy for these children.

Research has also shown that the outcome is better for adults with FAS/FAE when they have had appropriate services available (e.g., those offered by the Division of Developmental Disabilities [DDD]) (Streissguth et al., 1996). Advocates can be effective in lobbying for such services for their person with FAS/FAE, but they can also be effective in working to promote change in state policy that affects the protection of children in high-risk, alcohol- and other drug-abusing households and the promotion of long-lasting placements in homes of good quality. Community policies regarding the care and placement of dependent children are of great importance to the well-being of those with FAS/FAE because of the risks for secondary disabilities when the care is not adequate and appropriate services are not available.

Table 8.2. Advocacy strategies for preventing secondary disabilities in people with
FAS/FAE

Secondary disabilities	Advocate strategies	
Alcohol and other drug problems	Provide:	Knowledge of FAS/FAE diagnosis Knowledge that mother was alcoholic Knowledge of family vulnerability to alcoholism Stable and nurturant household Freedom from sexual/physical abuse Early diagnosis of FAS/FAE
	Don't:	Facilitate or encourage alcohol use/abuse Encourage friendships with alcohol abusers
	Do:	Encourage recreation and friendships not contingent on alcohol Discuss adverse consequences of alcohol use/abuse
Inappropriate sexual behaviors	Provide:	Freedom from sexual abuse Freedom from physical abuse Stable and nurturant household Early diagnosis of FAS/FAE
	Don't:	Overstimulate children Encourage out-of-control behaviors
	Do:	Provide feedback on inappropriate behaviors Give instruction on appropriate behaviors (sexual and otherwise) Give extra time and attention (not as a consequence of inappropriate behaviors) Teach good touch/bad touch Teach consideration for others
Disrupted school experience	Provide:	Diagnosis of FAS/FAE before 6 years of age Stable and nurturant home Good quality home
	Don't:	Facilitate alliances with gangs/groups of troublemakers Permit too much free, unstructured time
	Do:	Work closely with a school advocate Explain FAS/FAE diagnosis to school Work with school district to target help as needed Monitor tardiness, truancy, and resistance to attendance Apply for DDD services
Mental health problems	Provide:	Good quality homes of long duration Early diagnosis of FAS/FAE Stable and nurturant home
	Don't:	Permit physical/sexual abuse
	Do:	Apply for DDD services Get mental health treatment as needed Explain FAS/FAE to mental health worker

(continued)

Table 8.2. (*continued*)

Secondary disabilities	Advocate strategies	
Trouble with the law	Provide:	Stable and nurturant home Good quality home of long duration Diagnosis FAS/FAE before 6 years of age
	Don't:	Permit physical and sexual abuse Facilitate/encourage friendships with non–law-abiding people Facilitate/encourage alcohol or other drug use/abuse Permit too much free, unstructured time Ignore criminal activity
	Do:	Encourage healthy recreational activity Monitor friends and activities Apply for DDD services

ADVOCATING FOR ADVOCATES

In helping people with FAS/FAE achieve the best quality of life for every stage of development, much depends on successful advocacy at the interpersonal level. But successful advocacy also includes working to ensure that appropriate community services are available—not just for people with FAS/FAE, but for their advocates as well, including support groups (see Chapter 9) and focus groups (see Chapter 11). Advocates greatly benefit from services that let them discuss ideas about coping mechanisms, share effective problem-solving strategies, and learn the latest developments from research and service providers. As service providers may also be advocates, it is useful for them to be as familiar as possible with the day-to-day lives and needs of people with FAS/FAE and their families across the life span, knowledge that can be gleaned by meeting with other advocates and caregivers (see Lutke, 1997).

Advocates have many domains of operation, from the direct interpersonal to the implementation of sound public policy (see DeVries, 1997). Through understanding FAS/FAE, taking a life-span perspective, and effective advocacy at all levels, advocates help people with FAS/FAE to develop to the best of their abilities.

REFERENCES

Clarren, S., & Astley, S. (1997). The development of the FAS diagnostic and prevention network in Washington state. In A. Streissguth & J. Kanter (Eds.), *The challenge of fetal alcohol syndrome: Overcoming secondary disabilities* (pp. 38–49). Seattle: University of Washington Press.

DeVries, J., & Waller, A. (1997). Parent advocacy roles in FAS public policy change. In A. Streissguth & J. Kanter (Eds.), *The challenge of fetal alcohol syndrome: Overcoming secondary disabilities* (pp. 168–176). Seattle: University of Washington Press.

Lutke, J. (1997). Spider web walking: Hope for children with FAS through understanding. In A. Streissguth & J. Kanter (Eds.), *The challenge of fetal alcohol syndrome: Overcoming secondary disabilities* (pp. 177–184). Seattle: University of Washington Press.

Streissguth, A.P., Barr, H.M., Kogan, J., & Bookstein, F.L. (1996). *Understanding the occurrence of secondary disabilities in clients with fetal alcohol syndrome (FAS) and fetal alcohol effects (FAE): Final report to the Centers for Disease Control and Prevention on Grant No. RO4/CCR008515* (Tech. Report No. 96-06). Seattle: University of Washington, Fetal Alcohol and Drug Unit.

9

Families Speak Out

The final person of the three who waited to speak to me after one of my public lectures was a sparkling girl of 16. "I've always been bright and a good learner and have loved school," she said, "but my mother has fetal alcohol syndrome. She looks just like those pictures, and she's quite unable to function as an adult. She's always being victimized by men and really can't take care of herself. She couldn't take care of me either; that's why I was adopted. I found her only recently. The thing I'm really thankful for," she said, "is that she didn't drink during her pregnancy with me."

FAMILIES HAVE
DIVERSE BACKGROUNDS

The world of fetal alcohol syndrome (FAS) and fetal alcohol effects (FAE) can be topsy-turvy. The "patient" with FAS/FAE may be the child, the mother, or both. The "alcoholic" may be an upper–middle-class woman from a good family who is a Girl Scout administrator. The family may not be "dysfunctional" at all, yet the child may have many behavior problems. The family may know nothing about FAS or may deny that a drinking problem

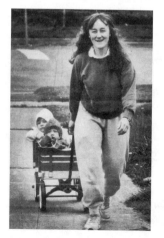

even exists. Or, the family may know more than their doctor about FAS/FAE. The "family" can include a biological mother in recovery, a biological mother still drinking, a biological father whose alcoholic wife has died, or a foster or adoptive family who thought they were raising a typical child who just needed a stable home.

Despite this diversity, approaches to intervention should still follow one simple rule—match the services to the individual's specific needs and concerns. No one who begins to advocate for someone with FAS—whether he or she is a family member or a professional in any one of the many relevant fields or community agencies—need fear he or she is not following the "established" protocol. In actuality, there is no universal intervention for individuals with FAS/FAE. There are only specific and unique solutions for the individual at hand. The better the individual's problem is understood by his or her advocate, the closer the two can work together and the more successful their efforts will be in identifying and addressing the problems and in considering the resources and constraints at hand. The most important thing an advocate can do is listen to the individual and his or her family. Listening to families reveals what they need and how they can best be helped.

FAMILIES ILLUSTRATE IMPORTANT ISSUES

Widespread Family Denial of FAS/FAE

Sylvia's mother: Sylvia, my 15-year-old daughter, has FAS because I drank alcohol heavily when I was pregnant with her. It doesn't seem to make much difference that I didn't know the alcohol I was drinking could harm her, that my doctor suggested an occasional cocktail might be good for me, or that I had the "disease" of alcoholism and wasn't "responsible" for my behavior. My feelings of guilt, shame, and grief have still been overwhelming.

Sylvia was born 2¹/₂ months early and weighed 2 pounds 8 ounces. She spent several weeks in an intensive care nursery for preemies. Her medical records included results of brain scans, a multitude of tests and procedures, and comments about my visits and phone calls to the nursery. There was no mention of my drinking habits. Who would have asked a middle-class professional woman who appeared to be successfully moving through the world, combining motherhood and a career as a Girl Scout executive, if she had a drinking problem?

When Sylvia was 4 years old, I was hospitalized with cirrhosis of the liver. A year later I was treated for alcoholism, and I have been abstinent since treatment. When I first heard about FAS, a cold, sick feeling lodged in the pit of my stomach. Sylvia was 6 years old. However, I was able to convince myself that Sylvia's small size, her immaturity (she was held back in kindergarten), her difficulties with memory, and her extremely short attention span were due to her prematurity (she must be slow catching up) and the stress of her dad's and my divorce.

When Sylvia started the seventh grade, a teacher friend suggested she be tested for learning disabilities because of her ups and downs in school. Despite her erratic progress and difficulties in school, she was denied testing because "she is not 2 years behind in her classwork." My quest for testing led us to the Fetal Alcohol and Drug Unit at the University of Washington and to Dr. Sterling Clarren at the Children's Hospital and Medical Center, where she was diagnosed with FAS. My response to the diagnosis was horror. Sylvia's response was "What a relief!"

That was 2 years ago. I told anyone who would listen that she was misdiagnosed. "She doesn't even look like an FAS kid. . . . She is on the honor roll in school. . . . She can play the piano!" At the same time, I was reading everything I could find about FAS and trying to parent "as if" she had the problem. Sylvia's tests at the University of Washington revealed her specific learning disabilities. Tests in hand, I went to her school counselor. He has been very concerned and helpful, carefully scheduling her for classes with those teachers whose techniques are most appropriate for her learning styles. He also indicated that her diagnosis of FAS would guarantee more in-depth help, should that become necessary.

The diagnosis also means that we, as a family, have been able to help Sylvia because we understand now what she can and cannot do. I have been able to temper my expectations, which previously had been either too high or too low, depending on each conflicting report from her teachers. I am sure Sylvia's many successes in junior high school have been the direct result of our family working hard with the school and now finally accepting, coming to grips with, and coping with the realities of her FAS. I think I began to truly accept her diagnosis about 6 months ago. Of course, with that acceptance came the necessity to deal with the same guilt, grief, and pain that it brought to the surface.

Since I accepted my alcoholism in 1980, a large part of my recovery has been focused on working through the shame, guilt, grief, and pain that the acceptance that saying "I am an alcoholic" brought. Sharing my story with others and reaching out to help them whenever I can has really helped me to work through these feelings and has played a big part in my recovery.

Part of the denial that many families experience in accepting that their children have FAS/FAE involves pointing out other potential causes for their children's disabilities. Prematurity, a difficult labor and delivery, low birth weight, early sickness, hospitalizations, family break-up, and remarriage are all part of the litany of "other possible causes" that families pour forth to account for their children's disabilities. Straightforward information about FAS/FAE, delivered with kindness and compassion, can help them understand the linkages to prenatal alcohol exposure and get earlier help for their children and themselves.

Chuck's mother: I started using alcohol at age 13. Once I started, there was no turning back. I drank about 3 beers per evening and 6–12 beers on weekend evenings. I got pregnant when I was 19. At that time, there was no information on FAS and my doctors never warned me against drinking, although they recommended not smoking. The doctor said that drinking a beer every evening would help me get rid of excess fluids. I was also taking prescription drugs. It never occurred to me that I was an alcoholic or that I had a drinking problem. I thought I got carried away with my drinking sometimes, and sometimes I couldn't remember things. Basically, I just drank to have a good time.

During my pregnancy, I had to go to the hospital every 2 weeks for a diuretic shot. Then I went into labor. I had a hard time birthing Chuck; I was under lots of ether, so Chuck got lots of ether too, and it was a forceps delivery. He weighed 6 pounds and was 19 inches long. I always intuitively thought there was something wrong with him—although physically he was okay. My first big indicator was at the start of first grade. The school said he was mentally retarded, needed testing, and had to go to special education classes. I was still drinking.

When he was 15, a high school psychologist first suggested he might have FAE. Looking back on it, it took me several attempts to get through this information. At first, I just didn't hear it. I had lots of guilt and remorse. I wanted to blame someone. It took several sessions for me to deal with this. After about a year of working through this, I helped Chuck get into a school for kids with behavior problems. Now he's 18½ years old. He is at about a fourth-grade level academically—like a 9- or 10-year-old. They think that maybe with daily tutoring he could get to a sixth-grade level. He gets into lots of trouble—10 days in jail this past year. It appears as though he has no gauge of danger; he does even life-threatening things. He has a strong need for acceptance; at the mere suggestion, he's up and doing what others want. He has many general behavior problems, but he's extremely personable. He has a wonderful sense of humor. He's like a chameleon—changes roles real fast. He really resents being placed among the retarded—he's not stupid.

Advocates and physicians need to persevere when telling parents about FAS/FAE. Parents often don't even hear the message the first time. Many need multiple sessions—to talk it over, to work through the other possible causes, to blame others, and so forth—before finally accepting the information. Considering the seriousness of the implications, who among us would not engage in some denial? Yet, because of the lag that so often occurs between the identification and acceptance of FAS, the earlier the diagnosis, the earlier the acceptance.

Knowing the risk of secondary disabilities, so clearly described by Chuck's mother, what professional would delay this discussion with the parents and risk letting any secondary disabilities become well-established? A family who doesn't receive appropriate diagnostic information until late in the child's life misses the opportunity to act as his or her advocate at school and work out special arrangements (e.g., those described by Sylvia's mother). Family members also may fail to appropriately parent their child with FAS/FAE, which diminishes any chance they have of possibly preventing the serious secondary disabilities that children with FAS/FAE all too commonly display as teenagers. Knowledge of how their drinking damaged their children, Sylvia and Chuck, did not immobilize these two mothers—quite the opposite: Knowledge empowered them to engage in positive advocacy for their children.

Widespread Professional Denial of FAS/FAE

Sometimes, professionals—including social workers, physicians, and school counselors—also deny the possibility of prenatal alcohol exposure. Lisa, a mid-life alcoholic, reports how the professionals' unwillingness to query her about her alcoholism fueled her own denial. Sobriety not only helped her understand the cause of her son's disability but also allowed her to become an effective advocate for her son at school and for all children with FAS through her community activities. Following are excerpts from a letter she sent me after I first met her at a conference at which I had lectured about FAS:

Denny's mother: I had my first baby at the age of 17; by the time I was 27, I had had five more. All were normal and healthy, except one stubborn breech. Although I did smoke during my pregnancies, I don't recall even one occasion that I drank any alcohol. It just wasn't part of my life at that time. Under the stress of managing the family and an increasingly successful restaurant business, my marriage fell apart. After the divorce, the children remained with me and so did my ever-escalating drinking. At 40, and in the midst of my 9-year slavery to the master [alcohol], I fell in love again and became pregnant. As my pregnancy progressed, so did my drinking. Although I had never heard of FAS,

I knew in my heart of hearts that drinking, especially as much as I was, was bound to carry some consequences. But I never thought it would cause mental retardation or deformities, an oversight that to this day confounds me. I recall visualizing a "little" baby, a "weak or frail" baby; but I pushed away my instincts with my own denial and my physical need to satisfy my alcohol craving. When my inner self would nag at me and fear and guilt would start to torment, I'd simply drown the feelings with another drink and make them retreat into silence, leaving me alone.

A severe kidney infection required hospitalization late in pregnancy, at which time I had a c-section. After 24 hours, I finally beheld the cutest little "funny baby" I had ever seen. It was love at first sight! Denny weighed in at 5 pounds, 9 ounces; and except for his baggy skin with no fat under it and a kind of an "E.T." facial appearance, he was a perfectly whole, perfectly lovable baby. The next day they told me that his Apgar scores were pitifully low. They unexpectedly placed him in my arms, saying that for him to "make it" he needed to be close to me. For 4 more days, I never let him out of my arms. He had very poor sucking ability, but I persisted in trying to breastfeed him as I had done with all his brothers and sisters, and he began to respond. He was sleeping for only an hour or so at a time, and his sleep was fitful, as though he were having a bad dream. I just kept holding him as tightly as I dared and rocking as I sang mommy love songs to him. Deeply enmeshed in the alcoholic's best weapon, denial, I consoled my fears and the haunting guilt that what was "not right" with my funny baby was all speculation and circumstantial. Even the doctors and nurses were busy playing out their parts in this psychological game of vindication. Their excuses included: He was 3½ weeks premature; he was probably overmedicated with anesthesia; he had oxygen therapy; he had a low birth weight; he had a mommy with a kidney infection. It was all so easy, it was all so easy.

When he was about 2 months old, I received a postcard from the county health department requesting that they be allowed to do a follow-up examination with regard to Denny's unusually low Apgar scores. Out of fear that my drinking problem be discovered and I'd have to hear the words I feared the most, I, as I had done all through my pregnancy, did not drink on the day of my appointment or on the night before. If I could hide my alcoholism, I could avoid the responsibility that went with it. It was a two-way street, though: If they also could hide my alcoholism, they could avoid confronting me.

When the examination was over, I was advised that Denny's scores on the Denver Developmental Test indicated a definite lag, but there was his prematurity to be considered. He also exhibited excessively rigid muscle tone that suggested the possibility of a congenital hip deformity. For several years, we received help through Crippled Children's Services, which offered the finest in physical therapy and taught Denny sign language. It was the general consen-

sus that he would never learn to speak normally. I was gently made aware that my funny baby would probably progress slowly to the age of 4–5 mentally and then continue to grow only physically. Through those years, many reasons for his developmental delays and hindrances were alluded to. He endured CAT scans, EEGs, a spinal tap, and constant blood tests. He was scrutinized by a team of world-renowned geneticists with regard to his facial features. Family photographs were studied; similarities were searched for and hours of detailed questioning endured. All without one single query about my alcohol intake. No one even seemed to suspect that his problems might be the result of alcohol abuse during my pregnancy. And far be it for me to bring up the subject. As it stood, no matter what the reason for his problems might have been, he was receiving the ultimate in medical attention, and I was conveniently able to remain hiding all snuggled up in the cozy blankets of excuses that were so freely given by those who surely had to have known the truth.

By the time my little funny baby was 5 years old, I am proud to say that he had surpassed even the most optimistic goals by leaps and bounds. That was also the year that I, at 45, found sobriety. Whether it was because of Denny or for Denny, I'll never know. It was, however, with Denny; and I have him to love and share and grow with for always. With my sobriety also came courage: courage to finally face the truth once and for all. More physical examinations, psychological testing, and IQ assessments were conducted—this time with an honest, contributing mother. I was, for the first time, prepared to hear and accept, if necessary, the truth. And so it was, my Denny was indeed a victim of my negligence. A condition known as fetal alcohol syndrome. It was the first time I had ever heard of it!

As for now, I have long since ceased to spend useless energy beating myself up over "the things I cannot change." I have accepted the responsibility for my son's limitations and a history, which I sadly regret I have no power to alter. It is in what the future can be for both of us that I find my strength and encouragement and the determination to carry on. It is in the smallest accomplishments and constant progress that I find a joy that is unequaled by any I've ever known. With love and patience and a daily dose of laughter (sometimes at ourselves), we are working together to help each other reach our highest levels of potential. Who can say what course our lives might have taken had someone early on had the integrity and conviction of purpose to chance offending me with the truth? On whom does the responsibility to ensure moral, ethical, and honest dissemination of facts from the medical community rest? It rests squarely on the shoulders of every individual member of the group. Not until each accountable representative takes a stand on his or her own, not allowing his or her principles to be compromised by fear or emotion, will these unfortunate children begin to receive a chance at life. They are only innocent victims of someone else's negligence or abuse. Without the recognition and care of those *who are in a position to offer assistance, they are prisoners in an invisible jail, chained by misconception and held captive by limitations they are unable to comprehend.*

Lisa did not mother Denny during the Middle Ages, not even during the 1960s, when there was no general awareness of FAS or the dangers of drinking during pregnancy. It was 1987—14 years after the first papers describing FAS appeared in the international medical literature and 6 years after the Surgeon General issued his warning about drinking during pregnancy (Surgeon General's Advisory on Alcohol and Pregnancy, 1981), in which abstinence was recommended.

Recognition of Maternal Alcohol Abuse and Appropriate Support for a New Mother Can Provoke Sobriety

Sobriety helps mothers to organize their own lives and build support systems around themselves. When mothers are able to find effective ways to deal with their grief and pain without drinking, they are better able to help their children and advocate for them. It is important to remember, however, that the pain, like the FAS/FAE, lasts a lifetime, and continuing supports are needed.

Alex's mother: I've been in recovery for 18 years. I drank from age 13 on—was a real wino. I've been married three times. After I married my last husband, I had three miscarriages before Alex was finally born. He was small—only 7 pounds at birth—compared with my girls who had all been 10 pounds. He was very fussy, was in and out of hospitals, and had a hard time digesting food. I started my recovery when he was 3 months old. I had to stay sober for 2 months to get the kids back. AA and Antabuse helped.

When Alex was 4 months, he sat up alone; at 6 months, he was walking. He never crawled. When he started walking, he'd run into walls and doors; he had no space perception at all. He was very hyperactive—always getting hurt. The social services were always investigating me. One time he had two black eyes; he ran right into a wall. He ran his tricycle into walls, too. When Alex was 2, I decided to go to college and finish what I had started earlier—a psych major. I got support from Alex's child care center; professionals there counseled me for 1½ years.

When Alex started school, they said he was dyslexic. He repeated first grade, and then we learned about FAS. "Oh my God, what have I done, what have I done?" I thought about AA and the serenity clause that says you must accept the things you cannot change. Four years later, Alex was finally diagnosed with FAE. By then, the school was giving up on him. They decided he was lazy and passed him on without learning. In junior high, the principal said, "Look for alternatives for Alex because the school can't handle him." I demanded more testing; he wanted to drop out. But he stayed with it on to high school: all Fs. In his sophomore year, he got all Ds three times and then dropped out. They opened an alternative school, and he goes there now. At 18, he likes school. He's got two certificates for good behavior. He says, "Mom, what a difference, I don't have all that stress any more. I can work at my own pace. When I don't get it straight, I can go outside and walk around a lot." He's such a joy. He's had some trouble with alcohol—been drunk three times in the past 3 years. He's a loner, stays by himself a lot or stays in his room listening to music. He's best friends with a few others who also have FAS/FAE.

What does he look like? He's kind of short and not so heavy. He looks just like other Indian kids. It's hard to realize that he has FAS, really. My daughter has been trying to teach him some things, and he just can't understand them— not at all. He finally got real angry and said, "I just don't get it. I just don't," and went to his room and slammed the door. I thought I'd dealt with all the pain and all the grief, but it was very hard for me. [Jackie, the mother, stopped talking as she sobbed heavily, then continued:] I just have to remember that I have to do the best I can with him as long as I have him.

Fathers Can Be Important Advocates

Husbands of alcoholic women often become the active parent, either through divorce, death, or the active alcoholism of their wives.

A couple of years ago, I received a phone call from a father in a small town in Europe who'd recently read an article on FAS for which I had been interviewed. This father told me that he'd been struggling for 4–5 years to find out what was wrong with his son. Then he'd read a National Geographic article (Steinmetz, 1992), and it occurred to him immediately that the symptoms associated with FAS described his son perfectly. He'd had many psychological tests performed on his son, but nothing had ever offered a definitive diagnosis. He said his son has memory impairments, but he's talkative and outgoing. He also has difficulty learning from his experience. This perplexed father wondered why, with all the medical advisors he'd had for his son, that this had never been a point of discussion. "He's a fine boy," the father said, "Absolutely tops. You'd estimate him to be very bright. It's the abstract things he just doesn't get. I cannot get him to read the clock, no matter what. At his football training, I notice a kind of reluctance—like they're really not working with him. When I finally asked them, they confessed that they thought he just didn't listen to them.

"They're so strict in their teaching over here," the father said, "I'd hoped you could give me some help with what to expect, how to handle these things as he grows up. He's always been extremely good with fine-motor things—played

since age 3 with very small things; but now he just can't handle abstract thought at all, even in describing things he can handle very well manually. He came by cesarean section and was in intensive care for the first 8 weeks with pneumonia. We always thought his early problems might have been related to this." "Was he prenatally exposed to alcohol?" I finally asked. "Oh yes," came the reply across the seas. "His mother has had five hospitalizations in two countries for her alcoholism; she's also been in AA for years. Things have gotten worse and worse; there seems to be no way to save her. The last doctor finally said, 'Let her go—you can't cope with it.' I am optimistic still; it's hard to give up. But for peace at home, I filed for a divorce but keep busy to find new programs as well."

I've heard this same story many times before from fathers struggling to care for their children with FAS/FAE born to mothers who had subsequently died of alcohol-related causes or been unable to conquer their alcoholism. These fathers, with incredible courage in advocating for their children, also experience grief and guilt: grief at the loss of the child they might have had and guilt for whatever their perceived role in the mother's alcoholism might have been. Still, biological fathers, with knowledge of their wives' drinking histories, are often able to experience the "A ha" phenomenon of awareness once they read or hear about FAS. Adoptive and foster parents, without knowledge of their children's prenatal alcohol exposure, often have a harder time making this association.

The Absence of an Appropriate Diagnosis Particularly Thwarts Appropriate Parenting by Adoptive and Foster Parents

Adoptive parents bring their own set of expectations to parenthood. Many who have only a desire to share their love and resources with a child are puzzled, dismayed, and often blamed when their children do not thrive. Michael Dorris (1989) eloquently described his first encounter with his adoptive son and his expectations.

> He looked up and met my eyes. His face was perfect, deeply etched, with dark narrow eyes, bright beneath thick, straight lashes and brows. Black hair feathered under the ruff of his snowsuit. His mouth was wide, his expression measuring. And then he lit with recognition.
> "Hi Daddy," he said, and without a beat of strangeness or doubt went back to his trucks. I stood—stunned, blessed, transported, forever changed—listening with rapt attention to his sounds of screeching brakes and revving engines. [The next day at the airport:] It was impossible to see his thin legs dominated by the thick balls of his knee joints, without making resolutions. He needed nourishment, care, encouragement, stability. I was determined that his development in every area would match his age before another year had passed.

Somewhere over the Great Lakes, he fell asleep in my lap, and in wonder and absolute contentment, I watched the ebb and flow of his breath, the movement beneath his lids as he dreamed, the sudden flutter of his fingertips. For the space of that flight, the world was in my arms.

For years I assumed I was fighting the effects of his medications, battering the barriers of his late start, scaling self-protective walls erected against the neglect he experienced as an infant. It was not until the following summer, when Adam was 5 years old, that I began to have an inkling that my real adversary was the lingering ghost of Adam's biological mother, already dead in 1973 of acute alcohol poisoning. (pp. 11–14, 45)

Adoptive and foster parents of young children with FAS/FAE are full of hope, almost always believing that their care and love can make a difference—can change a life. Of course, it *does* make a difference—a stable, loving home is clearly better than an abusive, neglectful, and unpredictable one. But love alone cannot reverse the brain damage caused by prenatal alcohol exposure, although a stable, loving home can reduce some of the secondary disabilities seen in individuals with FAS/FAE. There is still much to be learned about exactly how. So few systematic efforts at rehabilitation have been scientifically explored and reported. Early knowledge of the FAS/FAE diagnosis is clearly an important ingredient for the adoptive or foster family trying to mitigate the effects of earlier traumatic environments. Early knowledge of the diagnosis helps the family temper their expectations in accord with the emerging talents and disabilities of their child. One valuable lesson that a child with FAS/FAE can learn is to accept help without shame or anger.

Delaney died last week—scarcely 20 years old—from an overdose of heroin. He wasn't found in his rental room until 3 days later. With a score of 118, he had one of the highest IQ scores of any of our patients with full FAS. But he still couldn't tell time except with a digital watch. He was so ashamed of his disabilities, he'd never tell anyone. He tried to pretend they didn't exist.

Delaney had held more jobs then anyone could even remember. He just couldn't seem to keep them. His last job was in a submarine sandwich shop, but he couldn't remember the orders long enough to make up the sandwiches: "Swiss cheese and salami, no mayonnaise, double tomatoes. . . ." He never asked for special allowances or special help; he left when he got fired and went out into the night to look for another job. No one missed him when he didn't show up— no one was expecting him anywhere. His corrections officer finally found him.

Delaney had three families, and they all tried to help. No one actually knew the extent of his limitations, however, until his adoptive parents saw a rerun of the episode about FAS on 20/20 (Wenner, 1990) when Delaney was 15. They immediately figured out the problem and arranged for a diagnostic exam-

ination, which confirmed their suspicions: Delaney had FAS. But by then his behavior was out of control.

Delaney's biological mother was an alcoholic who had four children with four different fathers before contact with her was lost. From her pictures and history, it looked as though she also had FAS. She was frequently suicidal and had been diagnosed by a psychiatrist with borderline personality disorder. She was unable to cope with raising Delaney and often left him at the hospital emergency room when things got out of control. Her biological mother was also alcoholic and reportedly drank during all 12 of her pregnancies.

Delaney's second family adopted him when he was 3½ years old—they loved children and had three beautiful girls, but further pregnancies were contraindicated for medical reasons. So, they adopted Delaney—a "darling blond, blue-eyed boy" with the scars of cigarette burns on his legs. He had been abused and neglected and didn't talk. But with three older sisters playing school with him constantly, he did soon talk. His adoptive mother reports that a lot of the things he did didn't make sense. At 5 or 6 years: "Dee—go down and start the dryer for Mom, please." "Sure, Mom," said Dee, happily and willingly going off to the basement. Upon his return: "Did you start the dryer, Dee?" "Mom, which one's the dryer?" Mom took him down to the basement and explained, "Look, the dryer is the one with the big hole in the side. Later: "Dee, put these dirty clothes in the washer for Mom." "Sure, Mom." Mom finds the dirty clothes in the dryer—"Remember, Dee? The dryer is the one with a big hole in the side." "Oh, I forgot, Mom." Still cheerful, ready to help.

School got harder and harder, and Delaney started hanging out with a bad crowd. He couldn't understand why his parents were concerned when he started getting dope from kids at school: "But Mom, it was free. I didn't have to pay any money." By his teenage years, he was running away and out of control. His adoptive parents finally had to get him into a residential home. The state subsequently billed them $86,000 and demanded they mortgage their home to pay the bill. With the help of a lawyer, they settled out of court and agreed to pay half the cost of foster care until he turned 18 years old.

His third family, his foster family, was also devoted. They lived in the country and did all they could to help him. But at 18 he insisted on living on his own in the city with his girlfriend. He planned to finish high school but couldn't hold a job. He started hanging out on the streets at night with a bad crowd, using dope. His girlfriend had a job but just couldn't cope with his lifestyle. Eventually he went to prison for the rape of two girls at a party where people were high on drugs. He'd talked about killing himself for years—tried slashing his wrists and talked of drinking bleach. Yet, the police said his death was not a suicide, because no note was found.

If Delaney or even his biological mother had received an early diagnosis, it is easy to see how a better understanding of their problems could have resulted. Understanding should stimulate a more effective delivery of community services early in life, when individuals are less enmeshed in self-destructive activities and more receptive to interventions.

FAMILIES REVEAL SIMILAR NEEDS

Despite their obvious diversity, families with FAS/FAE concerns share many similar, pressing needs. Through understanding and advocacy, community professionals can do much to meet these needs, thereby improving life for people with FAS/FAE and their families.

Families Need Support and Opportunities for Sharing

Maternal sobriety and an early diagnosis are only the beginning of the long struggle that many families—both biological and adoptive/ foster—are engaged in on behalf of their children with FAS/FAE. The tremendous need for a support network of parents of other children with FAS/FAE is shared by all types of families. Working together, sharing ideas and solutions, educating and advocating for FAS, they can bring about increased understanding and services.

Lisa's quest: In mid-March of last year, I was in desperate need of finding a support group or even just one other parent who I could talk and relate to. Denny was being "overlooked" by his teacher; even after several attempts to communicate my child's educational needs, I felt we were getting the runaround. If only I'd known then what I know now! He has always been a very loving and eager-to-please little boy, but I could see a temperament change and almost daily signs of frustration. He was coming home from school with tears in his little eyes almost every day because his name was put on the board and he had to forfeit his recess. The homework he brought home was so far beyond what he was capable of that it was an impossibility—more defeat, more rejection. I even toyed with the idea of home tutoring for him to protect him from the embarrassment and ridicule that I knew by now were a matter of course. I called the health department; they gave me a couple of telephone numbers that proved to be dead ends. I called our local hospital to see if they could make a recommendation. They suggested I call AA. When I did, the woman who was in charge said, "Fetal what?" In all the referrals and suggestions and people who said they would get back to me, I heard from only one person. But it was the right one! She was a nurse in San Diego, and she had just received a flyer in the mail concerning a seminar on FAS and said she would mail it to me that very day. It was at that seminar (March 30, 1990) that I met Jan and all the other wonderful friends who have helped me more than words can ever say.

Now, everything is coming together perfectly. Denny is in a new school, in a special education class with a teacher who is familiar with FAS. My son now brings home awards for his spelling and reading. To say there's been a change in his self-worth would be an understatement of gross dimension.

Denny's problems didn't end that year; each year and in each new school district, Lisa has to continue her advocacy efforts. She has to seek out the best teachers, teach them about FAS, and keep monitoring the success of each school day by reading Denny's body language. Even as recently as last year, Denny was kept from going for recess for days on end because he hadn't earned enough "points" in his special education class. Once Lisa had to withdraw Denny from school until a satisfactory program could be worked out that would help Denny grow to the best of his abilities without sacrificing his sweet-tempered, compliant, and eager-to-please personality. When Lisa says she wants Denny to be the best that he can be, she isn't just referring to his academic performance; she is referring to his emotional well-being as well—a task that has provided the biggest challenge to the school. Still, Lisa continues to advocate, saying over and over, "I just want Denny to be the best Denny that Denny can be."

Families Need to Be Asked the Right Questions

Queries about maternal drinking during pregnancy are essential to circumvent denial and to ensure that any potential linkages between prenatal alcohol exposure and later developmental disabilities can be established. There are several essential times when professionals need to ask the family about the prenatal alcohol exposure history and record this information in the child's records. The first is around the time of the child's birth (during the pregnancy or at the delivery, especially if little or no prenatal care was obtained); at any postpartum contacts (either for medical concerns about the child or child protective concerns (e.g., abuse and neglect on the part of the community); and at any points at which adoption or foster care are being considered. If this critical information is not documented at these times when the biological family is still involved or available, it can jeopardize the ability of the child to ever receive an appropriate diagnosis. It is also important that professionals ask about prenatal alcohol exposure in the course of any evaluation of the child (whatever his or her age) for any medical problems or problem behaviors. If the doctors, nurses, and social workers dealing with the family around the time of delivery have done their jobs, this information will be part of the child's official record and part of the family's knowledge about this child, and available to permit a prenatal alcohol-related diagnosis if one is appropriate.

Families Need Straightforward Information About FAS/FAE, and They Need Understanding

Withholding information doesn't spare the family pain, it only incapacitates their ability to effectively solve problems. All relevant information about prenatal alcohol exposure should be transmitted to families. This information should be readily available for biological, foster, and adoptive families of all children suspected of having FAS/FAE. This information should always be tempered with understanding and consideration of the special needs and circumstances of the individual. Information about FAS/FAE is not a sentence—it is a building block. It is seldom possible for a clinician to make dire predictions about an individual—each child and each family holds an opportunity for hope, and each deserves encouragement in facing the future.

Professionals who believe that they are sparing a family pain by lack of an honest disclosure or by believing that the individuals in their practice couldn't have these problems haven't felt the lifelong pain of biological families of children disabled by prenatal alcohol. Professionals who believe that having this information will bias a family against a given child and thus thwart that child's development haven't heard the anguished pleas of adoptive and foster parents who are trying to figure out what is wrong with their children and desperately want to help their children but can't obtain this critical information. Although some states (like Washington) mandate full disclosure, others are bogged down in old confidentiality rulings. It is the children with FAE who are most hurt by such guidelines because, in the absence of FAS facial stigmata, the exposure history is essential to understanding that the observed behaviors may be related to prenatal alcohol exposure.

Children with FAS/FAE are not only more likely to be in foster or adoptive homes than other children, but they also are placed in an unusually high number of different foster homes. It seems likely that if more specific diagnostic and exposure history information accompanied each child, community agencies would achieve a better match between the child and the family and facilitate foster parent understanding.

As children grow, they too need information about FAS/FAE. An issue that often concerns professionals working with children with FAS/FAE is that the children will become dreadfully angry with their biological mothers if they are told about their FAS/FAE diagnosis. Compared with the importance of children and adolescents understanding their diagnosis and making some sense of their own disabilities, this is a smaller concern. By far the predominant reaction of children is simply one of relief at finally learning their own diagnosis. Sadness and perplexity, rather than anger, are the more usually expressed feelings in terms of the biological mother's alcoholism. "I wonder why she had to go and do that?" one young girl mused sadly. "I sure am not going to drink when I'm having a baby," said another.

Families Need to Be Heard

In the present research void of effective treatment modalities, the experience of other parents represents almost the only source of help and understanding regarding what is needed and what isn't needed, what works and what doesn't, and who understands FAS in each community and who doesn't (e.g., Caldwell, 1993; Dorris, 1989; Gere, 1993; Groves, 1993; King, 1993; Lutke, 1993, 1997; Malbin, 1993; Rathbun, 1993; Wortley, Wortley, & the grandparents, 1993). Working collectively and in conjunction with concerned and knowledgeable professionals, parents represent a powerful force for change in each community.

CONCLUSIONS

In their own words, the families in this chapter have clearly revealed their needs in terms of the community professionals with whom they interacted. Families of all types need clear information about alcohol and pregnancy. Pregnant women need honest, straightforward information about the adverse effects of alcohol on their developing children delivered in a forthright and nonjudgmental manner. The caring, sympathetic clinician is an important part of the process. Each in her own way, these mothers have revealed how dependent they were in the throes of their alcoholism on the integrity, sincerity, and understanding of the professionals from whom they sought help. Only later, in sobriety, were these mothers able to express their dismay at health care professionals unwilling or unable to respond to their needs, and their compassion for their children. Fathers have also shown how important they are to the advocacy process. Together families and professionals must build networks of support, hope, and advocacy to permit each child to be the best that child can be, across the many domains of life.

REFERENCES

Caldwell, S. (1993). Nurturing the delicate rose. In J.K. Kleinfeld & S. Wescott (Eds.), *Fantastic Antone succeeds! Experiences in educating children with fetal alcohol syndrome* (pp. 97–129). Fairbanks: University of Alaska Press.

Dorris, M. (1989). *The broken cord.* New York: HarperCollins.

Gere, A.R. (1993). Cindy's story. In J.K. Kleinfeld & S. Wescott (Eds.), *Fantastic Antone succeeds!: Experiences in educating children with fetal alcohol syndrome* (pp. 55–68). Fairbanks: University of Alaska Press.

Groves, P.G. (1993). Growing with FAS. In J.K. Kleinfeld & S. Wescott (Eds.), *Fantastic Antone succeeds! Experiences in educating children with fetal alcohol syndrome* (pp. 37–53). Fairbanks: University of Alaska Press.

King, C. (1993). Raising alcohol-affected twins. In J.K. Kleinfeld & S. Wescott (Eds.), *Fantastic Antone succeeds! Experiences in educating children with fetal alcohol syndrome* (pp. 161–170). Fairbanks: University of Alaska Press.

Lutke, J. (1993). Parental advocacy for alcohol-affected children. In J.K. Kleinfeld & S. Wescott (Eds.), *Fantastic Antone succeeds! Experiences in educating children with fetal alcohol syndrome* (pp. 71–95). Fairbanks: University of Alaska Press.

Lutke, J. (1997). Spider web walking: Hope for children with FAS through understanding. In A. Streissguth & J. Kanter (Eds.), *The challenge of fetal alcohol syndrome: Overcoming secondary disabilities* (pp. 284–294). Seattle: University of Washington Press.

Malbin, D.B. (1993). Stereotypes and realities: Positive outcomes with intervention. In J.K. Kleinfeld & S. Wescott (Eds.), *Fantastic Antone succeeds! Experiences in educating children with fetal alcohol syndrome* (pp. 253–271). Fairbanks: University of Alaska Press.

Rathbun, A. (1993). Overcoming the cycle of failure and frustration. In J.K. Kleinfeld & S. Wescott (Eds.), *Fantastic Antone succeeds!: Experiences in educating children with fetal alcohol syndrome* (pp. 295–313). Fairbanks: University of Alaska Press.

Steinmetz, G. (1992). The preventable tragedy: Fetal alcohol syndrome. *National Geographic, 18*(2).

Surgeon General's Advisory on Alcohol and Pregnancy. (1981). *FDA Drug Bulletin, 11*(2). Rockville, MD: Department of Health and Human Services.

Wenner, K. (Executive producer). (1990, March 30). What's wrong with my child? 20/20. Seattle: American Broadcasting Co.

Wortley, M., Wortley, D., & the grandparents. (1993). On raising Lisa. In J.K. Kleinfeld & S. Wescott (Eds.), *Fantastic Antone succeeds! Experiences in educating children with fetal alcohol syndrome* (pp. 270–283). Fairbanks: University of Alaska Press.

IV

Preparing People with FAS for Life in the Community

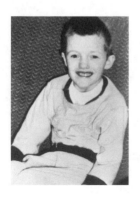
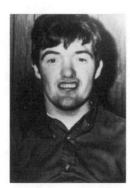
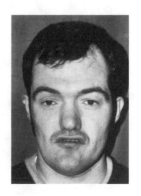

10

Preparing Children with FAS/FAE for Adulthood

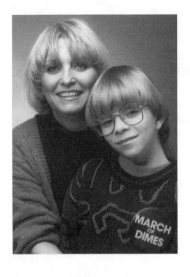

A 25-year-old man diagnosed with FAS as an adult: I always figured there was something wrong with me when I was growing up, but I never knew what it was. It was only after my mom sobered up that she talked about it with me, said I was an FAS child. At first I didn't want to believe it because I felt normal—but when I finally accepted it, I was relieved because I knew I had a lot of learning disabilities, too. My youngest brother also has FAS—he has more learning problems than I have and more troubles, too. I cry for him. How much more I could have been without alcohol as a part of my life. I am proud of what I've become in my life, but I cry every night when I go to sleep when I think of what I might have been if alcohol had not been an important part of my life.

PROBLEMS ENCOUNTERED BY PEOPLE WITH FAS/FAE

When I hear the sense of disabilities from my patients' own lips, over and over, from individuals from every walk of life, from many types of family backgrounds, and with varied intellectual abilities, it is clear that they are often much more disabled as adults than I would have estimated they would be when they were children. They don't just go out on their own and become independent once they're made to fend for themselves, face the music, or go through whatever rites of passage an uninformed community inflicts on them. They seem to make a better adjustment when they have been given supportive services; but, until now, little data have been available.

New Research

The secondary disabilities study described in Chapter 6 (Streissguth, Barr, Kogan, & Bookstein, 1996), demonstrates the scope and magnitude of employment and independent living problems that people with FAS/FAE experience as adults. By administering a Life History Interview (LHI) to caregivers or family members, this part of the study evaluated 90 adults, ranging in age from 21 to 52 years.

In terms of lifetime employment history, we found that most had some sort of work experience. Half were working at the time of the interview, but the median duration of the current job was only 9 months. Throughout their lifetimes (the average age was 28 years), only half of these adults with FAS/FAE had ever held a job for longer than 1 year. More than half had repeatedly had trouble getting hired or holding a job or were fired or lost a job without understanding why. Common problems experienced in the workplace were being easily frustrated, manifesting poor judgment, having difficulty understanding the task, and experiencing on-the-job social problems. More than one third had had problems with being unreliable as well as with anger, supervision, and lying.

In order to study independent living skills in adults with FAS/FAE, we examined 12 activities representing different levels of complexity. Almost no one needed help with dressing, but almost everyone needed help with managing money. Only one quarter needed help negotiating public transportation, but more than three fourths needed help with making decisions. Between one half and three fourths needed help obtaining medical care and social services, handling interpersonal relationships, and grocery shopping. Between one third and one half needed help with cooking meals, structuring leisure time, staying out of trouble, and maintaining personal hygiene.

Who provided the ongoing caregiving for the 90 adults with FAS/FAE in our study? More than one half still relied on their parents. One quarter were helped by other relatives, spouses, or partners, and another one quarter had a case manager or an advocate.

Even when parents, relatives, and friends are willing to take on this responsibility, it is often difficult for them to know how to proceed. Many of these young adults need specialized services provided by experienced professionals. Yet these services may not be readily available or may be available too late in life for maximal effectiveness. For example, in our study, the median age for starting to get job support services was 18, which is far too late for people with FAS/FAE to begin this important process. In order to overcome or intercept these problems with working and living independently, families must begin special planning efforts early in their children's lives; knowledge of the nature of the child's disability is a key factor in enabling parents to know how to proceed, and an early diagnosis of FAS/FAE is important in this process.

RECOGNIZING AND ACCEPTING DISABILITIES

At an FAS conference, I met two young adults, Stewart and Patsy, who were both recently diagnosed as having FAE and had never met anyone with FAS or FAE. The three of us sat in the foyer and talked for nearly an hour while the conference went on without us. They were eager to share their experiences and feelings with me and with each other and were enchanted with their own similarities.

When I asked them what it felt like to be diagnosed with FAE, Stewart said, "At first I thought it was some contagious disease or something. But then after my father explained what it was, I gradually came to accept it. . . . I always knew I was different because I don't make friends like normal people do. I never had friends hanging around me like other people do." Patsy had a different slant: "I've gone through life thinking, 'Is everyone as forgetful as I am?' In school, teachers reported I had a learning disability—but it's more than that. They just don't know how it affects your living. . . . [The diagnosis] explained a lot of things that were wrong with me. . . ."

At the end of the conversation, Stewart said, "This is so incredible. Listening to her and her experiences and her job history—it's just like looking at a twin. And I might get a friend out of it, too!" When I asked them if they had any words of advice to other young people with FAS/FAE, Patsy said, "Tell them there is help out there for people like us. Look for someone who can see you for what you are. Don't look down on your disability. Have a positive attitude. Learn from it. It's not your fault."

People with FAS/FAE almost always have some kind of behavioral disabilities because of the central nervous system (CNS) dysfunction that is part of the diagnostic criteria. Whether this means that they are "disabled" depends on what they are trying to do. They are certainly not disabled for all of life's activities—they often run like the wind, laugh with gusto, sing like birds, and work hard.

It's this patchwork of strengths and disabilities that is so perplexing to them and their families.

As my patients with FAS/FAE tell me over and over again in their own words and with their actions, it is hard enough having these disabilities. It is even harder living up to the totally unrealistic expectations of others. Although parents of children with many types of disabilities have appropriate expectations for their children, which set the stage for successful adulthood, the situation is far different for children with FAS/FAE for several reasons: 1) Their disabilities are often hidden (from both themselves and their parents) because of the subtle nature of the brain damage with which they've been living all of their lives; 2) most children do not get an appropriate FAS/FAE diagnosis until later in life, after problems have begun; and 3) most communities don't understand or provide for the specific needs of people with FAS/FAE at different ages. Disability, backed up by an official diagnosis, may well be the mediating condition for an improved outcome in people with FAS/FAE.

PLANNING EARLY FOR A HEALTHY LIFE

A number of years ago, after a conference at which I had spoken on FAS, an adoptive mother came up to talk. She shared her joy and her sorrow as she reflected on the two children she had raised. Her joy was that her adoptive son with FAS was in community college studying sheet metal work and doing fine. I remembered him well: He had been a typical small, charming, fearless lad brought onto the stage 15 years earlier to demonstrate FAS during a conference at which I spoke at a medical school in another state. He had been diagnosed shortly after birth. This mother had extrapolated from this knowledge an appropriate and successful rearing environment for him. She'd clearly done well.

"What's the sorrow?" I asked. She said that she had had absolutely no idea at the time that this little lad's older brother, whom she and her husband had also adopted, must have had FAE. (FAE wasn't even a term anyone was using in those days—we were just starting to use the term FAS). At any rate, she said that because the older brother was not growth deficient and didn't have the characteristic facial features associated with FAS, they had assumed that he was a normal child. This assumption led them to raise him with normal expectations. She said they'd made him keep his nose to the grindstone in terms of homework and studies and did everything they knew to help his life turn out well. They didn't budge an inch. They dedicated their lives to this project. They knew that if they just tried hard enough that this little child whom they had hoped to help by adopting would indeed be helped and be able to move on to a successful adult life as a result of their interventions. "Nothing could be further from the truth," she said sadly. "How I wish I had known. How I wish I had

given him the benefit of the doubt like I did his younger brother with FAS. Knowing that our younger son had FAS gave our parenting an entirely different pitch. Knowing that no one expected him to be exactly like everyone else got us off the hook as parents. It was no longer our fault if he wasn't behaving properly or learning enough. Everything he did learn was like a gift. Each day of good behavior, a pleasure. We had many opportunities to show him how much we loved him, and he reciprocated with his own love and appreciation. If only we had had the same insight into the problems of his older brother," she sighed.

"Where is he now?" I asked hesitantly. "In jail," she replied. "He dropped out of school, got in with the wrong crowd, got involved in alcohol and drugs, and got into trouble with the law. We were never able to turn things around once they started going downhill. Just too much history of bad feelings, mistrust, unmet expectations, frustrations. If only we had known."

An early diagnosis is one of the strongest factors associated with fewer secondary disabilities (Streissguth et al., 1996). In our study of 415 patients with FAS/FAE, those who had a diagnosis before age 6 had a lower rate of disrupted school experiences, inappropriate sexual behavior, trouble with the law, alcohol and other drug problems, and institutional care in psychiatric hospitals or prison (see Chapter 6). Early detection empowers parents to plan creatively for their children with FAS/FAE as individuals and to obtain the services necessary to allow those children to develop to their best potential.

In comparison with their peers, people with FAS/FAE seem to have more and more difficulties as they grow older, rather than more and more competencies. Somewhere around the time of adolescence, they seem to be "treading water" in their development—suddenly their peers are becoming independent and turning into adults while they're still stuck in child-like patterns of behavior. When they haven't yet been diagnosed, it's even more perplexing because nobody understands why their progress is arrested. The diagnosis helps the family and the individuals themselves put their behaviors into perspective: "Aha! It isn't just a motivational problem after all!" Actually, I've seldom seen a person with FAS/FAE at this age who didn't want to do more than he or she could. But it is easier for an adolescent to get excited about learning a trade when he or she hasn't been planning on going to college for 12 years.

An early diagnosis helps parents set appropriate expectations for each child based on that child's characteristics, rather than on the parents' dreams of what they had hoped their child would become. It is easier to relate to a child one knows has disabilities than to a child one thinks is merely ungrateful, lazy, or behaving ridiculously. An early diagnosis helps people with FAS/FAE grow up enjoying the skills they do have and striving for the goals they can achieve.

BUILDING PERSONAL STRENGTHS AT HOME

When they are young, many children with FAS/FAE have an enthusiastic, sparkly, upbeat manner. They may love going to school—until they are unable to keep up academically. As they begin to fall behind in their classes (and if their disabilities go unrecognized), and as the premiums for academic success exceed their best efforts, discouragement and poor self-esteem may ensue.

Alert families, taking a life-span approach and listening to the needs of children with FAS/FAE through their behaviors as well as their words, realize that the real goal is a healthy emotional life, not just academic achievement. Children with FAS/FAE often need to be taught things that other children learn by "osmosis," just by observing. Some of the most important things a child with FAS/FAE can be taught at home to prepare for life after school are:

- To be a friend and to behave in a socially appropriate manner
- To be alone and to find constructive, solitary things to do
- To work and to enjoy working

Families are important learning centers for all of these activities. The family may well be the center of the universe for the individual with FAS/FAE, the ultimate caregivers and overseers. Families can model, reward, encourage, and facilitate behaviors and activities that are important ingredients of adult successful living—and they can do this within a comfortable context, without lesson plans or homework. Families can also help by ensuring that these individuals' learning needs are explicit rather than assuming that they will be intuitively recognized by others. Grandparents, siblings, friends, and neighbors can easily join in this undertaking once they understand that the individual has a disability and needs special help.

A cohesive family and its solidarity gives a person with FAS/FAE something exciting to belong to and something important to talk about. Family rules, rituals, festivals, and celebrations become extraordinarily important to children who are not winning science medals, being selected for the football team, or being asked out on dates. A close family is a haven of protection and a source of social intercourse that helps compensate for the peer group rebuffs that otherwise may lead to depression or to dependence on an undesirable peer group. Family values such as kindness, respect, and concern for others; learning to make choices; learning to take appropriate steps toward independence without being overwhelmed with freedom; and learning to feel good about oneself, including both one's strengths and limitations, are valuable assets to possess, regardless of the individual's ultimate level of independent functioning, job performance, or salary.

Learning to Be a Friend and to Behave in a Socially Appropriate Manner

Families with prosocial values are likely to find it easy to teach their children to befriend others and behave in a socially appropriate manner. Clearly, a family that teaches their child to stand up for his or her rights at any cost will be jeopardizing the life and safety of the child with FAS/FAE. But even families that consciously endorse values of love, respect, and compassion can have a hard time parenting a child with FAS/FAE when that child manifests behaviors that are incomprehensible to them and that violate their family values. When a child has FAS/FAE but the family doesn't know it, family members often misguidedly try to use the same teaching techniques they've used with other children or believe are appropriate. When they try and try to keep the child out of trouble without knowing the cause of the trouble (perhaps getting bad advice from the professionals to whom they go for help because no one has thought to ask about possible prenatal alcohol exposure), it is no wonder they are confused and desperate. Sometimes the child becomes scapegoated as the "bad" child in the family. Sometimes the child is ostracized from the family's church or social group, which only further alienates him or her from support.

Helping children with FAS/FAE grow up observing normal social conventions is a good investment for future socialization and maintenance of friends. Learning to listen as well as to talk, learning to ask polite questions, learning to use acceptable table manners, learning to write letters, say "please" and "thank you," and to express appropriate feelings of friendship when young are all part of the social armamentarium that a concerned family can teach a child with FAS/FAE. It is best to teach these skills when children are young and eager to please, not after they're teenagers and the peer culture expects them to be cool, disdainful, and noncompliant. The way to teach these skills is by demonstration, expectation, recognition, and reminders.

As social rejection can be an important trigger for maladaptive behaviors in people with FAS/FAE who want desperately to fit in, families can actually teach prosocial behaviors in many explicit ways in the course of daily living. Nowicki and Duke (1992) describe techniques that can be used both by families and therapists for helping children who are deficient in receiving and sending nonverbal messages and who have difficulty in recognizing and expressing particular emotional signals. Although these authors do not discuss using these techniques for children with FAS/FAE, they focus on many topics with which children with FAS/FAE have difficulties (see also Antonello, 1996).

Noncompliance and sexually inappropriate behaviors are two lightning rods for families raising children with FAS/FAE. Both can be approached by seeking to understand the meaning of the behaviors. The roots of noncompliance in people with FAS/FAE can often be traced to cognitive disabilities (see Chapters 6 and 7). Understanding this can help parents to develop appropriate remedial strategies. Lutke (1997), an insightful parent and FAS/FAE educator who has raised many children with FAS/FAE says, "At the heart of all compliance issues is a competence issue. We have to move from seeing behavior as non-compliance to seeing it as non-competence" (p. 184).

Some sexually inappropriate behaviors have the same origins in children with FAS/FAE. Inappropriate sexual touching and advances are two of the most frequent sexually inappropriate behaviors reported among people with FAS/FAE (Streissguth et al., 1996). Not understanding and respecting personal space, for example, and needing multisensory input for learning can result in young children with FAS/FAE needing to be taught about personal boundaries that other children in the family may pick up through implicit learning. In addition, many people with FAS/FAE have experienced sexual or physical abuse or domestic violence (a total of 72% of those older than 12 in our 1996 secondary disabilities study). Having experienced violations of their own personal space was a clear risk factor for these individuals themselves having inappropriate sexual behaviors. Furthermore, we found large differences in how families and society responded to these behaviors: Girls who engaged in inappropriate sexual behaviors were more likely to be sent to treatment; boys were more likely to be sent to jail or to get into legal trouble (Streissguth et al., 1996). As entry into the criminal justice system is seldom therapeutic and often involves other risks and liaisons, it would be more useful if both males and females with FAS/FAE were given opportunities to be helped by appropriate professionals when their inappropriate behaviors are too extreme to be effectively dealt with in the family.

Novick (1997) recommended the use of cognitive behavioral therapy for people with FAS/FAE because it is more concrete and directive than other therapeutic approaches for inappropriate sexual behaviors. She also describes many techniques and constructs that parents can use at home to explicitly teach respect for boundaries and personal space among children with FAS/FAE in order to avert problems around inappropriate sexual behaviors.

Two children with FAS from two savvy families had visited back and forth a lot during their younger years—neither had made true friends at school. Their families had often joked that they'd get married some day, living one week with one family and the next week with the other. "It won't work, Mom," the boy said while fastening his seatbelt for the drive home one day. "What won't work?" asked his mother. "Me and Annie," he replied. "She's just too FAS for me!"

Learning to Be Alone and Finding Constructive Solitary Things to Do

Children with FAS/FAE desperately need extracurricular venues of success in their lives in order to develop pleasurable skills for a lifetime of healthful recreation and for learning the satisfaction and self-worth of goal-directed behavior. Such activities can include positive experiences with dance, music, art, sports, gardening, cooking, knitting, or computers, depending on the interests and inclinations of the family. A medal in the Special Olympics, for example, can go a long way toward offsetting difficulties with the multiplication tables. Whatever the activity, family support and organizational help will be an important ingredient of success.

Kyle, who has shared many insights with me on growing up with FAS/FAE, once said, "The trouble with school is that you spend all of your time doing things you do poorly and no time doing the things you do well." Families can make up the difference, but it doesn't happen automatically.

Ralph was a Special Olympics medalist—his greatest achievement and the source of much family and community pride. "How did he ever do it?" I asked innocently one day, thinking about the attentional problems that Ralph was born with. "Well, we trained him ourselves by riding our bicycles on either side of him," said his mother, "while he just ran, which he does naturally, right between us. Then, on race days, we station family members and friends all along the course and as he approaches, they yell out, 'Keep on running, Ralph!'"

Learning to Work and to Enjoy Working

Training for being a good worker should begin not at age 14 or 18 but when a child is 4–5 years old. Capitalizing on the desire of young children to please the people they like helps them build repetition, order, and organization into their lives. Paying children for performing piecemeal household jobs that are repetitive, cumulative, and easily under their control (e.g., pulling up weeds, picking up pine cones) can help to build good work skills. Working beside a parent or an older sibling can also enhance the enjoyment of work while also teaching the child that work is not a banishment but an enjoyable communal activity.

The key to a successful work experience is a good instructor. Careful instructions, tireless demonstrations, and tangible rewards are the glue that unifies the work experience for individuals with FAS/FAE and leads to the internalization of the activity. Good work habits (e.g., being methodical, learning to work at a reasonable pace, keeping focused, keeping tools in order) are best taught by imitation. Good job skills (e.g., how you go about gathering pine cones, pulling specific weeds, making Jell-O, picking apples, sweeping the sidewalk) are best taught by demonstration. When the child is young, family members can learn to be effective trainers—especially if they are cognizant of the child's "hidden disabilities" and do not expend all of their energies on traditional homework. Instructors are most successful when they give clear, simple instructions; enumerate only one or two steps at a time; demonstrate the job as they speak; and pace the work/reward ratio appropriately. With increasing age, more complex job skills are appropriate, but the same techniques will still be necessary.

As the child matures, families should be on the lookout for job experiences that might eventually have some value in the marketplace. Volunteer work where the supervisors are willing to learn how to work with people with FAS/FAE is also useful. But best of all are opportunities to learn a specific skill that can then be an entry ticket for a paying job. Some such skills can be learned in special programs at school or through extracurricular activities, summer experiences, or volunteer work.

Riley had a special skill in his "back pocket," having learned printing in junior high school. When he graduated from high school, he started out working in fast-food chains, like the rest of his friends. He had failed repeatedly in these jobs and become exceedingly discouraged when a friend remembered that Riley had printing skills and told him about an apprenticeship opportunity. The kindly owner of a small printing company let him serve an apprenticeship for several years, then hired him to work in the print shop. The predictable nature of the work, the patience and kindness of the master printer, and the relaxed pace of the shop all combined in a successful employment experience for Riley for many years.

Most individuals with FAS/FAE don't have opportunities like Riley did—very few have learned any specific skills while growing up that are of any use in the workplace. Very few chance into appropriately paced and supervised work experiences even after getting training. Compare Riley's experience with Sylvia's:

Sylvia was no slouch. She attended general classes at her local high school, where she got good grades and earned a high school diploma. She even held a job for a short time while in high school. After she graduated, she obtained assistance from a vocational training consultant who helped her to choose a career as a dental hygienist. Sylvia, however, failed the entry exam. She spent the next 3 months and $1,200 getting a dog-grooming certificate. Although a good student, she was unable to continue this work in the competitive employment market, and the school had no job supervision program. Despite all of Sylvia's early promise, success in coping with school, and good family support, she has had repeated difficulties in the workplace. She herself says, "Well, I start out okay, then things build up, and then even the thought of work brings stress."

When I met with Sylvia to see if I could help her, she itemized in explicit detail and with much emotion, the exact nature of her work-related stress: "First of all: Directions and understanding what's expected of me. When someone explains something to me, the words get all mixed up in my head. When they give me lots of directions, I seek a detour, an easier solution, or I eliminate something to simplify—both make problems at work. Like, at one job, I had to learn the cash register. They explained it all to me in just a few minutes. I kept asking them to say it slower and write it down. I finally said, 'I just don't understand.'

"Then there's communications. I get panicked and feel I can't find the right word. Or if two things are happening at once, like a telephone call comes in while I'm waiting on a customer—I just can't handle it. I tried to explain to my boss about when things were overwhelming me, and she just said, 'Read a stress management book or go to a yoga class.' She just didn't understand.

"Then there's the fast pace—it terrifies me. You just gotta keep going— you just never do enough. Then there's lots of people and confusion. I just get boggled and lose concentration. When there are too many people and too much to do at one time, I just go on overload. A fast-food restaurant is the last place I could work—the fast pace, the cash register—I'd just lose my mind. That's why

I think I'd be a better dog trainer than I am a dog groomer, which demands a fast pace for the profits. I'm not sluggish. I completed the [dog-grooming] course okay and didn't quit. But I was a student then and my job was learning, so the pace was different."

"And then, I don't like to ask for help. That's how I hurt my back. The dog was too heavy. I tried to lift him anyway. I didn't ask for help, and I should have. It's hard for me to ask for help. I know it's my fault, but that's just the way I am."

At one point, Sylvia sobbed openly as she described one particularly stressful time when she ultimately quit by walking off the job and never returning. Although she recognized that this was unacceptable behavior and repeatedly stated how she hated to let anybody down, in the intense stress of the situation, she apparently saw no alternatives. She felt desperate at the time, but even months later felt ashamed of her behavior.

Even with savvy parents acting as advocates, the transition from high school to unsupported employment is often too overwhelming for people with FAS/FAE. To be successful, Sylvia needs the kind of job training and long-term, on-the-job supervision that are available only through a disability training program. Sylvia has many areas of perfectly normal functioning, yet she clearly has cognitive impairments as well as a result of her prenatal alcohol exposure. On a 5-hour battery of neuropsychological tests, she functions well within expectations in some areas but has significant impairment in others, particularly mathematical abilities, auditorially mediated attention, and memory. In the typical work environment, these cognitive disabilities make it almost impossible for her to function effectively. She is overwhelmed by expectations she is unable to meet. Intense internal stress makes her even more dysfunctional and eventually incapacitates her.

The search for meaningful work is a driving force in the lives of many young adults with FAS/FAE, but, unfortunately, this search almost always ends in disappointment and frustration.

Patsy: "I was in special ed all through school. Then, in high school, I was in vocational training for the last couple of classes of the day—intensive job training—but the teacher wouldn't find me a job. All the other kids got a job, but not me. He'd put those kids in jobs, but not me. I finally resigned because I said the teachers weren't doing their jobs. They really weren't giving me attention and helping me find a job. Then, finally, they gave me a job I wasn't trained for. On-the-job-training is hard. I said, 'I need to be told exactly what to do. Write it down so I know exactly what to do.' But my new boss said, 'I don't think I need to be a parent to my employees.' He gave me the job but refused to explain things. I had the job only 3 weeks; he complained that I didn't do more than what he'd tell me. I didn't know how to figure out what to do. So I just quit. Then they took money out of my paycheck for expenses. I've only had two jobs. At my other jobs I worked with someone with Alzheimer's disease. I left high school at 17 in the junior year, after I had that bad voc rehab [vocational rehabilitation] experience. I didn't work from [ages] 17 to 22. I raised my sister's baby for 4 years and took the GED [graduate equivalency diploma] eight times. We [people with FAS/FAE] need a training program on how to keep a job and stay at it without losing it."

Stewart: "Most employees don't have the patience to work with us. I worked at a bike shop for 3 months. They said I was a great worker but not consistent. I assembled 85 bikes in 3 months. One time I did it right, another time I'd forget to fasten something. Speed was another thing; other workers did 2½ times as many bikes. I couldn't work at McDonald's either—I just have no sense about things. One time when I wasn't thinking, I poured a milkshake on the griddle instead of butter."

Patsy, in a strong statement of empathy and compassion, responded, "On the other side, if I wanted someone to do a long, hard, nasty job for long hours, you'd do it. I know you would!"

For students with FAS/FAE, the traditional system of school-to-job transition is simply not appropriate. These students do not learn well from books or classroom exercises. An apprenticeship with a supportive trainer who individually trains and supervises one trainee at a time is much more effective at preparing these students for life beyond the classroom. The learning process is enhanced when the supervisor is liked and admired by the trainee, offers plenty of hands-on experience, repeats instructions as needed, provides supportive feedback, and shows that he or she is pleased with the apprentice's progress. These, however, are not duties that can always be expected of regular employers; special instructors are needed for ongoing on-the-job supervision.

Clearly, some type of specialized job training program is needed to equip most people with FAS/FAE for appropriate and sustained employment. Professionals frequently provide training similar to that given to individuals with Down syndrome, yet many people with FAS/FAE require training that is more specific to their needs. Even those who do not have mental retardation often have biologically based problems with memory, attention, and information processing. Some have recommended using the training programs developed for people with traumatic brain injury (TBI). But individuals with TBI usually have a lifetime of normal functioning before their trauma. Individuals with FAS/FAE have been coping with their disabilities all of their lives and don't usually have the same insight into their problems.

Dana, a young man with FAS, had some good "survival skills" but keeping a job wasn't one of them: "I've had lots of jobs, but I have trouble with my memory. I can remember long strings of numbers but still have trouble on the job. I've been trying so hard to get along with people and trying to hold a job, but the people are always the problem. I've had 20 or 30 jobs—what I'd like is to be able to hold a job. I haven't succeeded in holding jobs because I can't find the kind of jobs I like. The kind of jobs I'd like, I'm not trained for. I've tried to train myself, on my own, but it's hard to concentrate—really hard. One time I took a 6-month training program and found a job right away. But usually I get fired pretty quickly. People get really annoyed with me. Sometimes I see some problem that needs fixing or something and I make a suggestion and people really get bent out of shape about that. I just can't ever seem to pin down what makes them so pissed off. I feel really frustrated."

People with FAS/FAE often fail in the workplace because of the social aspects of the work. Social skills training and continuing job coaching are frequently needed. Even when people with FAS/FAE have job training (e.g., Sylvia), actually finding a job; getting matched with the right job; and obtaining appropriate and ongoing help, supervision, and support on the job all present problems.

After several years of trying to get Donald, a patient of mine with FAS, into a widely known behavior modification program that trains those with mental retardation to work in the food industry, Donald's brother finally got him in. He lasted 1 month. He was too social and talkative with the restaurant clients when he was clearing the tables but not gracious enough to his co-workers with Down syndrome. He resisted spending hours scrubbing pots in the kitchen because he wanted to work in the restaurant, and he was too flirtatious with his female supervisor. His main problem essentially involved the fact that he behaved like a person with FAS/FAE instead of like a person with Down syndrome. Since then, he has been kicked out of a sheltered workshop for stealing a tape recorder and then denying it when confronted with the evidence.

Donald is eager to work to fill his days with meaningful activity, to have a sense of dignity about himself, and to have a sense of community with other adults. He could not get into the forestry vocational training program he really wanted because his IQ score was too high. The program is for individuals with mental retardation, and Donald's IQ score is 78 (8 IQ points above the thresh-

old). Donald receives numerous community services and even qualifies for Supplemental Security Income (SSI). But without meaningful work to fill his days, he is always on the brink of disaster and often has conflicts with the law. His brother has helped him to obtain many jobs that seemed appropriate (e.g., bagging groceries at a supermarket that hires a small quota of people with disabilities, doing cleanup at a veterinary hospital). But without ongoing outside supervision, his jobs were all short-lived. In high school, Donald was permanently expelled for having a consenting sexual encounter on the school grounds with a female classmate and thus lost access to any school-based vocational training. He now lives alone in a trailer, and his adult "friends" frequently victimize him by stealing his possessions. He is lonely. Children in the trailer park like to play with him, but he can't play with them anymore because he's on probation for two felony charges after having sexual encounters with teenage girls. If Donald commits another felony, he will go to prison for the rest of his life. Donald is an adult man in his early 20s who longs for the dignity of working and of being part of a community. He is cheerful, helpful, and energetic. He wants to be of help, but nobody wants him.

HOW SOCIETY CAN HELP

Families, understanding the problems that people with FAS/FAE face as they mature, can do much to ensure that their children are as ready as they can be for the challenges they will face as adults. But, important as they are, early therapeutic experiences are not inoculations. Unless families have unlimited resources and are willing and able to take on the responsibility, there are several arenas of responsibility that society must assume in order to adequately prepare the child with FAS/FAE for adulthood. Society needs to provide:

- Diagnostic services for FAS/FAE evaluations
- Apprenticeship or appropriate job training
- Ongoing supervision in appropriate job placements
- Safe shelter, with a sense of community

Additional services are, of course, provided through the schools (see Chapter 11) and through the community institutions that serve the main secondary disabilities of people with FAS/FAE—mental illness, alcohol and other drug problems, and trouble with the law (see Chapter 5).

Diagnostic Services for FAS/FAE Evaluations

It is incumbent on society to provide more available and effective diagnostic services for people with FAS/FAE and their families. In most communities, it is still difficult to get a diagnostic evaluation. Although some physicians are comfortable making this diagnosis, many are not, especially for adolescents and adults. Multidisciplinary teams are most appropriate for the diagnostic process because of the multidisciplinary needs of the individuals with FAS/FAE and their families. Even traditional teams evaluating other types of disabilities, including learning disabilities, mental retardation, and mental health problems, are not reliably making this diagnosis, although it is obvious that individuals with FAS/FAE are among their clientele. Although a state center for FAS diagnosis is a possibility, these are usually less than optimal for linking the family with appropriate services. Some communities have used the model developed in the 1970s by the Indian Health Service—namely, flying in a diagnostic expert to the community at regular intervals to examine individuals who have been prescreened by community health teams (May & Hymbaugh, 1983). In the 1970s, when the FAS diagnosis was first described, this system was all that was available; it is still useful in communities without diagnosticians. A model funded by the Washington State legislature and run by Dr. Sterling Clarren places experts at the University of Washington in charge of training community diagnostic and intervention teams who then become home-town experts, available in the community not only to diagnose and refer but also to become involved in FAS education efforts and prevention (Clarren & Astley, 1997).

Apprenticeships and Appropriate Job Training

Individuals with FAS/FAE often fail to qualify for special job training programs, or when they do gain entry, as Patsy and Stewart so eloquently describe it, the training often fails to meet their needs. As Dana describes, they often do not receive training in the kinds of social interactions that are problematic for them, even though behavior modification techniques can effectively correct these kinds of behaviors. In the absence of an individual diagnosis and of an understanding of the FAS diagnosis, training programs generally, but understandably, fail to comprehend the depth of the cognitive disabilities these individuals possess and the corresponding, frustrations, discrimination, and sense of injustice. Peter McKee (1997), a Seattle lawyer specializing in Social Security disability issues, sees two methods of solving these problems and bringing about change: group and individual advocacy.

Group Advocacy Group advocacy can be carried out by active parent–professional organizations working at the local, state, or national level to change guidelines for eligibility and policy among the organizations responsible for providing services to people with disabilities. These agencies include the Division of Developmental Disabilities (DDD), which provides job training, shelter, and counseling for individuals with disabilities acquired prior to adulthood; the Social Security Administration, which provides SSI for individuals deemed unable to work at a particular time in their lives; and vocational rehabilitation (VR), which provides job training for qualified participants. It is interesting to note that only 32 out of 415 people with FAS/FAE had ever received services from DDD (Streissguth et al., 1996), and only 40 out of 130 adults with FAS/FAE had ever received VR services. Although our secondary disabilities study (Streissguth et al., 1996) found that receiving DDD services was a protective factor against some secondary disabilities, not all DDD programs are sufficiently aware of the special needs of people with FAS/FAE.

In Washington State, a large, active parent organization called the FAS Family Resources Institute (FAS-FRI) has been an effective lobbying force on behalf of individuals with FAS/FAE and their families (see DeVries & Waller, 1997). Three of the members, two adoptive mothers and one biological mother in recovery, have been particularly active, visiting the Washington State superintendent of schools, the newly elected Washington State attorney general on her very first day in office, state representatives and senators, and even the governor's wife. These three women speak of the plight of children with FAS/FAE, including the difficulties they have in obtaining diagnoses, services, and appropriate consideration. FAS-FRI has succeeded in getting some experimental wrap-around (multilevel) services for a few adolescents with FAS on a trial basis. Members are hopeful that policy change will follow. This work is a small but important beginning. In many states, even gaining entry into DDD services remains a major hurdle, especially for people with FAE.

Individual Advocacy   In a second form of advocacy, parents and other advocates (or the individuals with FAS/FAE themselves) work to obtain services on an individual basis. Repeated telephone calls to local services agencies can sometimes obtain services for an individual without any actual change in policy. The effective advocate strives to find a person at the agency who will listen and perhaps provide help. Effective advocates are not daunted by the pat responses such as "People with FAS aren't covered by our policy guidelines" or "I'm sorry, that category isn't on my computer." McKee (1996) also recommended that people with FAS/FAE and their advocates seek help from institutionalized advocacy organizations, such as the National Organization of Social Service Claimants Representatives (NOSSCR) or local chapters of the Arc (formerly the Association for Retarded Citizens) and the National Association on Mental Illness (NAMI) (see Appendix).

I believe the kind of job training programs most effective for people with FAS/FAE will focus on developing useful job skills in junior high school, when academic work is reaching a plateau and will then involve an apprenticeship model during the high school years. As Riley's experience demonstrates, both of these combined not only to prevent secondary disabilities but also to contribute to successful satisfying lifetime employment that enhanced his feelings of self-worth and made him a productive citizen. Among many adolescents with FAS/FAE, there is a strong drive to succeed in life and an ambition to "make something of themselves." By keeping them captive in an educational system that focuses their energies on classes they will never remember, they are deprived of putting their energies into productive learning experiences to succeed in the workplace as adults. Research on innovative and appropriate early vocational programs for this population is greatly needed.

McKee (1997) described how the Social Security system works from the standpoint of people with FAS/FAE and their families and clarified what to many has seemed a capricious process in terms of obtaining income for those unable to work full time at some point in their lives.

Ongoing Supervision in Appropriate Job Placements and Ongoing Case Management and/or Advocacy

Once job training is achieved, many people with FAS/FAE will need ongoing supervision to troubleshoot the many day-to-day difficulties that arise. A big mistake is to consider this supervision as "transitional." In our experience, an advocate at work is necessary on an ongoing basis. In addition, an advocate or case manager is also important for the rest of life's activities.

Charles recently received his 20-year pin for janitorial work at a local school. Although he wasn't diagnosed with FAS until adulthood, his family had recognized his need for assistance early on. Before their death, they set up a trust fund that provides both case management and financial support. When Charles began his job 20 years ago, he was fortunate to have an apprentice-like relationship with a supervisor who for years provided direct and compassionate feedback on his day-to-day activities in the workplace. He also was fortunate to have had a sensitive, flexible, and experienced case manager who recognized that he was quite different in his needs from the usual developmentally delayed people whose lives she managed. As she became Charles's advocate, she helped organize the nonwork parts of his life, buffer his work experience, and, in essence, make it possible for him to be successful in the workplace (see Schmucker, 1997).

Having productive work is an anchor for people with FAS/FAE. Work gives structure to the days that they are unable to schedule or plan on their own. Work gives a focus to life, verifies one's status as an adult, and enhances self-worth immeasurably. There should be work opportunities appropriate to the needs and capabilities of each person with FAS/FAE.

Sonny was diagnosed with FAS in late adolescence, just in time for his father to plan effectively for his adult life. Sonny's family had obtained much help and support for him since his early years, although they never knew the source of his hyperactivity and learning disabilities. After graduating from high school in special education classes, he went immediately into a sheltered workshop experience, where he entered readily into the social activities of the center. Sonny has many social skills, largely because of the strong social support he received at home. His father was his primary advocate and companion. After years in the sheltered work environment and after a long period of supervised on-the-job training, Sonny now runs a big vacuum cleaner at a local office building; he gets paid the minimum wage. He has never been in trouble with the law or victimized by others. He has always had a roof over his head and has never proved to be disruptive in school or had problems with substance abuse. He doesn't have any children (he really wouldn't be able to care for them). He appears to be living to the best of his abilities, which is all we can ask of anyone.

Safe Shelter with a Sense of Community

Safe housing for young adults with FAS/FAE is a continuing problem in every community, although those with active and resourceful advocates or independent family resources seem to make a better adjustment than others. Living alone in an apartment or house, even when subsidized by parents or public funds, is usually not a satisfactory solution for these individuals. Their strong needs for socialization and community involvement are not adequately met in solitary housing, and they are often victimized or get into trouble during their unsupervised time. Residences for people with FAS/FAE are best not viewed as "transitional" housing; rather, structured or supervised housing is appropriate for most throughout their lives. I know of no successful models of a residential facility for people with FAS/FAE, although the Bancroft School in New

Jersey has a broad-based program to suit people of all ages and levels of disability and has a special interest in effective programming for people with FAS/FAE (Dyer, Alberts, & Nieman, 1997; Hess & Nieman, 1997). The Delancey House project in San Francisco appears to have many appropriate characteristics, but administrators at this facility haven't specifically noted their interest in this population.

As with employment, the housing needs of adults with FAS/FAE will not replicate those of people with other chronic mental illnesses, such as schizophrenia or autism, nor will they replicate those of people with mental retardation, such as those with Down syndrome or even those of people with other birth defects such as cerebral palsy. The gregarious nature of most people with FAS/FAE, coupled with their attentional problems and poor judgment, suggests to me that a structured small-group living setting with communal meals and responsibilities and some ongoing supervision, advocacy, and vocational counseling would be ideal. I dream of developing such a model group home somewhere.

I see no reason to assume that the high rate of secondary disabilities and unemployment among people with FAS/FAE is an inevitable consequence of the diagnosis. Now, with an understanding of the cognitive disabilities inherent in the FAS/FAE diagnosis, it should be possible for public and private partnerships to develop the model programs for children, adolescents, and adults with this disability that will facilitate their development across the life span.

REFERENCES

Antoello, S.J. (1996). *Social skills development: Practical strategies for adolescents and adults with developmental disabilities.* Needham, MA: Allyn & Bacon.

Clarren, S.K., & Astley, S. (1997). The development of the fetal alcohol syndrome diagnostic and prevention network in Washington State. In A. Streissguth & J. Kanter (Eds.), *The challenge of fetal alcohol syndrome: Overcoming secondary disabilities* (pp. 38–49). Seattle: University of Washington Press.

DeVries, J., & Waller, A. (1997). Parent advocacy and FAS public policy change. In A.P. Streissguth & J. Kanter (Eds.), *The challenge of fetal alcohol syndrome: Overcoming secondary disabilities* (pp. 168–176). Seattle: University of Washington Press.

Dyer, K., Alberts, G., & Nieman, G. (1997). Assessment and treatment of an adult with FAS: Neuropsychological and behavioral considerations. In A. Streissguth & J. Kanter (Eds.), *The challenge of fetal alcohol syndrome: Overcoming secondary disabilities* (pp. 50–61). Seattle: University of Washington Press.

Hess, J., & Nieman, G. (1997). FAS: Residential programming and economics. In A. Streissguth & J. Kanter (Eds.), *The challenge of fetal alcohol syndrome: Overcoming secondary disabilities* (pp. 185–193). Seattle: University of Washington Press.

Lutke, J. (1997). Spider web walking: Hope for children with FAS through understanding. In A. Streissguth & J. Kanter (Eds.), *The challenge of fetal alcohol syndrome: Overcoming secondary disabilities* (pp. 177–184). Seattle: University of Washington Press.

May, P.A., & Hymbaugh, K.J. (1983). A pilot project on fetal alcohol syndrome among American Indians. *Alcohol Health and Research World, 7,* 3–9.

McKee, P. (1996). Maneuvering the maze: Social Security for people with FAS. *Iceberg, 6*(3), 5–7.

McKee, P. (1997). FAS and the Social Security process. In A. Streissguth & J. Kanter (Eds.), *The challenge of fetal alcohol syndrome: Overcoming secondary disabilities* (pp. 107–118). Seattle: University of Washington Press.

Novick, N. (1997). FAS: Preventing and treating sexual deviancy. In A. Streissguth & J. Kanter (Eds.), *The challenge of fetal alcohol syndrome: Overcoming secondary disabilities* (pp. 159–169). Seattle: University of Washington Press.

Nowicki, S., Jr., & Duke, M.P. (1992). *Helping the child who doesn't fit in.* Atlanta, GA: Peachtree.

Schmucker, C.A. (1997). Case management of adults with FAS: Practical hints and suggestions. In A. Streissguth & J. Kanter (Eds.), *The challenge of fetal alcohol syndrome: Overcoming secondary disabilities* (pp. 91–96). Seattle: University of Washington Press.

Streissguth, A.P., Barr, H.M., Kogan, J., & Bookstein, F.L. (1996). *Understanding the occurrence of secondary disabilities in clients with fetal alcohol syndrome (FAS) and fetal alcohol effects (FAE): Final report to the Centers for Disease Control and Prevention on Grant No. RO4/CCR008515* (Tech. Report No. 96-06). Seattle: University of Washington, Fetal Alcohol and Drug Unit.

11

Guidelines for Schools

Janey had FAS and was diagnosed when she was 10 years old. Her adoptive parents, who were attuned to her needs, had been pleased with her academic success up through the fourth grade. As she entered the fifth grade at a new school, however, she seemed to be at psychosocial risk because of her maladaptive behaviors, which isolated her socially. Although Janey had an IQ score in the normal range and was passing all her subjects (particularly favoring science), she'd been kicked out of Girl Scouts and made a laughingstock among her classmates because of the "whoppers" she told—unbelievable stories with sexy, gory details.

The school nurse, recognizing Janey's need, became her advocate. Every day from then on, Janey took her sack lunch into the nurse's office and ate with her. This allowed the nurse to carefully monitor the day's activities, assess Janey's stress level in relation to her various academic subjects, and provide Janey with some respite from her most stressful activity—peer interactions. The nurse, her advocate at school, was also in close touch with her parents, her advocates at home. Working together, they gave her enough support

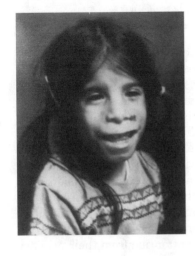

to get her through her first year at the new school while she brought her social behaviors under better control.

In August of 1990, I received a telephone call from a school psychologist in a small school, asking for information on FAS and FAE. A local dysmorphologist had just diagnosed one of his students, a teenage girl named Marcy, as having FAS. He wanted to engage her in the appropriate counseling but needed direction. Marcy was described as usually pleasant but, at times, very unpleasant. She was impulsive and sometimes did unusual things, such as drawing obscene pictures on windows. She was very manipulative of new teachers, and although she formed intense attachments with adults, she often got into arguments with the other kids. Marcy had been adopted at 5 months of age. Although she did not have microcephaly, she did have a variety of major and minor congenital anomalies. She had been on the varsity softball team as a freshman. Her overall IQ score was in the normal range, but she had considerable scatter among subtests, with particularly poor verbal memory. Her performance IQ score was considerably higher than her verbal IQ score.

I spoke with the school psychologist for some time about my ideas of how schools could help children with FAS/FAE. This made me think, specifically, about how a concerned psychologist, educator, or any member of the school team could become an advocate for students with FAS/FAE. I began to visualize how the advocate could serve as the missing link in interpreting the seemingly illogical behaviors of the student with FAS/FAE for the rest of the school and in helping the student to understand and modulate her own behaviors. It seemed obvious that once school personnel understood that students with FAS/FAE are different from students with other types of learning disabilities or mental retardation, each district could set up appropriate educational experiences that were more responsive to the needs of these perplexing students.

Of all the community's institutions, the schools are most advantageously situated to influence the lives of people with FAS/FAE. If schools are responsive to the challenges presented by these students, the students' lives can be greatly enhanced. If the schools fail to respond appropriately, these students can face tremendous obstacles.

The primary challenge that children with FAS/FAE present at school is their disruptive, unpredictable, or uninterpretable behavior. Although neuropsychological testing often reveals attentional impairments, memory impairments, auditory comprehension difficulties, information processing disturbances, and other organically based cognitive impairments, these are typically not identified as the cause of their behavior problems at school. Students with FAS/FAE tend to inadvertently detract attention from their primary disabilities by their inappropriate behaviors. For example, social interaction difficulties may hide serious communication impairments. Noncompliance may reflect a failure to understand. In addition, their neurological limitations may be masked by their various strengths. For example, their adequate reading and spelling skills may obscure difficulty with arithmetic and math; their knack for accumulating facts may mask their difficulty with comprehension.

Students with FAS/FAE may need to be taught things that other students simply learn through experience. Although children with FAS/FAE can learn, they require more repetition, less distracting environments, more specialized techniques, and more encouragement. They are often highly motivated to please teachers they like but may have difficulty relating to teachers who don't give clear commands, say too many things at once, or are inconsistent even though friendly and effusive. Students with FAS/FAE may be an enigma to school personnel, particularly when they have not yet been diagnosed or when their diagnosis is not known to the educational team. Students with FAS/FAE have special needs at school (see Table 11.1) that are inferred from their behaviors. There has been almost no systematic research on the educational needs of people with FAS/FAE or on best educational strategies.

In a 1996 study of secondary disabilities in 415 people with FAS/FAE, which involved a life history interview administered to parents and caregivers, 61% of those 12 years and older and 14% of those ages 6–11 had had a disrupted school experience, defined as being suspended or expelled from school or dropping out. Among those 12–20 years old, 29% had been expelled and 26% had dropped out. Among those 21 years and older, 19% had been expelled and 37% had dropped out—disconcerting findings for people born with a birth defect (Streissguth, Barr, Kogan, & Bookstein, 1996).

Gorman (1995) conducted a study in which she personally interviewed 20 individuals with FAS/FAE between the ages of 15 and 20 to learn more about their perceptions of school. The majority of

Table 11.1.   What students with FAS/FAE need at school

- An advocate for trust, availability, concern, and action
- Gentle guidance: understanding what is expected of them and when and how to act
- Realistic goals, structure, and supervision with constructive feedback, both academic and social
- More time, more repetitions, and fewer distractions
- Something to feel good about; some successes somewhere
- Some friends, even if older or younger, including teachers and advocates
- A school that coordinates with parents

these individuals (80%) reported having disrupted school experiences: nine students had been suspended, six had dropped out, and one had been expelled. The four who reported no disrupted school experiences expressed the feeling that someone at school had really cared about them. These four also reported that they had a friend whose school experience was not disrupted and that they had participated in extracurricular activities, both of which seemed to be related to high self-esteem (Gorman, 1995).

Staying in the structured school setting is beneficial for students with FAS/FAE. Once a student is suspended, expelled, or drops out, the stakes are high for additional secondary disabilities (e.g., alcohol and other drug problems, trouble with the law). Being disconnected from school also cuts them off from school-related job and vocational training and much-needed associated services such as job placement, job coaching, and life-skills training programs.

Schools should be challenged first to identify students with FAS/FAE and then to determine how to detect and best serve their needs. Beyond increasing awareness of FAS/FAE among school personnel, there should be a school-based process for identifying and effectively designing programs for students who are affected by fetal alcohol exposure. There should also be a school-based advocacy system for working directly with these students to understand and interpret their behaviors to school personnel and to themselves. Any effort devoted to these two undertakings will surely pay off by comparison with the chaos of dealing with an individual with FAS/FAE on a crisis-by-crisis basis.

AN FAS/FAE PLAN FOR SCHOOL DISTRICTS

In a 1992 study of educators and school personnel throughout Washington State, 97% of the respondents believed that understanding and dealing with students prenatally exposed to alcohol or other drugs are important educational issues, 96% of the respondents reported having direct personal experience with such children, and 94% believed these students had more problems in school than other students (Streissguth & Burgess, 1992). Almost half of the respondents (46%) felt overwhelmed by the challenges presented by these students. More than 90% agreed that they needed more information on appropriate educational and behavior management strategies as well as instruction on how best to work with the families of these students (Streissguth & Burgess, 1992).

Although educators have indicated that they would like support and training regarding educating students with FAS/FAE, a 1995 survey of special education divisions in each of the 50 states revealed that none recognized or specifically served the needs of students based on a diagnosis of FAS, nor did they have plans to do so (Wentz, 1997). This study suggests that state special education divisions may not be aware of the needs of educators regarding students with FAS/FAE.

School personnel who feel overwhelmed by thinking that, on top of everything else, they have to worry about FAS/FAE too should consider that they are already spending a disproportionate amount of time and energy on students with FAS/FAE without achieving satisfactory results. Children with FAS/FAE are among those in any school that the staff is already worrying about and wondering how to help. Diagnosis of the problem is a positive step toward solutions. Understanding the special needs and problems of children with FAS/FAE should help prevent school disruptions and enable the school team to prevent problems from erupting or escalating.

Students with FAS/FAE are not all alike: They are not all retarded or learning disabled nor do they all have behavior problems. They are spread throughout the schools in both general and special education classrooms. Because FAS/FAE has lifetime implications for the affected individual, educational planning must encompass a life-span approach. Therefore, the ideal unit for organizing around the topic of FAS/FAE is the school district. Preschool is the easiest time to begin a healthy working relationship with the families of children with FAS/FAE. The earlier affected children are identified, the better their long-term outcomes. This is not a coincidence: The knowledge that a child has a disabling condition helps educators utilize their resources in assisting the child as needed, rather than puzzling over why the child doesn't behave better. Understanding that children have special needs galvanizes help to meet those needs.

By organizing for FAS/FAE at the district level, a coherent system of planning can take place for individuals suspected of having FAS/FAE as they move through the various schools and programs of the district. District-wide, there can be an interlocking system of communication across schools to manage children with special needs. Of all the children with special needs, children with FAS/FAE are probably most in need of appropriate management because on the surface they may not appear to be disabled. Districts are in a better position than individual schools to ensure that every member of the school team understands what it means to have FAS/FAE and that students with FAS/FAE aren't hopeless. If the needs of these students are not met, they are at high risk of costly, sometimes irreparable, disruptions of schooling.

Finally, school districts are in a favorable position to incorporate concepts of both prevention and intervention. Referring children for FAS diagnostic exams can help in preventing subsequent children from being born with FAS/FAE, as mothers in Chapter 9 related. FAS prevention can also be taught through science and health classes. FAS outreach can be incorporated into school-based alcohol and other drug programs, student health care programs, and into home schooling programs.

To address the problem of increased FAS awareness and programming, districts should

- Establish a district-level FAS task force
- Set up an FAS support team at each school in the district
- Develop a plan for serving the needs of individual students who have, or are suspected of having, FAS/FAE

The District-Level FAS Task Force

District-level FAS task forces can develop policies and serve an administrative role. Tasks of the force include 1) formulating district policy on FAS/FAE-related identification and intervention activities; 2) developing an FAS/FAE resource/information center for the district and disseminating appropriate materials; 3) coordinating ongoing in-service training on FAS/FAE; and 4) implementing plans for incorporating FAS/FAE prevention units into existing science, health, and extracurricular programs and activities at school.

One of the most important policy issues districts must address involves improved identification of students with FAS/FAE within the schools. One course of action is to modify the school entrance health questionnaire to include individual histories of prenatal exposure to alcohol and other drugs and to include FAS and FAE among the list of possible or suspected diagnoses. Some districts may opt to keep systematic records for all children suspected of having FAS/FAE in their jurisdiction in order to evaluate the children's progress and provide additional help as needed. Districts may also choose to coordinate their efforts with the parent–teacher association (PTA), which can increase awareness and lead to collaboration between educators and parents. Legislation in some states requires pre-adoption disclosure of prenatal exposure to alcohol and other drugs. Often adoptive or foster care parents are eager for the opportunity to coordinate planning with their children's teachers.

Other important district activities for dealing with FAS include a district plan for regular, ongoing in-service training and development of specific policies for improving services for students suspected of being affected by fetal alcohol exposure. For example, by understanding the life-span needs of individuals with FAS/FAE, districts could opt to put more emphasis on early intervention programs. These would involve parents by establishing early working relationships with families and facilitate early diagnostic referrals. Likewise, districts could opt to develop earlier and more specific vocational training programs for students with FAS/FAE as they enter middle school and are less able to meet academic demands.

Of equal importance are specific policies for improving transitions. Important transitions are among schools in the district; among programs with a special focus on vocational, basic skills, social skills, and job training; and between alcohol and other drug treatment and school health care programs. Transitions relevant to the individual child with FAS/FAE can also include changes in the teaching staff and even in the classroom roster so that students can be matched with teachers compatible with their needs.

The FAS Support Team at School

The FAS support team at each school should be oriented around the needs of individual students who have or are suspected of having FAS/FAE. This team would hold regular meetings to discuss the progress and needs of the child. The support team would also assign a school-based advocate for each student under consideration who would be willing to collaborate with parents and design an individual action plan for the student. Gradually, the FAS support team at each school would become a source of local expertise on the special characteristics and service needs of this population and be able to provide consultation to other school personnel. In evaluating individual students, the support team would obtain useful information from school records, from talking with school personnel who know the student, and from systematically observing the student in various school settings such as recess, the lunch room, before and after school, and in a variety of classroom experiences. Helpful information can also be obtained from parents and from talking with the students themselves. School is a marvelous greenhouse in which to study the many facets of the daily lives and stressors of children with FAS/FAE and the growing conditions that enhance their development, to help students cope more effectively.

The support team would also develop a liaison between the student's parents or guardians and a representative from the school, preferably a designated advocate, to work out an individual plan for the student. If possible, the plan should include an evaluation of the child at a local diagnostic facility familiar with the diagnosis and service needs of individuals with FAS/FAE. However, not all families will instantly feel comfortable with this idea, unless they have already had similar concerns. If families are hesitant, school personnel can begin by listening to any concerns the parents have about their child or the school. Maintaining a supportive attitude rather than one that is accusatory or defensive will encourage parents to participate in the partnership. Facilitating the parent–school relationship is important as this alliance will allow schools to better serve the needs of the student.

The support team, in conjunction with the student's advocate and family, should also develop an individual action plan, with both short-term and long-term goals, for each child having or suspected of having FAS/FAE. This will include plans to understand and work around the student's individual cognitive strengths and impairments, to foster success and enhance self-esteem, to monitor problem behaviors closely in order to understand the antecedent conditions, to reduce maladaptive behaviors and teach social skills, to develop appropriate basic skills and job skills at each age, and to design appropriate transitions and supports to the next programs.

Finally, the FAS support team at each school will provide back-up support, encouragement, and help with problem solving for members who are active advocates for specific students with FAS/FAE. In this way, the students' needs are better met, advocates are spared "burn-out," and the whole group increases their knowledge about FAS.

The School-Based Advocate

Each child under consideration by the support team should have a designated advocate at school who works on the student's behalf. Advocates can be classroom teachers, school psychologists, nurses, administrators—anyone at school who feels comfortable and enthusiastic about this role. The advocate is a key player in support team activities involving the students in question. Some tasks of a school advocate are listed in Table 11.2.

A 10-Step School Plan for Students Suspected of Having FAS/FAE

Because many children have not had an opportunity to be evaluated for FAS/FAE, these guidelines presume that this will be one of the tasks with which the task force will be involved. The student's advocate will play a key role in developing and carrying out the individual plan. The FAS support team at the student's school would provide support for the advocate and facilitate the implementation of the plan (see Table 11.3). Regular psychological evaluation can

Table 11.2.   Tasks of the school advocate of a student with FAS/FAE

- Befriend the student in an advocacy relationship.
- Provide a safe haven where the student can stop in and chat.
- Talk to the student regarding concerns, confusion, misperceptions, and perceived injustices going on in his or her everyday life at school. The initial goal is to understand the student's perspective—to try to feel how the world feels to this student. The goal is not to uncover historical data, to interpret or criticize past behaviors, or (initially) to give unsolicited advice.
- Become a clearinghouse of information on the student, receiving complaints, crisis reports, and compliments from teachers and school personnel.
- Initiate observations of the student in problem settings, such as a functional analysis of behavior to determine factors related to problem behaviors (see Dyer, Alberts, & Nieman, 1997).
- Mediate as needed between the student and teachers and between the student and other students.
- Coordinate between school and parents with respect to the student's needs, perceptions, and misperceptions. Defuse potential parent/teacher misunderstandings by establishing direct links of communication such as regular telephone calls and notes.
- Give direct help. After the relationship is established, it is possible to give quite a bit of direct advice and feedback to the student with FAS/FAE.

help a knowledgeable advocate evaluate a child's progress and current status.

SCHOOL–PARENT COLLABORATION

Working together, the schools and the family can effectively provide the network of support that children with FAS/FAE need. Teachers and parents can help each other to understand and monitor these children who are unusually dependent on external support to frame their own behavior. A child whose behavior is out of control or who appears irrational at school is at high risk of a disrupted school experience, which will only further complicate the problem. The school-based advocate, with the help of the FAS support team at school and working in conjunction with the parents at home, can be instrumental in averting crises at school for children with FAS/FAE by bringing about understanding of their seemingly irrational behaviors (see Figure 11.1 for an example of how the scholastic abilities of children with FAS/FAE don't always correspond with their social abilities and adaptive behavior skills).

After a year of successful home schooling and few behavior problems, Tara re-entered general education high school classes at age 15. Pressures at school mounted. She experienced both inappropriately high academic standards and increasing social isolation from peers, and her family had nowhere to turn for sup-

Table 11.3.   A 10-step school plan for students suspected of having FAS/FAE

1. Refer the name of any student suspected of having FAS or ARND to the FAS support team.

2. Gather information about the student from all school sources.

3. Select a person from the support team to be a personal advocate for this student and have the advocate meet with the student to understand his or her perspective and goals.

4. Arrange for the advocate to meet with the parents to hear their concerns and to understand how they view the child and the child's relationship to the school. This is a team-building informational meeting, not a feedback session. A brief, informal medical and social history can be obtained at this time if it seems comfortable for the parents; if not, postpone it for a later meeting.

5. Identify and summarize the behavior and academic problems that are of concern to the school, the parents, and the student.

6. Make appropriate in-school referrals. This usually involves a direct psychological evaluation of the child and a secondary evaluation by the parents, using a tool such as the Vineland Adaptive Behavior Scale (Sparrow, Bella, & Cicchetti, 1984). Referrals to school counselor, school nurse, and other in-school personnel may also be in order.

7. Develop an individual action plan for the student, incorporating information from all of these sources addressing the problems or problem behaviors. Local consultants interested in FAS/FAE could be brought in at this point, or other schools experienced with students with FAS/FAE could be consulted by phone. The action plan should involve a strategy for obtaining a diagnostic evaluation if this has not already been done.

8. Meet with the parents to report the in-school evaluations, discuss the individual action plan for this student, and enlist the parents' support and help in carrying it out. In the short term, the school and parents can work together to cope effectively with the specific behavior/academic/social problems the child may have without attributing them to a specific cause. In the long term, understanding the cause of the dysfunctional behaviors will help student and family cope more effectively and make more realistic plans. Working within the parent's timetable on etiology issues, the advocate could suggest joining a parent support group or reading some literature about FAS/FAE.

9. Monitor the child's behavior regularly. It is important that the advocate receive input from the other teachers and school personnel who are in close contact with the student. Much can be learned by studying the specific situations that prove problematic for the student. Parents and advocates should be in close communication regarding topics of mutual concern such as homework, tardiness, missed classes, absences from school, reluctance to attend school, distress upon returning home from school, and school bus problems.

10. Evaluate progress through regular support team meetings, and modify the therapeutic plan in accordance with observations.

port because her therapist was unexpectedly out of town for an extended period. Tara began stealing from classmates' backpacks and lying when confronted with the evidence. Viewing this as a lapse in moral development, a misguided plan was proposed that would supposedly teach her honesty by embarrassing her in front of her classmates. When we [at the Fetal Alcohol and Drug Unit] were consulted by the family and the teacher independently, we advised against this plan, suggesting that her "out of control" behavior was a cry for help. When expectations were lowered and a support network developed at school through the collaboration of her teacher-advocate and her parent-advocates, Tara's stealing and

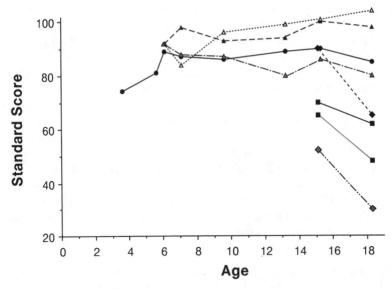

Figure 11.1. Dolly's test scores over time. These data show the good reading and spelling scores of a girl with FAS relative to her IQ level and arithmetic performance. Note her poor adaptive behaviors as measured by the Vineland Adaptive Behavior Scales (VABS; Sparrow, Bella, & Cicchetti, 1984). (Key: ●—● = full-scale IQ score; ▲– – = Wide Range Achievement Test–Revised (WRAT–R; Jastak & Wilkinson, 1984) reading score; – –△– – = WRAT–R spelling score; •–•▲•–• = WRAT–R arithmetic score; ■– – – – –■ = VABS communication domain; ■———■ = VABS daily living skills domain; ■–••–••–••■ = VABS socialization domain; ■•••••••••■ = VABS adaptive behavior composite.)

lying subsided. In this instance, her teacher became her important school-based advocate and helped resolve the crisis and set the stage for increased collaboration with the family. But had an advocate been in place at the beginning of the school year, this escalation might have been averted.

Collaboration means that parents and schools work together for the best interest of the child. In some instances, the school advocate may guide the parent in understanding; but, in other instances, it is the parent who can help interpret the child's behaviors so that the child's needs are better met at school.

From an early age, Denny had loved to learn. His mother had always helped him to learn to the best of his ability. Denny loved attending school. He and his mother had developed a routine for going to school each morning. Denny would follow this routine systematically as he had been taught, arriving at school smiling and ready to begin the day. One autumn, his mother noticed that Denny was resisting his pre-school routine, his smile was waning, and he was dragging his feet about leaving for school. In the afternoons, when he re-turned, his cheery smile was a nervous twitch; sometimes he'd be in tears.

His mother discussed this behavior change with his special education teacher and learned that the teacher was running the class on a point system, which she believed to be a successful educational strategy to enhance perfor-mance. When a student earned a certain number of points for good behavior, he or she got to use the computer. Denny adored working on the computer but couldn't possibly master the level of behavioral control necessary to earn com-puter privileges. Recess posed a similar problem. Recess had to be earned by an accumulation of points for work accomplished. Denny could never achieve the level of performance necessary for recess, so he never got to go out with the other children. Unable to bring about positive change in the classroom from speaking with his teacher, Denny's mother finally pulled him out of school and home-schooled him until the school could help the teacher develop a more effective classroom management strategy.

The problem here wasn't the teacher's attempts to use positive be-havioral management principles, but her failure to set the rein-forcement level so it was attainable and to "listen" to the child's needs as expressed through his behaviors rather than his words. Positive behavioral support strategies utilize a well-researched method of improving performance and behavior (see Alberto & Troutman, 1990; O'Neill, Horner, Albin, Storey, & Sprague, 1990; Sulzer-Azaroff & Mayer, 1991) but depend upon the student receiv-ing positive (not negative) rewards to reinforce the behavior. Posi-tive behavioral support strategies have proven effective with chil-dren who have FAS/FAE, especially when parents and teachers can work together to determine the most effective rewards (Dyer, 1995). Additional strategies for working with children with FAS/FAE are described by parents and educators in Kleinfeld and Wescott (1993) and in FAS newsletters such as *Iceberg, Fen Pen,* and *FAS Times* (see Appendix).

Although school–parent collaboration is the ideal, it isn't al-ways possible. For example, the school may provide the primary support and structure for those children with FAS/FAE from trou-bled homes. In these situations, the school can become more than an institution of learning—it can become a haven of understanding and sound advice.

FAS OVERVIEW FOR CLASSROOM TEACHERS

Educators can facilitate the overall development of children with FAS/FAE by realizing that some of the behaviors that appear most challenging are actually misguided attempts at communication by the student (see Burgess, Lasswell & Streissguth, 1992; Burgess & Streissguth, 1992). For example, crumpling up a math paper can be the student's way of expressing that the task is too hard, that the time allotted for the task is too short, or that he or she cannot figure out how to get started on the task. By recognizing the message behind the behavior, the educator can respond more effectively to these needs and also help the student learn appropriate methods of communicating his or her needs. Students who inappropriately express their needs are often misunderstood and ridiculed or goaded by fellow students and viewed as troublemakers by administrators and teachers. Teaching these students to shape their inappropriate behaviors into appropriate words and actions is perhaps even more useful to the student's success in life than a specific math concept or lesson in grammar. Effective educators using a life-span orientation will look for ways to generalize these social and functional learning skills outside of the classroom and eventually to facilitate adaptive behavior in the workplace.

One of the problems many teachers face in developing expertise in working with children with FAS/FAE is that most do not get this experience while in training, nor do they work with enough students already identified as having FAS/FAE in their classrooms to develop and refine their own strategies with this population. In 1993, with the publication of *Fantastic Antone Succeeds! Experiences in Educating Children with Fetal Alcohol Syndrome* (Kleinfeld & Wescott, 1993), educators, parents, and mental health specialists who had each had considerable experience with a number of children with FAS/FAE described what works based on their personal experiences. In sharing her "wisdom of practice," Murphy (1993) espoused the importance of early intervention. Tanner-Halverson (1993, 1997) described a successful elementary school classroom she funded with a grant for children with FAS/FAE. She developed specific strategies for dealing with hyperactivity, impulsivity, and the agitational problems manifested by these students. Winick (1993) described how mainstreaming works in a small rural school in which the focus is on individual needs and on the development of cooperation and work experience. Philpot and Harrison (1993) described how parents and teachers work together to meet the needs of students with FAS/FAE in a one-room schoolhouse, which is a learning center for students of all ages and how their community funded this creative effort. Lutke (1993) emphasized parental advocacy as well as close and frequent communication between parents and school. Through raising eight adopted children with FAS/FAE who span the ages from preschool to adulthood, Lutke, a keen observer and indefatigable advocate for her children, is rich in advice for both classroom teachers and other parents. For example, she recommended using short sentences, precise language, and avoiding idiomatic expressions like "step on it." Also, she claimed that saying "put your feet on the floor" works better than "get your feet off the wall" (Lutke, 1993, p. 84).

In 1986, in developing a manual on adolescents and adults with FAS/FAE, we wrote that an essential environmental component was "structure, structure, structure" (Streissguth, LaDue, & Randels, 1986/1988). This message applies not only to the general environmental milieu but also to the manner of communication by the teacher. In a paper on conducting a functional analysis of problem behaviors with an adolescent with FAS, Dyer, Alberts, and Nieman (1997) described the dramatic rise in problem behaviors when Michael was told, "I want you to practice your volleyball skills today" compared with when he was told, "Throw the volleyball so it hits above the line on the wall." In a more global context, Michael engaged in low rates of problem behaviors when he had a high degree of structure. When he lived in a structured group home with constant supervision, he was able to attend school successfully and to work 30 hours per week with lots of site supervision. When these supervisory experiences were terminated by the state on his 18th birthday, he was in jail within a few weeks for having taken a recreational vehicle on a joy ride (while on probation). Michael illustrates the success that students with FAS/FAE can experience in settings that are sensitive to their needs and also how fragile and vulnerable they are when their basic needs are disregarded.

Guidelines for Educators of Students with FAS/FAE

It helps to listen and watch, be accessible, earn respect, and be consistently fair with students with FAS/FAE. These students (perhaps owing to the magnitude of their daily struggles) are often sensitive to perceived slights and do not respond well to embarrassment or condescension. Feelings of resentment for perceived inconsistencies or unfairness can trigger bizarre behaviors. Avoid assigning timed or long tasks that are beyond reach. Instead, break tasks into smaller pieces with frequent feedback. Monitor progress on tasks and provide assistance as needed. Intervene before behavioral control is lost. Keep in touch with parents, other teachers, and the student's advocate regarding how the student is faring elsewhere; coordinate activities as needed. Get to know the parents so you're working together for the student. Vigorously pursue absences, tardiness, and any other deviations from the student's routine behavior. As students with FAS/FAE age and become more isolated from peers, they often become emotionally needy and more reliant upon the adults in their lives. A good teacher will give students with FAS/FAE plenty of time, encouragement, and praise. Good teachers will also give students responsibility, as much and as often as the student can handle on a regular daily basis. However, they will be aware that continued monitoring and supervision is needed and that responsibility doesn't mean freedom from supervision.

The classroom teacher may be the most important person in the life of a child with FAS/FAE and can make an enormous difference to his or her life-long quest for self-esteem. Some adults with FAS/FAE remember a particular teacher as the crucial force that saved them from despair at a critical time in their lives (see Table 11.4).

The vignette that follows describes an innovative approach used by a 15-year-old student with FAS, at her counselor's recommendation, as she approached the transition from middle school to ninth grade. She distributed this letter [original spelling preserved] to all of her teachers and had a successful high school career, graduating at age 19:

When I first found out that I had the symtoms of fetal alcohol syndrome, I was confused and angry. I thought that I was different from everyone else and that I would be known for what I have. Since then I have learned that the symptoms vary from individual to individual due to what state of the pregnancy the mother drank and the amount of alcohol consumed.

Some of my symtoms are understanding instructions. When a teacher explains a certain topic, I can understand. Visual contact is a very important way of learning for me. Following instructions sometimes confuses me. When I'm

Table 11.4. Guidelines for the classroom teacher working with students with FAS/FAE

- Maintain a calm, orderly environment.
- Establish clear, consistent rules.
- Use simple, concrete instructions.
- Help the student set realistic goals.
- Monitor performance to facilitate success, avoid repeated failures, and prevent loss of control.
- Balance structure with responsibility, starting with structure.
- Plan ahead for change, and supervise transitions.
- Teach functional and social skills in the classroom.
- Work closely with the family.
- Take a life-span approach—develop good work habits and skills for now and for the future.

asked or told to do something like take out the garbage, I won't understand or the words will get all mixed up in my mind. Some other symtoms are, not being able to follow oral or written instructions. Example: Teacher giving an assignment instructions orally, not being able to remember or follow correctly. Not hearing exactly what has been said to me. Example: My stepfather giving me a command to do and not hearing him clearly even in the same room. It's like I block out words or phrases. Impulses, doing or acting on excitement, and not able to focus on reality if disaster strikes. Most of the time I worry a lot and make problems seem impossible to handle. When I worry, I make myself sick.

These symtoms are very small to some of the other symtoms I've heard of. Some people think when I explain my problem they find it impossible to believe, since I don't show the signs. This letter is to help me guide myself and others. [signed] Sylvia

GUIDELINES FOR USING THE ADVOCACY
MODEL WITH A STUDENT WITH FAS/FAE AT SCHOOL

I originally developed these guidelines in 1990 for the school psychologist who called me about how to keep the girl with an FAS diagnosis at school, but they can be used by anyone who decides to be an advocate—a teacher, a school nurse, a coach, an administrator. Because the point of entry for the advocacy relationship is variable, the following items are not necessarily consecutive. They may need modification for children not yet formally diagnosed.

1. **Establish the advocacy relationship when the time is ripe.** Get to know the student and be available to chat with her, observe her interactions, listen to the problems she is facing, and hear what others say about her. At a time when she is facing some challenge or problem, offer to be her advocate at school. Explain that an advocate is somebody who helps students clarify and achieve their goals. Explain that an advocate is willing and able to listen; an advocate is a friend.

2. **Build a relationship with the student by establishing periodic meetings.** Meet with the student regularly and have fun at the meetings. Become his confidante. Ask him how you can be of help. Establish yourself as a sounding board. Tell him you will be available when crises occur but will also meet on a regular basis just to talk about things. Explain that meeting together can actually help to prevent crises from occurring because you'll have a chance to understand together when trouble is brewing and take preventive action. Develop a friendly relationship. Be structured and clear in giving advice, but not rigid.

Use humor and commiseration to plan strategies. Remember that positive reinforcement and a common-sense approach are more effective than punishment, shaming, lecturing, demanding, or offering insight. It is useful, however, to point out what does and does not work, especially in the context of a friendly advocacy relationship.

3. **Troubleshoot problems and crises at school as they emerge.** The problems encountered will mostly be behavior problems, not described as academic problems per se. However, these behavior problems may be triggered by unrealistic academic expectations, social misperceptions; unpredictable events (e.g., a substitute teacher); or misguided attempts to gain friendships or acclaim. Advocates must develop a clear understanding of what actually transpires when a crisis or problem occurs. If the student does something that seems bizarre or gets into trouble, find out the precipitating circumstances, then determine how the student perceived (or misperceived) the environment and what environmental situations drove her behavior out of control. Use this information to gently help the student develop better coping skills, including how to manipulate the environment as necessary to prevent crises and how to avoid situations in which the student is likely to lose behavioral control.

4. **Monitor and modify inappropriate sexual behaviors.** Sexual issues can be a major source of concern for adolescents with FAS/FAE. Inappropriate sexually explicit behaviors can often prompt scapegoating, victimization, and escalation of behavior problems that can isolate these students from their peers. For example, a student's lack of judgment may surface in his or her attempts to be noticed by the opposite sex and his often childlike trust in those who express interest in him, regardless of whether he is being mistreated or misled. The school-based advocate is often in a much better position to observe this process than the family at home. The magnitude of the problem will determine whether these are behaviors that come within the realm of the advocate's socialization activities or that require an appropriate community or mental health referral.

5. **Teach functional skills at every opportunity**. Enroll the student in programs that explicitly teach functional skills, particularly those involving organizational skills, such as handling money, managing time, developing hobbies and recreational activities, solving social problems, and coping with anger. Teach and model good problem-solving skills during the regular advocacy meetings.

6. **Facilitate practical work skills and appropriate supervision.** Even people who are lonely and isolated can get personal satisfaction out of productive work. Help the student find meaningful work activities as part of the school program. Programs that teach specific job skills are the most useful, especially when combined with appropriate on-the-job supervision. Ensure that supervision is continued throughout the work experience and that the work is appropriate to the student's capabilities.

7. **Establish teamwork between school and home on the student's behalf.** By keeping in close contact with all three parties—the student, the school, and the home—the advocate seeks to resolve misperceptions and promote adaptive problem solving and crisis resolution. After the advocacy relationship is established with the student, a home visit to meet the family is useful, especially if there are not yet any specific problems to be resolved. Students with FAS/FAE often unknowingly create a web of confusion around them—a quick phone call between the advocate and the parents can often provide a needed reality check.

8. **Help the student complete school and plan beyond school.** Help to prevent suspension, expulsion, or drop-out by actively troubleshooting for the student. Work with parents to coordinate goal-setting, and work with the student to establish postschool goals that are realistic, attainable, and satisfying.

9. **Help make school a pleasurable experience.** Monitor school activities to include those that highlight the student's strengths, not merely those that focus on remediating the impairments. Encourage sports activity, but be ready to monitor social conflicts that might interfere with success in this realm. Children and adolescents with FAS/FAE seem to have a real need for physical activity. Those who are relatively well-coordinated and socially aware can put such skills to work in a team sport. However, if team sports are not feasible, encourage participation in more solitary sports alternatives like swimming, running, or biking. Be sure the student gets involved in activities that will enhance self-esteem and make school more satisfying.

10. **Help everyone understand FAS better.** Explain to the student that a diagnosis of FAS/FAE does not necessarily mean he has mental retardation, cannot finish school, or is a hopeless case. Using a basic common-sense approach and providing an atmosphere of support, demonstrate good problem-solving approaches to any problems the student identifies. Anyone who is

a successful advocate with a student with FAS/FAE becomes a local expert and can help explain the condition to people in the school and community, thereby helping other children who are affected by prenatal alcohol exposure.

SUMMARY

The school is the most important institution in the community to intervene effectively in the lives of children with FAS/FAE and their families. To do this most successfully, a district-based plan is proposed that involves an FAS task force at each school. This serves as a support and coordination center for school-based advocates for each student with FAS/FAE and for development and implementation of an individual action plan for each. By taking a life-span approach, each district can begin early intervention, achieve smooth transitions between schools and programs, and begin planning early for successful life work, with supervision appropriate to the individual. Increased in-service and preservice education about FAS/FAE is urgently needed for the entire educational team, including administrators, as well as increased research on effective programs. The societal costs once the schools lose a child with FAS/FAE are high; the costs of effective prevention and intervention are a bargain.

REFERENCES

Alberto, P.A., & Troutman, A.C. (1990). *Applied behavior analysis for teachers* (3rd ed.). Columbus, OH: Charles E. Merrill.

Burgess, D.M., Lasswell, S.L., & Streissguth, A.P. (1992). *Educating children prenatally exposed to alcohol and other drugs* [Booklet developed for the Planning for Learning Project]. Seattle: Washington State Legislature and the University of Washington, Fetal Alcohol and Drug Unit.

Burgess, D.M., & Streissguth, A.P. (1992). A special section on children at risk: Fetal alcohol syndrome and fetal alcohol effects: Principles for educators. *Phi Delta Kappan, 74*(1), 24–30.

Dyer, K. (1995). Using structure and consistency with high activity toddlers. *Iceberg, 5*(1), 3–4.

Dyer, K., Alberts, G., & Nieman, G. (1997). Neuropsychology and behavior: A case study. In A. Streissguth & J. Kanter (Eds.), *The challenge of fetal alcohol syndrome: Overcoming secondary disabilities* (pp. 50–61). Seattle: University of Washington Press.

Gorman, A. (1995). *Factors associated with disrupted school experiences in subjects with fetal alcohol syndrome and fetal alcohol effects* (Tech. Report No. 95-02). Seattle: University of Washington, Fetal Alcohol and Drug Unit.

Jastak, S., & Wilkinson, G.S. (1984). *Wide Range Achievement Test–Revised.* Wilmington, DE: Jastak Associates.

Kleinfeld, J.S., & Wescott, S. (Eds.). (1993). *Fantastic Antone succeeds! Experiences in educating children with fetal alcohol syndrome*. Fairbanks: University of Alaska Press.

Lutke, J. (1993). Parental advocacy for alcohol-affected children. In J.K. Kleinfeld & S. Wescott (Eds.), *Fantastic Antone succeeds! Experiences in educating children with fetal alcohol syndrome* (pp. 71–95). Fairbanks: University of Alaska Press.

Murphy, M. (1993). Shut up and talk to me. In J.K. Kleinfeld & S. Wescott (Eds.), *Fantastic Antone succeeds! Experiences in educating children with fetal alcohol syndrome* (pp. 189–199). Fairbanks: University of Alaska Press.

O'Neill, R.E., Horner, R.H., Albin, R.W., Storey, K., & Sprague, J.R. (1990). *Functional analysis of problem behavior: A practical assessment guide*. Sycamore, IL: Sycamore Press.

Philpot, B., & Harrison, N. (1993). A one-room schoolhouse for children with FAS/FAE. In J.K. Kleinfeld & S. Wescott (Eds.), *Fantastic Antone succeeds! Experiences in educating children with fetal alcohol syndrome* (pp. 233–244). Fairbanks: University of Alaska Press.

Sparrow, J.S., Bella, D.A., & Cicchetti, D.V. (1984). *A manual for the Vineland Adaptive Behavior Scales*. Circle Pines, MN: American Guidance Services.

Streissguth, A.P., & Burgess, D.M., (1992). *Final report to Washington State Legislature: The Planning for Learning Project* (Tech. Report No. 92-04). Seattle: University of Washington, Pregnancy and Health Study.

Streissguth, A.P., Barr, H.M., Kogan, J., & Bookstein, F.L. (1996). *Understanding the occurrence of secondary disabilities in clients with fetal alcohol syndrome (FAS) and fetal alcohol effects (FAE): Final report to the Centers for Disease Control and Prevention on Grant No. RO4/CCR008515* (Tech. Report No. 96-06). Seattle: University of Washington, Fetal Alcohol and Drug Unit.

Streissguth, A.P., LaDue, R.A., & Randels, S.P. (1986/1988). *A manual on adolescents and adults with fetal alcohol syndrome with special reference to American Indians*. (Available free from National Clearing House for Alcohol and Drug Information [Inventory No. IHS002]; 1-800-729-6686.)

Sulzer-Azaroff, B., & Mayer, G.R. (1991). *Behavior analysis for lasting change*. New York: Holt, Rinehart, & Winston.

Tanner-Halverson, P. (1993). Snagging the kite string. In J.K. Kleinfeld & S. Wescott (Eds.), *Fantastic Antone succeeds! Experiences in educating children with fetal alcohol syndrome* (pp. 201–222). Fairbanks: University of Alaska Press.

Tanner-Halverson, P. (1997). A demonstration classroom for young children with FAS. In A. Streissguth & J. Kanter (Eds.), *The challenge of fetal alcohol syndrome: Overcoming secondary disabilities* (pp. 73–83). Seattle: University of Washington Press.

Wentz, T.L. (1997). A national survey of state directors of special education concerning FAS students. In A. Streissguth & J. Kanter (Eds.), *The challenge of fetal alcohol syndrome: Overcoming secondary disabilities* (pp. 84–90). Seattle: University of Washington Press.

Winick, P. (1993). Mainstreaming children with FAS in a small rural school. In J.K. Kleinfeld & S. Wescott (Eds.), *Fantastic Antone succeeds! Experiences in educating children with fetal alcohol syndrome* (pp. 223–231). Fairbanks: University of Alaska Press.

12

Guidelines for Human Services

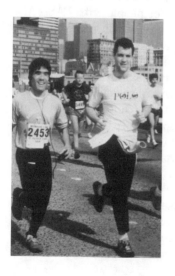

Irving called one morning. He'd been hospitalized the day before and wanted to see me. I went up to the psychiatric ward wondering what had gone wrong. I thought we had him all settled into a good group home and that his job clearing tables at the restaurant was going well. "What happened, Irving?" I asked. "Oh, I don't know—nothing, he replied." "How come you're up on the psychiatric ward?" I persisted. "What happened, Irving?" "Oh, I don't know. Nothing." "Well, how come you're up on the psychiatric ward?" "Oh, I just got all riled up." "Well, what exactly happened before you came in?" "I don't know. I just lost it and smashed a bunch of stuff."

Repeated questioning with concrete questions and offering a sense of rapport with my concern, I eventually understood what had happened. Actually, it was the cash register's fault that Irving was hospitalized. It's a typical story for people with FAS/FAE whose work placements are not adequately supervised. He was moved up from the job that he did comfortably and well (clearing tables) to a new job on the cash register, on which he got insufficient training. In the extreme stress that ensued, he lost control, became agitated and assaultive, and he was hospitalized.

Of the many secondary disabilities that afflict people with fetal alcohol syndrome (FAS) or fetal alcohol effects (FAE), three are most prevalent: 1) mental health problems, 2) alcohol and other drug problems, and 3) trouble with the law. The behaviors that accompany these conditions are often inappropriate or dysfunctional and tend to elicit the attention of various community services, which then attempt to modify or treat the individuals who display these behaviors. Many of these services, however, fail to provide the best management strategies or treatment alternatives to these individuals, primarily because they often treat only the behaviors without comprehending the nature of the underlying organic brain dysfunction. Direct services staff are hardly to blame, though. The damage that arises from prenatal alcohol exposure is not a familiar construct to staff members. In fact, the terms FAS and FAE are not even identified in the *Diagnostic and Statistical Manual of Mental Disorders, Fourth Edition* (DSM-IV) (American Psychiatric Association, 1995)—the handbook responsible for setting policy for diagnosis and treatment of mental disorders in the United States.

Furthermore, the behaviors of people with FAS/FAE are often an enigma, failing to make sense according to commonplace theories of eccentric or defective behavior. The behaviors of people with FAS/FAE often seem bizarre and unpredictable, and their explanations may shed little light on the problem. For example, it is not uncommon for these individuals to engage in some action without knowing why or to deny an action, even when they know they have been caught. Just as an accurate diagnosis and an understanding of what that diagnosis implies can help individuals to better understand these behaviors, an accurate diagnosis is also the key to providing more effective community services for people with FAS/FAE. In fact, the earlier that individuals are diagnosed in the treatment or incarceration process, the more effectively human services staff can use available resources to promote behavior change, encourage improved well-being, and reduce secondary disabilities.

Yet, community service agencies often fail to detect or diagnose FAS/FAE, even though individuals with these conditions are being served. In fact, our study of a large group of individuals with FAS/FAE revealed that 50% of those who were 12 years of age and older had been confined in some type of community institution: 35% have been incarcerated for criminal activity, 23% have been in residential mental health treatment, and 15% have been in residential treatment for alcohol or other drug abuse problems. Of individuals ages 6–51, 86% have received mental health treatment in outpatient treatment settings or residential programs (Streissguth, Barr,

Kogan, & Bookstein, 1996). Even those under the age of 12, 8% have been confined in mental health residential treatment centers.

IDENTIFYING AND SERVING INDIVIDUALS
WITH FAS/FAE WITH COMMUNITY SERVICES

In order to better serve individuals with FAS/FAE, some basic changes are needed in each of the three main phases of community service delivery: intake, management or treatment plan, and aftercare. These guidelines apply to any of the three primary agencies serving people with FAS/FAE: mental health, corrections, and alcohol and other drug treatment.

Intake

All human services agencies, whether public or private, have some type of regular intake procedure that can easily be adapted to identify those individuals who may have FAS/FAE. By making the intake a two-part process, consisting of an intake interview and a brief examination, human services personnel can establish whether individuals have a history of prenatal alcohol exposure and whether they have characteristics suggestive of FAS/FAE.

The Intake Interview   The intake interview obviously involves the individual but will be more helpful when supplemented by information from knowledgeable family members or other informants. Specifically, the intake interview should establish the family's history of alcohol use and identify any signs of central nervous system (CNS) dysfunction, growth deficiency, or other birth defects in the identified individual.

It is useful for the interviewer to probe not only for the family history of alcohol problems but also for the alcohol history of the biological mother: Did she have a drinking problem? How frequently did she drink? How many drinks per occasion? Was she drinking around the time of the patient's birth? (It is usually not possible to obtain an exact retrospective drinking history of the pregnancy unless the biological mother is available and in recovery.) Nevertheless, careful questioning can often reveal rich qualitative data (see Novick & Streissguth, 1996; Streissguth & Novick, 1995).

A number of circumstances warrant more careful questioning. For example, if the biological mother admits to having used illegal drugs while pregnant, this may indicate heavy alcohol use. Drug addicts often discount the sizable amounts of alcohol that frequently accompany their use of illegal drugs. In addition, if the biological father had a drinking problem, the mother's drinking may be underestimated in comparison. If a child has been raised by someone else, this may be suggestive because often a mother's alcohol problems render her unable to meet maternal responsibilities. If the biological mother died at a young age, this may have been due to an alcohol-related disease or accident. Any of these circumstances call for further questioning. Interviewers should also remember that the absence of a notation about maternal alcohol problems in the birth record is not the same as a negative exposure history.

Interviewers should probe for any signs of CNS dysfunction that might reflect prenatal brain damage, including seizure disorders; developmental delays; gross or fine motor problems; intellectual impairments; learning disabilities; attentional, memory, or language problems; and microcephaly (see Chapter 2). It is important to evaluate the individual's grasp on reality by asking open-ended questions (e.g., How did you arrive at this agency? What happened to bring you here [i.e., their perception of the precipitating event]?). Individuals with FAS/FAE may give answers that do not quite make sense and seem vaguely illogical. As LaDue and Dunne (1997) pointed out, an understanding of someone's thinking process cannot be obtained from questionnaires, checklists, or strict question-and-answer interviewing formats; open-ended questions are better.

Questions about early manifestations of growth deficiency, particularly family legends about birth size and general size in relationship to other children during the early childhood years, are especially important when no early records are available. Also of importance are questions about other birth defects and diagnoses (e.g., heart defects, central or peripheral auditory impairments, cleft lips and palates, joint problems). In particular, staff members should always ask, with every intake, whether FAS or FAE has ever been suspected in the past and, if so, by whom and for what reasons (see Kopera-Frye et al., in press).

Brief Intake Examination During the intake examination, staff should systematically obtain and record the individual's height, weight, and head circumference and compare with normative charts. An individual's face can be quickly scanned for any signs of the facial features of FAS. Facial photographs from the early preschool period or early school portraits can be very useful when examining adults. An in-service training on FAS screening will be useful to develop both screening and diagnostic referral procedures.

Interpreting the Intake Data and Taking Action The information obtained in the intake and brief examination should be summarized and organized in the computerized database so that it is readily available for treatment and after-care staff and for institutional population statistics and referral purposes. (Data not in the database will not readily become part of the full gamut of planning for an individual.) For individuals who are not diagnosed but are suspected of having FAS/FAE (see Chapter 2 for diagnostic guidelines), three important steps are necessary: 1) refer the individual to a credible diagnostician, 2) establish an advocate for the individual, and 3) order a psychological evaluation. The individual should be referred for a diagnostic evaluation as soon as possible so that appropriate measures can be built into the treatment or management plan early. Local child development/mental retardation centers or the State Genetics Office (part of the Department of Health) can usually provide referrals to diagnosticians in the area (see Appendix). Increasing awareness of FAS diagnostic and prevention networks should become available in many states and communities, as they are now in Washington State (see Clarren & Astley, 1997). Lack of easy access to diagnostic and treatment information specifically regarding FAS/FAE is a great barrier to effective service delivery to this population in communities.

Staff members should also query the individual with FAS/FAE about his or her advocate. To convey the concept of an advocate, staff can make this inquiry in simpler terms (e.g., Is there a special friend or relative who helps you when you find yourself in trouble?). Once the advocate has been identified, staff members should involve this person in the treatment process in order to devise a more comprehensive, applicable plan of action. Parents, in particular, often have valuable insights into the needs and concerns of the individual, even though they may not be able to provide sufficient supervision and structure to maintain the individual at home.

A psychological evaluation should be ordered for the individual. Understanding the general intellectual and academic level at which the individual is operating as well as the general level of adaptive functioning will facilitate planning for after-care. The psychological evaluation is especially important because individuals with FAS/FAE often appear more competent than they actually are because of their superficially good verbal skills and their sociability. Depending on available resources, neuropsychological evaluations are useful to uncover primary cognitive disabilities and strengths (see also Dyer, Alberts, & Nieman, 1997). The treatment team can also initiate the planning and paperwork necessary for the individual to obtain appropriate supports and services, such as those through the Division of Developmental Disabilities (DDD) and through the Social Services Disability system (see McKee, 1997).

The Management or Treatment Plan

It will be useful to designate an institutional advocate for individuals with FAS/FAE soon after his or her arrival at the institution. Whereas some people with FAS/FAE easily adapt to the institutional environment, appreciating the structure and predictability, others find the close interpersonal interactions in confined settings to be stressful. These individuals can quickly become victimized or viewed as troublemakers, and their inappropriate remarks and behaviors can result in their being ostracized, scapegoated, or castigated. Feelings of isolation, indignation, frustration, and/or outrage in response to perceived isolation, infringement, or slights can trigger increasingly inappropriate behaviors.

In these situations, an advocate is an invaluable ally who can work to change the system to better accommodate the individual and negotiate plausible controls and compromises. Advocates can defuse potentially explosive interpersonal situations and improve the individual's experience with the service system. If an individual requires residential treatment, the advocate can act as a liaison to develop useful linkages. Many people with FAS/FAE are pleased by this assistance and typically like having the help of an advocate once they understand the concept.

After-Care

After-care is the phase of institutionalization that follows the residential phase. In mental health or alcohol and other drug treatment programs, after-care usually consists of outpatient treatment after discharge. In the corrections system, after-care usually involves a parole or supervision period that follows incarceration in prison or jail. Most after-care programming is based on the concept that the care will be temporary and transitional. For individuals with FAS/FAE, after-care usually involves planning for some type of ongoing supervisory system and someone who will orchestrate the ongoing multiple needs of these individuals. When planning after-care for individuals with FAS/FAE, human services staff must include permanent planning for safe shelter, appropriate job skills training and workplace supervision, and a sense of community. Halfway houses offer a compromise between institutionalization and independent living in the community. However, halfway houses usually don't meet the long-term needs of individuals who cannot assume typical community roles, even with supportive outpatient assistance.

Society expects that most mental health patients, alcohol and other drug treatment patients, and offenders will resume their typical community roles, having to some extent been helped or rehabilitated by the institutional experience, and that they will function effectively with a minimum of supportive outpatient help. The situation is fundamentally different for people with FAS/FAE who are institutionalized when their behavior deteriorates to the point that it is no longer tolerable in the community or when they or their families recognize their need for "treatment." Although as of 1997 there is no specific treatment protocol per se for individuals with FAS/FAE, there is a great need for both research and practice. The institutional experience serves as a time to avert the immediate crisis, get off alcohol and other drugs, regain control of behavior that has gotten out of control, re-evaluate medications, and perhaps get away from unhealthy environmental influences—a respite from facing overwhelming life challenges and an opportunity to get help making more reasonable plans for the future. Ideally, some new skills will be learned in the institutional setting—interpersonal relations, anger management, basic life skills acquisition, recreational interests, vocational training. But, ultimately, it is the success of the after-care planning that influences the successful re-integration of the individual into the community. Communities should have some residential programs available and suitable for the needs of people with FAS/FAE, on both a short- and long-term basis (see Hess & Nieman, 1997), and case managers available who are knowledgeable about people with these diagnoses (see Schmucker, 1997). The almost total absence of writing in professional journals and books about the treatment and management needs of people with FAS/FAE across the life span is simply unacceptable and must be remedied.

The following letter is from a family that struggled for more than 20 years to help Penn, their adopted son with FAS. Penn wasn't diagnosed, however, until he was an adult. He again and again battled his alcoholism; yet each time he finished a treatment program, he found himself without any safe place in which to live and work. He was too lonely to live alone and always ended up with people who took advantage of him. When Penn's friends stole things, they sat in the car while Penn took the "goods" into the pawn shop. When the police came, the "friends" drove away, leaving Penn with the stolen merchandise. His mother wrote:

"I am sending you this narrative to include in Penn's file. It is very long and detailed, but I think it points up very well the difficulties FAS victims and their families have in dealing with adult life. It also illustrates the kind of people with whom FAS individuals are often involved.

"Although we seem to be able to provide Penn with the kind of structured work situation that will allow him to succeed, it is virtually impossible to pro-

vide him with an appropriately structured sheltered living situation that will keep his personal life together. When that falls apart, everything else goes down the toilet, so to speak.

"We are ready to get an unlisted telephone number and to find a disinterested party to administer his funds. After 20-plus years, the struggle has become too much. Perhaps 15 years from now the kind of living situation Penn needs will be available to FAS victims. It seems that everything has been about 15 years too late for Penn and for us."

Now, with greater community awareness about the needs of individuals with FAS/FAE and a better understanding of how communities, through their institutions, can meet these needs, people like Penn and their families may soon receive the help they need. Penn's family was capable of raising healthy, productive children. They did so with their other three sons. Their problem was in not knowing until adulthood that the son they adopted had a "hidden" birth defect. A single knowledgeable professional in all the institutions he encountered (a woman who had done a school report on FAS during her training) finally had the "A ha" experience of recognition during Penn's residential alcohol treatment. In my view, it is the community's responsibility to provide information on FAS/FAE to service providers and to provide the appropriate services that families will need to help their children.

ALCOHOL AND OTHER DRUG TREATMENTS

In a large study of secondary disabilities in individuals with FAS/FAE, we (Streissguth, Barr, et al., 1996) found that 30% of those older than 12 years of age experienced problems with alcohol and other drugs. Alcohol problems were more prevalent than were illicit drug problems, although it is interesting to note that the majority of individuals reported that they do not drink alcohol at all, particularly those who were raised by parents in recovery. This decision was often a personal rule of conduct that they had developed, either independently or from growing up in families in recovery or in families, for one reason or another, in which, members did not drink alcohol.

Sam, a 24-year-old man, sought residential treatment for alcohol and other drug problems at a community agency. At intake, Sam was fairly pleasant and cooperative, appearing to be of normal intelligence with occasional periods of clear insight into his problems. He said he drank alcohol regularly until he blacked out. Since 18 years of age, he had become increasingly violent at home.

He told his parents he thought of killing them and himself and had attempted suicide once by overdosing. Sam had been seeing an outpatient psychiatrist regularly for several years who had diagnosed him as having a panic disorder. He had been to Alcoholics Anonymous (AA) but had been unsuccessful in his attempts to quit drinking. At age 23, he entered an Indian alcoholism treatment program, but (according to his report) was expelled for dishonesty—a fact that angered him greatly. He reported recent memory problems and the desire to stop drinking. He was single, had no visible means of support, had moved four to five times during the past year, and reported concern that he could not pay his bills.

While in the alcohol treatment program, Sam was transferred twice to a psychiatric hospital because of increased suicidal ideation, increasing depression, and the possibility of a primary thought disorder. Vigorous attempts to involve him in group therapy at the alcohol treatment program led to his being overwhelmed with childhood memories. He began to regress and was frequently found sobbing in the corner or wandering aimlessly about the grounds weeping. One night Sam wandered off the grounds and became lost. He was again charged with being manipulative and was sent to a different psychiatric hospital. He was agitated and frightened, feeling that he would surely die of alcoholism as his mother had if he couldn't overcome his problem. He was overwhelmed with feelings of inadequacy and of being unable to cope. He was fearful about what would happen when he left the unit and anxious about his future living arrangements and lack of finances. When his insurance ran out, his adoptive parents refused to accept him home, and he was released to the streets without a follow-up plan. The absence of a psychiatric diagnosis disqualified him from placement in an appropriately sheltered facility upon discharge.

At discharge, Sam was referred to the University of Washington for a diagnostic examination. Once he was diagnosed with FAS, an advocacy network was formed. One advocate, the interested staff member from the treatment program, was all Sam needed to reorganize his life. His parents, finally understanding his plight, took him home temporarily while an after-care plan was designed to meet his needs. Once Sam understood that he had real cognitive disabilities and needed special supports, it was easy for him to comply.

Sam's story is typical of individuals with FAS who leave the structured environment of school and home in an attempt to live independently. It is likely that, although his alcoholism certainly reduced his ability to cope, the prenatal brain damage associated with FAS was the main cause of his dysfunctional life. Alcoholism, however, does present special problems for people with developmental disabilities, igniting more major behavior and disruptive problems than if these individuals abstained from alcohol (Westermeyer, Phaobtong, & Neider, 1988). Feelings of worthlessness, anger, depression, and panic as well as suicidal ideation are typical of young men with FAS. Yet treating these individuals for their secondary symptoms rather than their primary disability only proves to be problematic. In Sam's case, a treatment strategy oriented toward helping him cope with these seemingly insurmountable problems (i.e., housing, employment, social isolation) would have been far more therapeutic than "insight-oriented" psychotherapy or group therapy. In addition, if staff had recognized that his primary symptoms (i.e., memory problems, disorientation in time and space, impaired judgment) arose from a specific organic etiology, perhaps they would not have interpreted his actions as "manipulative."

In addition to the advocacy model, feasible alternatives include network therapy for alcohol and other drug abuse, a treatment model that involves active utilization of designated family members or friends who become an important part of the treatment team under the guidance of the therapist (Galanter, 1993a, b, c), and a harm-reduction model, which teaches individuals to invent rules to keep themselves out of harm's way (Marlatt & Gordon, 1985). Rules, especially when self-imposed, are a great strategy for individuals with FAS/FAE to employ and often provide the structure they need to function effectively.

After discharge, Sam stayed 1 month with his parents while plans were made for him to move to a new city so he could "start again." Once settled in his new home, he attended AA meetings regularly, was assigned a protective payee, qualified for Supplemental Security Income (SSI) as a result of his disability, and enrolled in a year of intensive counseling with long-term follow-up—all supports not available to him before. A counselor also began actively serving as his advocate. These institutionalized supports, key factors in the success of his after-care plan, were possible only after his diagnosis of FAS.

Sam worked at a number of jobs, gradually learned to take responsibility for his finances, and lived in a house on church grounds in exchange for grounds maintenance. Except for one relapse, he has been sober for 4½ years, and his family feels he continues to "get his life in order." He has developed a hobby—crocheting—that he does beautifully. However, he lives "on the edge of panic" every day and is vulnerable to any slight changes in his regular routine. At last contact, he was feeling discouraged and very frustrated because he desperately wanted a regular job in order to "get on with his life." He can work but needs close and appropriate supervision. At present, his situation is still precarious. Unemployment leaves him too much free time; there isn't enough structure or satisfaction in his day. (Part of Sam's story, along with the stories of several other adults with undiagnosed FAS/FAE, were published in Streissguth, Moon-Jordan, & Clarren [1995]; reprinted by permission of Hayworth Press, Inc.)

Clearly, being diagnosed with FAS was the turning point in Sam's life. The successful web of services and supports set in place as a result of the recognition of his organic brain damage permitted him to break out of the pattern of dysfunctional behaviors that had previously made it impossible for him to get his life under control. It seems hard to believe that Sam was not diagnosed as having FAS until adulthood. As a child, he had had major problems in school, seen three psychiatrists (one regularly for several years), and had two inpatient psychiatric evaluations in conjunction with alcohol treatment. Even as an adult, Sam has a classic FAS face and short stature (5 feet, 3 inches). He has short palpebral fissures (2.6 centimeters bilaterally with an inner canthal distance of 3.4 centimeters), a short nose, a flat philtrum, a marginally thick upper lip and flat midface, crowding of the front teeth, and unilateral ptosis. Sam's story shows that a seemingly hopeless situation can be turned around by an astute intake worker at an alcohol or other drug treatment program who takes responsibility for getting the person with FAS/FAE through the diagnostic process and for using this information to structure after-care needs with a permanent case manager rather than taking a "transition" approach to after-care.

MENTAL HEALTH TREATMENT

Even though diagnoses of FAS and FAE are not common in the mental health field, mental health problems are the most prevalent secondary disability that afflict individuals with FAS. In our study, more than 90% of 415 individuals with FAS/FAE of all ages and both sexes had some type of mental health problem according to the reports of their caregivers (Streissguth, Barr, et al., 1996). Overall, 58% of the individuals had attention-deficit/hyperactivity disorder; almost a third had panic attacks. More than one half of adults had experienced serious depression, more than 40% had threatened suicide, almost a quarter had attempted suicide, and 30% were reported as having displayed psychotic behavior (seeing visions and/or hearing things). In fact, 70 individuals had been detained in a psychiatric hospital, most frequently for depression, a suicide threat, or a suicide attempt. The median age for the first psychiatric hospitalization was 13 years, and the median duration was 4 weeks. Most individuals had only one psychiatric hospitalization, although a few like Irving had been hospitalized many times. The median age for the onset of mental health problems was 7 years.

Unfortunately, many of the treatment providers, including these individuals' psychiatrists, psychologists, social workers, and counselors, did not realize that these individuals had FAS/FAE.

A recent study of 330 consecutive medical records at a child psychiatry inpatient unit in Seattle, Washington, revealed that 81% had a notation that maternal alcohol use had been queried (Kopera-Frye et al., in press). Three individuals had been admitted with diagnoses of FAS/FAE, and 37 more were referred for an FAS diagnostic evaluation. Altogether, eight were diagnosed with FAS, a rate that is 15 times higher than the general population rate (using a 2 per 1,000 estimate). In addition, 11 individuals were thought to have FAE. Clearly, mental health facilities, both inpatient and outpatient, are important sites for the diagnosis and evaluation of people with FAS/FAE. Those serving children will be in a particularly important position in terms of getting this information to families when the children are still young. (See also the following additional mental health publications pertaining to FAS/FAE: Dyer, Alberts, & Nieman, 1997; Malbin, 1993; Novick, 1997; Snyder, Nanson, Snyder, & Block, 1997. Special issues involving mothers who themselves have FAS/FAE are discussed in Grant, Ernst, Streissguth, & Porter, 1997).

Using the Advocacy Model within the Mental Health System

Just as individuals with FAS/FAE display a diverse group of mental disorders, they have received a variety of therapeutic interventions. As of 1997, there is no indication that any treatment modalities are more effective than others; further research and treatment models are urgently needed. However, in the meantime, mental health hospitals and outpatient programs can institute policies for identifying and advocating for individuals with FAS/FAE and planning for their after-care needs in the community. Mental health professionals can use the advocacy model as an important adjunct to the therapeutic regimes initiated to treat the symptoms of mental illness that the individual with FAS/FAE manifests.

JUVENILE JUSTICE AND CORRECTIONS

When we interviewed the caregivers of 415 individuals with FAS/FAE, we found that 60% of those older than 12 years of age had been in trouble with the law. The rates were equivalent for those 12–17 years of age and for those 18 years and older. Among younger children, ages 6–11 years, only 20% had been in trouble with the law. The most frequent crimes were theft and shoplifting, although the whole gamut of criminal activity was represented to some extent (Streissguth, Barr, et al., 1996). These data are surprising. Criminality is not a typical behavior profile for people with Down syndrome, for example (Harris, 1988), and intentional premeditated criminal activity is not characteristic of people with FAS/FAE either, despite their high rate of trouble with the law. Many seem to slip into trouble with the law as a result of their maladaptive behaviors (impulsivity, difficulty sorting out cause and effect, trouble understanding consequences). When they have time on their hands due to unstructured days, disrupted schooling, poor family supervision, and unhealthy peer groups, and compound their problems with judgment with the use of alcohol and other drugs, they are more likely to get into trouble with the law.

As of 1997, society is not well-equipped to handle these individuals. Some of their behaviors that are labeled as criminal are really symptoms of the brain disease that accompanies FAS/FAE—symptoms that are best treated therapeutically rather than punitively. Not surprisingly, an early diagnosis of FAS/FAE appears to be associated with a lower rate of trouble with the law (Streissguth, Barr, et al., 1996). When families of young children understand the cause of the dysfunctional behaviors of their children, they are able to develop better educational and remedial strategies in response to the strengths and impairments they observe in their children. Early brushes with the law should serve as an opportunity to correct the situational factors that contribute to people with FAS/FAE getting into trouble. This will involve a better understanding of the nature of the primary disabilities in the individual and the interplay with the specific environment in which he or she lives. Such an understanding will be facilitated by a diagnostic evaluation for FAS/FAE, a psychological evaluation of the offender, and intensive interviews with the offender and with his or her family and/or advocate. But this information alone will protect neither society nor the offender if it isn't incorporated into a realistic sentence that takes into consideration both the individual's cognitive disabilities and the opportunities in his or her environment for structure and supervision. The corrections officer doing the presentence investigation, the defense attorney, the parents or family, and the judge all play important roles in using early incidents to protect against more serious later criminal behavior.

In every community, the corrections and juvenile justice systems will likely encounter individuals with FAS/FAE; whether they are identified as such is a different story. When they are not identified, their behavior is often viewed as bizarre, "off the wall," or manipulative. Why would someone knock over a street sign while a cop was watching? Why would someone pull out a gun and shoot at someone just because somebody told him to? Why would a girl get into a car with a guy she'd never met before and drive off to another state with him? Why would someone in prison steal a cookie when he knew it would count as an infraction? Behaviors such as these are hard to figure out unless the offender's brain damage is taken into consideration. Four case studies of adolescents with FAS, taken in the context of their psychological test profiles and maladaptive behaviors, help explicate their problem behaviors (LaDue, Streissguth, & Randels, 1992).

In carrying out an unpublished study in a Washington State prison, we became aware that the profile of behaviors characteristic of adults with FAS/FAE was well known to the corrections officers and counselors. However, until we worked together, they hadn't known what to call this profile, they hadn't known it was associated with brain damage, and they hadn't known it was caused by fetal alcohol exposure. A year and a half after we did the study, we found that two of the men with the behavioral profile of FAS had suddenly stopped all infractions even though we had never identified these men to the staff as explicitly having FAS/FAE. How had this happened? Figuring out that the behaviors that were getting these prisoners into trouble were indicative of prenatal alcohol exposure and not simply manipulative behaviors, the staff spontaneously figured out how to solve the problem. They set up one man with twice-weekly meetings with a counselor. With this kind of attention and monitoring, his infractions ceased. The other man was sent to a special training program of a mental health unit, where he also had no infractions. Infractions can be expensive because they are punishable by days or weeks in the intensive management unit (IMU), many times more expensive than prison time in "regular population" care.

Appropriate identification and management of people with FAS/FAE at all levels of the criminal and juvenile justice systems would be cost-effective. It is considerably less expensive to take preventive measures against infractions than it is to punish offenders once infractions occur. It is more cost-effective to provide adequate ongoing help and supervision after confinement than to keep readmitting people with FAS/FAE to jails, prisons, or mental hospitals. To this end, every person in a corrections center should be evaluated for FAS/FAE upon intake. Those individuals found to have FAS/FAE should receive an advocate and the appropriate vocational training, job and social skills training, and alcohol and other drug treatment. Improving state records to include notations about any maternal alcoholism, diagnostic information on FAS/FAE, and a tracking system for individuals with FAS/FAE across multiple agencies will greatly improve the plight of this population in the correctional system. In addition, initiating immediate and ongoing in-service training for all juvenile justice personnel, corrections officers, judges, and police officers will also prove useful. As of 1997, several authors have described FAS/FAE from a criminal justice perspective (see Barnett, 1997; Dagher-Margosian, 1997; Fehr, 1995; LaDue & Dunne, 1997; and Novick, 1997). Finally, more creativity in programming is needed to use the incarceration experience to teach skills that will truly enhance adaptive living.

Rothwell (1994) has been carrying out an innovative, "hands-on" school program in one of the juvenile justice facilities in Washington State for many years that is particularly effective with youthful offenders with FAS/FAE. Instead of sitting at desks, struggling to memorize their multiplication tables or improve their reading skills, the classes focus on active collaborative job- and skill-oriented projects that surreptitiously teach a wide variety of needed social and organizational skills. For example, a project to grow potted bulbs and plants to sell to employees and visitors for Mother's Day involved hands-on horticultural experience and research. The experiences included nurturing fragile plants, developing sales skills, taking orders, collecting money, making change, keeping records, and producing an attractively packaged product that enhances self-esteem and rewards community activism.

Bert was sent to prison for an unprovoked assault on an older woman. He admitted to the assault. When asked why he did it, Bert said, "Well, she snubbed me; she wouldn't speak to me."

Bert used to hang out at the bus stop in front of the house where he lived. It was a friendly neighborhood scene, a place where he could socialize and perhaps feel more integrated into the community. This particular woman was always friendly with him, and they usually chatted while she waited for her bus. One morning she arrived late and for some reason didn't speak to him. He just lost it.

Jim, a corrections officer interested in FAS/FAE, told me the following story one day after we'd done some in-service training at a corrections facility: Bert made an excellent adjustment to prison life and obtained a job folding laundry, which he did exceptionally well. He was very industrious and worked at this repetitive job for 4 months without problems. One day they told him he was promoted, but Bert didn't want to change jobs. Gradually, his superiors talked him into it by telling him he had a choice and giving him a 3-day trial with the option of returning to the laundry if he wished. Bert found he liked the new job, which involved working by himself with an electric sander, sanding new furniture. He learned to check his own work for quality control and again did an excellent job.

After 4 months, with no warning, they removed him from the sanding job and placed him directly on an assembly line job for another promotion. Bert went berserk. In his cell house, he became belligerent and pushy and shoved a staff member into a chain link fence (an action with extremely serious consequences in a prison). Prison officers then called Jim, who calmed Bert down. Jim explained that it was wrong to shove people but acknowledged that Correctional Industries was wrong to interfere with Bert's job. Jim contacted Correctional Industries and negotiated for Bert to get his old job back. He also told Bert to take the rest of the day off work and go see the prison psychologist to talk things over. Jim told Bert to take the night to consider whether he wanted to report to his old job in the laundry or report to segregation (IMU) because of the pushing and shoving of other inmates and officers.

Bert chose to return to his old job. Jim wanted to extend the good rapport he had established with Bert, so he visited him occasionally, making a point of facilitating conversation between Bert and his supervisor in order to build Bert's confidence in the supervisor. After about 9 months, Bert accepted a promotion to the assembly line. Jim then visited Bert on the assembly line, bringing Bert's supervisor as well. He let Bert ask questions as he and the supervisor demonstrated Bert's new job. Jim explained that the job was not time-sensitive and that Bert should feel no need to rush. Bert's new job worked out fine. With Jim's help as an advocate and the supervisor's understanding of Bert's needs (difficulty with changes, trouble with transitions, need for clear repetitive demonstrations, plenty of time for supportive practice, etc.), Bert acquired the skills needed for the new job and carried it out without further blow-ups or infractions. However, a success is not an inoculation that will prevent Bert from "falling apart" the next time a change that to Bert is horrendous is shoved on him without proper explanation. When the institution staff learns what to do and how to understand FAS-associated behaviors, then these individuals can function better in that setting. To the extent that the staff can teach this, as Jim did, they can expand each inmate's repertoire of adaptive behavior.

CONCLUSIONS

People with FAS/FAE, because of their inherent brain dysfunction, place certain demands on their environments. When these demands are understood and met, they can function fairly well. When their needs are not met, their behaviors can become out of control, bizarre, impulsive, desperate, and dysfunctional. Whether they end up in the corrections system, the mental health system, or an alcohol and other drug treatment program depends on a variety of circumstances. What is most important for their welfare and for society as a whole, however, is that whichever institution they end up in will take the responsibility for three things:

1. Screening for possible prenatal alcohol effects and obtaining diagnostic evaluations and psychological assessments
2. Designing individualized treatment/management plans that consider their individual needs as people with FAS/FAE
3. Setting in motion a realistic after-care program that takes into consideration both their FAS/FAE diagnoses and their own individual levels of development and specific skills, impairments, and desires

The identification of an advocate at the time the diagnosis is made (or even suspected) will enhance the success of this three-step plan, thereby extending as far as possible the periods of successful functioning of each individual with FAS/FAE. Without help and support, people with FAS/FAE through the ages have undoubtedly ended up in a variety of institutions and settings where their needs were not met (see Figure 12.1). Now, with awareness, advocacy, and appropriate community planning, this no longer need happen.

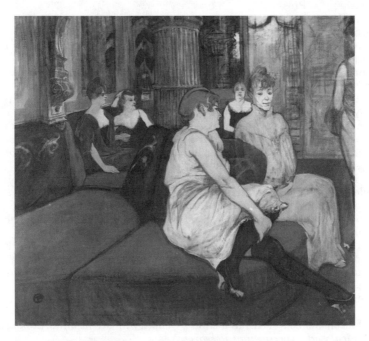

Figure 12.1. *Au salon de la rue des Moulins* [In the Moulins Street salon] by Henri de Toulouse-Lautrec. This prostitute (in long gown), immortalized by Toulouse-Lautrec in 1894, appeared on the cover of *Le Concours Médical* on April 23, 1994, with this question: "Quel est votre diagnostic? [What is your diagnosis?]." The answer, fetal alcohol syndrome, was supplied by Dehaene and Streissguth (1994, pp. 1271–1273). (Photograph courtesy of Musée Toulouse-Lautrec in Albi, France.)

REFERENCES

American Psychiatric Association. (1995). *Diagnostic and statistical manual of mental disorders* (4th ed.). Washington, DC: Author.

Barnett, C.C. (1997). A judicial perspective on FAS: Memories of the making of Nanook of the North. In A. Streissguth & J. Kanter (Eds.), *The challenge of fetal alcohol syndrome: Overcoming secondary disabilities* (pp. 131–140). Seattle: University of Washington Press.

Clarren, S., & Astley, S. (1997). Development of the FAS diagnostic and prevention network in Washington state. In A. Streissguth & J. Kanter (Eds.), *The challenge of fetal alcohol syndrome: Overcoming secondary disabilities* (pp. 38–49). Seattle: University of Washington Press.

Dagher-Margosian, J. (1997). Representing the FAS client in a criminal case. In A.P. Streissguth & J. Kanter (Eds.), *The challenge of fetal alcohol syndrome: Overcoming secondary disabilities* (pp. 119–130). Seattle: University of Washington Press.

Dehaene, P., & Streissguth, A.P. (1994). Quel est votre diagnostic? Le voir en peinture. [What is your diagnosis? Look at the picture]. *Le Concours Médical, 116*(15), 1271–1273.

Dyer, K., Alberts, G., & Nieman, G. (1997). Assessment and treatment of an adult with FAS: Neuropsychological and behavioral consideration. In A. Streissguth & J. Kanter (Eds.), *The challenge of fetal alcohol syndrome: Overcoming secondary disabilities* (pp. 50–61). Seattle: University of Washington Press.

Fehr, L.M. (1995, May–June). The criminal justice system and fetal alcohol syndrome. *Counselor, 13*(3), 33.

Galanter, M. (1993a). Network therapy for addiction: A model for office practice. *American Journal of Psychiatry, 150*(1), 28–36.

Galanter, M. (1993b). *Network therapy for alcohol and drug abuse: A new approach in practice.* New York: Basic Books.

Galanter, M. (1993c). Network therapy for substance abuse: A clinical trial. *Psychotherapy, 30*(2), 251–258.

Grant, T., Ernst, C., Streissguth, A., & Porter, J. (1997). An advocacy program for mothers with FAS/FAE. In A. Streissguth & J. Kanter (Eds.), *The challenge of fetal alcohol syndrome: Overcoming secondary disabilities* (pp. 99–109). Seattle: University of Washington Press.

Harris, J.C. (1988). Psychological adaptation and psychiatric disorders in adolescents and young adults with Down Syndrome. In S.M. Pueschel (Ed.), *The young person with Down syndrome: Transition from adolescence to adulthood* (pp. 35–51). Baltimore: Paul H. Brookes Publishing Co.

Hess, J., & Nieman, G. (1997). Residential programs for persons with FAS: Programming and economics. In A. Streissguth & J. Kanter (Eds.), *The challenge of fetal alcohol syndrome: Overcoming secondary disabilities* (pp. 185–193). Seattle: University of Washington Press.

Kopera-Frye, K., Streissguth, A.P., Clarren, S.K., Barr, H.M., Cadena, C., & Unis, A. (in press). Identification of fetal alcohol syndrome (FAS) and fetal alcohol effects (FAE) in a child psychiatry inpatient unit. *Alcoholism: Clinical and Experimental Research.*

LaDue, R.A., & Dunne, T. (1997). Legal issues and FAS. In A. Streissguth & J. Kanter (Eds.), *The challenge of fetal alcohol syndrome: Overcoming secondary disabilities* (pp. 141–158). Seattle: University of Washington Press.

LaDue, R.A., Streissguth, A.P., & Randels, S.P. (1992). Clinical considerations pertaining to adolescents and adults with fetal alcohol syndrome. In T.B. Sonderegger (Ed.), *Perinatal substance abuse: Research findings and clinical implications* (pp. 104–131). Baltimore: Johns Hopkins University Press.

Malbin, D. (1993). *Fetal alcohol syndrome and fetal alcohol effects: Strategies for professionals.* Center City, MN: Hazelden.

Marlatt, G.A., & Gordon, J.R. (1985). *Relapse prevention: Maintenance strategies in the treatment of addictive behaviors.* New York: Guilford Press.

McKee, P. (1997). FAS and the Social Security disability process: Navigating the system. In A. Streissguth & J. Kanter (Eds.), *The challenge of fetal alcohol syndrome: Overcoming secondary disabilities* (pp. 107–118). Seattle: University of Washington Press.

Novick, N. (1997). FAS: Preventing and treating sexual deviancy. In A. Streissguth & J. Kanter (Eds.), *The challenge of fetal alcohol syndrome: Overcoming secondary disabilities* (pp. 159–167). Seattle: University of Washington Press.

Novick, N.J., & Streissguth, A.P. (1996). Thoughts on treatment of adults and adolescents impaired by fetal alcohol exposure. *Treatment Today, 7*(4), 20–21.

Rothwell, M.A. (1994). Facing the challenge: Meeting special education needs of incarcerated youth. *Iceberg, 4*(4), 1–2.

Schmucker, C.A. (1997). Case managers and independent living instructors: Practical hints and suggestions for FAS. In A. Streissguth & J. Kanter (Eds.), *The challenge of fetal alcohol syndrome: Overcoming secondary disabilities* (pp. 91–96). Seattle: University of Washington Press.

Snyder, J., Nanson, J., Snyder, R., & Block, G. (1997). A study of Ritalin in children with FAS. In A.P. Streissguth & J. Kanter (Eds.), *The challenge of fetal alcohol syndrome: Overcoming secondary disabilities* (pp. 62–72). Seattle: University of Washington Press.

Streissguth, A.P., Barr, H.M., Kogan, J., & Bookstein, F.L. (1996). *Understanding the occurrence of secondary disabilities in clients with fetal alcohol syndrome (FAS) and fetal alcohol effects (FAE): Final report to the Centers for Disease Control and Prevention on Grant No. RO4/CCR008515* (Tech. Report No. 96-06). Seattle: University of Washington, Fetal Alcohol and Drug Unit.

Streissguth, A.P., Moon-Jordan, A., & Clarren, S.K. (1995). Alcoholism in four patients with fetal alcohol syndrome: Recommendations for treatment. *Alcoholism Treatment Quarterly, 13*(2), 89–103.

Streissguth, A.P., & Novick, N.J. (1995). Identifying clients with possible fetal alcohol syndrome: Fetal alcohol effects in the treatment setting. *Treatment Today, 7*(3), 14–15.

Westermeyer, J., Phaobtong, T., & Neider, J. (1988). Substance use and abuse among mentally retarded persons: A comparison of patients and a survey population. *American Journal of Drug and Alcohol Abuse, 14*(1), 109–123.

V

Preventing Fetal
Alcohol Damage

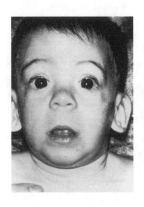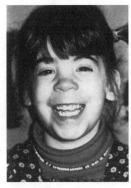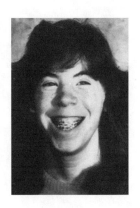

13

Education,
Training,
and
Public
Policy

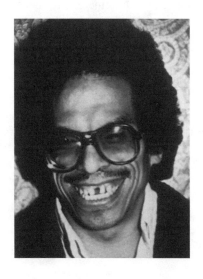

The Surgeon General advises women who are pregnant (or considering a pregnancy) not to drink alcoholic beverages and to be aware of the alcoholic content of foods and drugs (Surgeon General's Advisory on Alcohol and Pregnancy, 1981).

A pregnant woman never drinks alone (a sign from the Washington State Pregnancy and Health Program).

For baby's sake, don't drink (a sign from the Washington State Pregnancy and Health Program).

1) According to the Surgeon General, women should not drink alcoholic beverages during pregnancy because of the risk of birth defects; 2) consumption of alcoholic beverages impairs your ability to drive a car or operate machinery and may cause health problems (Alcoholic Beverage Labeling Act of 1988, PL 100-690).

No alcohol for our baby (a sign from the Washington State Pregnancy and Health Program)

When you're pregnant, the best drink is no drink at all (a slogan from the Washington State Pregnancy and Health Program).

249

Many steps have been taken to reduce FAS since its identification in the early 1970s. As Smith (1979) said, "If we can simply foster the concept of mothering from conception, this will be a major philosophic advance toward prenatal preventive medicine" (p. 2). Yet thousands of infants are born with FAS and fetal alcohol effects (FAE) in the United States each year. Considering the primary and secondary disabilities that accompany this birth defect and the lifelong implications of the diagnosis, this is a huge and compounding public health problem. Strategies for prevention are of grave concern—to individual families, to communities, to states, and to the federal government.

Prevention efforts for both FAS and FAE, however, are quite complex and much more involved than those for other birth defects. For example, iodine deficiency, which can cause mental retardation, is easily remedied by adding iodine to salt, as has been done for decades in the United States. Folate deficiency in pregnant women, which has been identified as increasing the risk of neural tube defects, can be reduced by adding folate supplements to familiar foodstuffs such as bread. Thalidomide, a sedative, was found to produce severe limb defects in children when taken during a specific stage of pregnancy. Once this connection was established, thalidomide was removed from the international market. Alcohol, however, is a legal drug used voluntarily by a majority of the U.S. population. It is associated with many pleasurable traditions and rituals, and forbidding its production, sale, or distribution was tried in the 18th amendment but repealed in the 21st.

The only way to prevent alcohol-related birth defects is to motivate women to abstain from consuming alcoholic beverages during their pregnancies. Even this solution is fraught with problems. Many women who inadvertently become pregnant continue to drink for the first month or two of the pregnancy (a particularly risky period for the developing fetus), before they realize that they are pregnant. Some women are never told that drinking during pregnancy is dangerous; others know but cannot stop drinking.

In order to protect children from the toxic effects of prenatal alcohol exposure, an entire network of activities is needed, organized around the five Ps of prevention:

1. Public education
2. Professional training
3. Public policy
4. Programs and services (see Chapter 14)
5. Parent and citizen activism

No one of these prevention arenas can, by itself, prevent all alcohol-related birth defects. Yet, together they can work to substantially reduce the risk of FAS and other types of prenatal alcohol damage to children. Decisions made at the levels of federal, state, and local governments with their varied resources and authorities will play an important role in initiating change. At all of these levels, citizen participation will be important and consortia of professionals, parents, and concerned citizens will be instrumental in the initiation and implementation of enlightened policy for the public good.

It is particularly important to incorporate these prevention efforts into long-term public health spending plans, instead of temporary "add-ons." The necessity of this has been demonstrated by our own experience at the University of Washington, where in 1978, we received a 3-year grant from the National Institute on Alcohol Abuse and Alcoholism (NIAAA) entitled *A Demonstration Grant to Prevent Fetal Alcohol Syndrome and Intervene in Female Alcohol Abuse During Pregnancy*. Under this grant, researchers and clinicians (Little, Streissguth, & Guzinski, 1980; Little et al., 1985; Little, Young, Streissguth, & Uhl, 1984) began the Pregnancy and Health Program (PHP), which encompassed a variety of focused projects aimed at providing public education, professional training, and services. We had a broad vision of what needed to be done, and the list we compiled would be much the same today for any community undertaking this challenge. We developed a variety of focused projects under the headings of public education, professional training, and providing services. We thought we'd done our job. It was only in retrospect that we recognized the importance of public policy.

Our community benefited greatly from the services provided by the demonstration program, but we did not realize then how important it was to ensure that the programs endured after the federal research dollars were spent. After our 3-year program closed, the warning signs at the liquor stores faded or were swept away and the mothers with whom we had worked seemed to vanish into the shadows. We now realize that plans for community implementation need to be developed at the outset and made an inherent objective of research demonstration programs from the start. Even for successful programs, policy change at some level will be essential if communities are to derive sustained benefits.

PUBLIC EDUCATION

Public education can be considered the cornerstone of all FAS prevention efforts. Only an informed public will support the focused activities of professional training and services required for a public health program of the magnitude necessary to prevent fetal alcohol damage in contemporary society.

In 1978, at the inception of the PHP demonstration project, we realized we'd need a good slogan. At that time, there were experimental animal studies demonstrating that alcohol was teratogenic, and hundreds of children with FAS had been reported in the medical literature. In view of the available evidence, it seemed plausible to advise citizens to abstain from drinking during pregnancy:

When you're pregnant, the best drink is no drink at all.

This slogan headed PHP's public education efforts, which included a massive campaign of warning signs and 220,000 brochures distributed in doctors' offices, liquor stores, buses, laundromats, libraries, and various other public places. We developed public service announcements for radio and television and generated frequent newspaper coverage of events relating to alcohol and pregnancy. Public awareness campaigns like these have been undertaken in part by a parent consortium group, the FAS Family Resource Institute, and other public service and philanthropic organizations (see Appendix).

In addition, the PHP, which was advertised in all the informational brochures, posters, and medical offices, operated a dedicated hot line (5-HEALTH)—a line concerned only with alcohol and pregnancy—to provide additional information. The hot line was staffed 12–24 hours a day by trained volunteers and by PHP health care professionals (see Little, Streissguth, Uhl, Young, & Durand, 1981; Little et al., 1984; and Rogan, 1985, for details). During its 2 years of operation, 5-HEALTH received almost 4,500 calls, half of these from pregnant women. One in every 44 pregnant women in the community called 5-HEALTH, almost two thirds of them during their first trimester. The interactive aspect of the informational campaign was an important component. Callers could get information, but they could also come by to talk with a specially trained health care professional and get help with their own drinking. The cost of 5-HEALTH was estimated to be $36,900, which averages approximately $14.50 per call or $429 per caller who became a PHP client. Women were much more likely to call in to a dedicated hot line than to a more general community information service. In Washington State, callers can still call in on an alcohol-and-other-drug 24-hour hot line and talk to a real person about alcohol and pregnancy concerns. Funded primarily by the Washington State Division of Alcohol and Substance Abuse, this service is provided by a corps of trained volunteers and a small professional staff. They not only recommend not drinking during pregnancy, but also, if asked directly for help, provide names and telephone numbers of physicians with special training in alcohol and substance abuse in the caller's area. This service, a direct legacy of our PHP, has operated continuously in Washington State since 1978.

In 1982, after the Surgeon General's (1981) advisory about not drinking during pregnancy, the NIAAA mounted a nationwide public education campaign that included local, state, and regional collaborative public education activities. The funding and organization of the accompanying state and local information campaigns on alcohol and pregnancy varied from state to state. Sponsors included an Alcohol and Drug Abuse Division; a Governor's Commission; a local affiliate of the National Council on Alcoholism; a categorically funded FAS prevention program; state health departments (e.g., Vermont); and state councils on developmental disabilities (e.g., Nebraska, Maine, North Carolina) (see Ronan, 1985). Several community organizations have also been active in disseminating alcohol and pregnancy information throughout Washington State, including the Western Washington Chapter of the March of Dimes (which has developed an award-winning video on FAS for junior high school students); the Arc (formerly the Association for Retarded Citizens, which has developed curriculum materials to educate school children); and the Washington State chapter of Healthy Mothers–Healthy Babies (which receives state health department and private local funding to produce educational materials in several languages and operates a toll-free information and referral line). In other states, chapters of these groups may also be a resource for local public education campaigns (see Appendix). Because every new generation of mothers needs to be educated about alcohol and pregnancy, communities must continue to promote public awareness.

A 1990 nationwide survey of more than 50,000 U.S. women showed that about 90% knew that heavy drinking during pregnancy could increase the chances of miscarriage, low birth weight, mental retardation, and birth defects; yet, only 73% had ever heard of FAS (Dufour, Williams, Campbell, & Aitken, 1994). Only 29% of all women of childbearing age could correctly identify FAS as a birth defect (an improvement from 1985, when only 16% of comparable women could identify FAS as a birth defect). The majority of the women surveyed in 1990 who had heard of FAS, however, thought it meant that the baby was born addicted to alcohol. Continuing ongoing campaigns of public awareness are clearly needed.

Although public awareness is probably not enough to stop most addicted women from drinking, it can yield direct results among those who drink socially. Public awareness can also help to set the stage for more comprehensive programs. Research data by Kaskutas and Graves (1994) indicate that one determinant of behavior change is the number of different types of messages a woman actually sees or hears.

PROFESSIONAL TRAINING

Prevention efforts should also concentrate on educating a wide range of community professionals about the risks associated with maternal alcohol use and abuse during pregnancy. Health care professionals, educators, school personnel, and social service workers are especially important to target.

PHP staff trained more than 6,000 professionals and distributed more than 7,000 brochures and professional packets in the late 1970s. An important measured outcome of these efforts was a substantial increase in the proportion of professionals who recommend abstinence during pregnancy (Blumhagen, 1985; Little et al., 1983, 1984, 1985). We also found that professional training was best accomplished by trainers from the same profession as those being trained.

Molly was an alcoholic, drinking heavily at the time she became pregnant. Although she'd heard of FAS, two pregnancy tests came back negative, and she continued to drink. When she finally learned she was pregnant, she told me this story of how her obstetrician helped her. He said, "Molly, I don't want you to drink any more during this pregnancy. Drinking can really hurt your baby, and it is very important not to drink. If you feel like you need someone to help you not drink anymore during this pregnancy, you just come right back in here and sit in my waiting room, Molly, and talk to my nurse and talk to me, and we'll get more help for you if you need it." Molly told me it was so comforting to know that she didn't have to stop drinking all on her own and that she could get help and support from her doctor and his nurse any time she felt she needed it. She said just knowing that made her stronger. She was able to stop drinking and was very glad that she did.

Professionals should be taught to capitalize on the fact that during pregnancy women can be highly motivated to stop drinking for the sake of their unborn children. The techniques of "motivational interviewing" described by Miller (1989) and adapted for the prenatal clinic by Handmaker (1993) are often effective. It is important to maintain an atmosphere of empathy, to endorse individual concerns about quitting or cutting down, and to actively support the individual's decision to modify her drinking behavior. Instead of just giving the individual a telephone number for a referral, for example, during the interview, the interviewer might actually call and schedule a referral appointment. Professionals should also be apprised of the misconceptions that pregnant women have about drinking during pregnancy in order to learn to respond appropriately to them in order to bring about behavioral change:

1. Alcohol cannot be bad because women have been drinking for thousands of years.
   Counterpoint: Cautions against drinking during pregnancy have existed since the earliest times.
2. It is safer to drink beer or wine than hard alcohol or liquor.
   Counterpoint: A standard drink of any of these has the same amount of absolute alcohol.
3. The placenta protects the fetus from danger.
   Counterpoint: Drugs such as alcohol easily cross the placenta.
4. Alcohol cannot hurt a fetus because some very smart people have been born to alcoholic mothers.
   Counterpoint: Twin studies and the experimental animal research show that individuals vary in their vulnerability to prenatal alcohol.
5. It is pointless to stop drinking if one has been drinking throughout the first trimester.
   Counterpoint: There is plenty of evidence to show that it is better to stop drinking any time during the pregnancy than not to stop at all.

The PHP personnel trained nurses and physicians caring for pregnant women to detect and respond to those with alcohol problems. For example, they prepared pregnancy care workers to 1) ask appropriately about a woman's history of alcohol use and current drinking level, 2) accurately inform women of the reasons why they should not drink during pregnancy, 3) follow up this advice with appropriate referrals to counseling or rehabilitation as needed, and 4) schedule women for regular prenatal visits and hold follow-up discussions as necessary. The PHP also trained alcoholism counselors to 1) consider the possibility that a female client could be pregnant, 2) ask about the possibility of a pregnancy in a non-threatening manner, 3) talk about the reasons for not drinking during pregnancy, and 4) make appropriate referrals as necessary. For both of these groups, detection of mothers at risk and appropriate referral were primary objectives.

Other Public Education and Professional Training Programs

Already by the mid-1970s, there was recognition that the prenatal clinic was an important site for preventing FAS; the earliest program was developed by Rosett and colleagues at Boston University (Rosett, Ouelette, Weiner, & Owens, 1977, 1978). Additional professional training programs related to alcohol and pregnancy are described in the following (see also those described in Chapter 14): Blumhagen (1985); Bolario, Nanson, and Chapman (1994); Casiro, Stanwick, Pelech, and Taylor (1994); Donovan (1991); Funkouser and Denniston (1985); Institute of Medicine, Stratton, Howe, and Battaglia (1996); Masis and May (1991); Morse, Idelson, Sachs, Weiner, and Kaplan (1992); NIAAA (1987); Robinson and Armstrong (1988); Rosett, Weiner, and Edelin (1981); Scharling (1993); Smith and Coles (1991); Streissguth and Little (1994); and Weiner, Rosett, and Mason (1985).

By 1988, when an international FAS prevention conference was held in Vancouver, British Columbia, Canada (Robinson & Armstrong, 1988), numerous programs were under way involving public education, professional training, and services to educate all women about the risks associated with drinking during pregnancy and to detect and treat pregnant women at high risk. The programs were centered on a common theme: abstinence during pregnancy. Popular slogans included "No alcohol for our baby," "For baby's sake, don't drink," "Building better babies," "Healthiest babies possible," "Healthy start," and "A pregnant woman never drinks alone."

May and Hymbaugh (1989) developed an inexpensive, macro-level FAS prevention program for Native Americans and Alaskan Natives that educated trainers in local communities across the United States in comprehensive FAS prevention skills and provided technical assistance for the development of local programs. For a little more than $300,000, May and Hymbaugh trained almost 2,000 people in 92 Indian Health Service Units. Using 8-hour workshops and resource materials developed and provided by a central source, the prevention program capitalized on local talent, enthusiasm, and commitment. A substantial amount of knowledge was retained by the various groups trained; and in at least one instance, May and Hymbaugh were able to effectively measure the diffusion of information to school children who were not part of the centralized program. This model could easily be replicated for statewide programs aimed at FAS awareness and prevention.

In Sweden, an FAS prevention program was built into existing, widely used district maternal and child health clinics throughout the country. District social service offices monitor child welfare and provide financial, housing, and psychological support as needed to 99% of all Swedish women (Olegård, 1988). For each regional clinic, the Swedish FAS program includes a pediatrician, an obstetrician, a child psychologist, and a coordinator responsible for continuing education of professionals. Confidentiality rules, which had perpetuated secrecy and prevented sharing of critical information among professionals, were changed to permit professionals and authorities to exchange information in the interest of the unborn child. Emphasis is placed on providing midwives with plenty of time to discuss alcohol use and abuse patterns with women at their first prenatal visit and list the availability of suitable alcohol treatment programs. Olegård (1988) noted that the estimated incidence of FAS in Sweden dropped from 1 in 600 infants in the mid-1970s to 1 in 2,400 infants by the mid-1980s.

PUBLIC POLICY

In the United States, several national public policy decisions have alerted the public to the risks of mixing alcohol and pregnancy. In 1981, Acting Surgeon General Edward N. Brandt, Jr., advised women who are pregnant (or planning a pregnancy) not to drink alcoholic beverages and to be aware of the alcoholic content of foods and drugs when pregnant or when planning a pregnancy (Surgeon General's Advisory on Alcohol and Pregnancy, 1981). Then, in 1988, the Alcoholic Beverage Labeling Act, PL 100-690, was passed, which mandates a warning on the label of each alcoholic beverage container sold in the United States:

1) According to the Surgeon General, women should not drink alcoholic beverages during pregnancy because of the risk of birth defects; 2) consumption of alcoholic beverages impairs your ability to drive a car or operate machinery and may cause health problems.

This law went into effect in 1989, exactly 10 years after the first hearings on bottle labeling of alcoholic beverages were held by the Bureau of Alcohol, Tobacco, and Firearms—the federal regulatory agency for alcohol.

State-level public policy decisions have also been instrumental in professional training on alcohol and pregnancy. Missouri, for example, has mandated that health care workers providing services to pregnant women must be appropriately trained and has described what this training should include. Missouri State Senate Bill No. 190—Pregnancy, prenatal and postnatal care, and education for women and children (on alcohol, cigarettes, and drugs)—went into effect July 1, 1992. At one point, however, alcohol was reportedly dropped from the bill altogether but was salvaged by a coalition of professionals and concerned citizens. As of May 1997, 17 states (Alaska, Arizona, California, Delaware, Georgia, Illinois, Kentucky, Maine, Minnesota, Nebraska, New Jersey, New Mexico, New York, Rhode Island, South Dakota, Utah, and Washington), legislative actions, executive orders, statewide propositions, or liquor control board mandates now require alcohol and pregnancy warning signs to be posted. Florida has a voluntary posting law, and Michigan has legislation pending for mandatory posting.

In Washington State, a citizens committee convinced the state legislature to pass a mandate requiring warning signs to be posted in all state liquor stores. Afterward, with encouragement from the governor, the Liquor Control Board worked with various citizens, business groups, and scientists to design a more attractive, less unwieldy sign and to make policies for posting by all alcohol vendors. Through a number of working meetings and public hearings, three signs (see Figure 13.1 for one example) were developed, allowing each proprietor a choice. Two signs must be posted in all places in Washington State at which liquor can be purchased, either by bottle, can, or glass, including grocery stores and restaurants. This state law went into effect October 5, 1994.

Mandatory signs to be posted warning of the possible dangers of consumption of alcohol during pregnancy. (Washington State Liquor Control Board, 1993)

The toll-free telephone number links the caller with the 24-hour alcohol-and-other-drug hot line. Other effective Washington State activities include the appointment of state FAS coordinators, situated in both the Department of Health and the Division of Alcohol and Substance Abuse. The coordinators become central coordinating figures for statewide FAS activities.

In addition, some cities including New York City, and counties, have mandated warning signs. Typically, these signs say that alcohol use during pregnancy can cause birth defects, recommend that women avoid alcohol during pregnancy and when planning a pregnancy, and offer a telephone number for more information or for services. The Center for Science in the Public Interest (1991) has published an informative booklet to help communities institute these mandates (see Appendix).

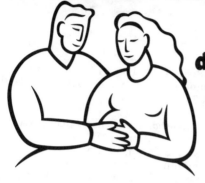

W A R N I N G

Avoid alcohol during pregnancy.

Alcohol use during pregnancy may cause birth defects such as Fetal Alcohol Syndrome.

For more information call 1-800-662-9111
Washington State Substance Abuse Coalition

AAP-9

Figure 13.1. Washington State warning sign about prenatal alcohol exposure. Posting is mandatory in two locations wherever liquor is sold. (From Washington State Liquor Control Board, 1993; reprinted by permission.)

CONCLUSIONS

Prevention, in all its multidimensional aspects, is an important state and local activity, as is the coordination of services for children with FAS and their families. The importance of interagency cooperation cannot be overemphasized, as alcohol and pregnancy activities cross all normal service delivery channels. Two Washington State governors (Booth Gardner in 1991 and Michael Lowry in 1995) established FAS advisory panels, whose reports outlined policy recommendations, and a "Washington State Needs Assessment Survey on Fetal Alcohol Syndrome/Effects" (James Bowman Associates, 1994) was funded through a Centers for Disease Control State-Based Capacity Building Project for the Prevention of Primary and Secondary Disabilities. FAS legislation passed in Washington State (Substitute State Senate Bill No. 5688 in 1995) mandated the establishment of an official interagency task force on FAS and the funding to begin a statewide network of FAS diagnostic clinics, tied in with the existing University of Washington FAS Diagnostic Clinic (Clarren & Astley, 1997). Activities like these could be ongoing in all states, involving health care professionals, parents, scientists, and concerned citizens, working together to ensure that the needs of our existing citizens with FAS/FAE are met and that future children are not born with this preventable disability.

Just 25 years after FAS was first identified and named, there has been a remarkable change in public and professional awareness about FAS and other prenatal effects of alcohol. Yet in order to achieve maximum efficacy, public education, professional training, and public policy must be coupled with programs for reaching those hard-to-reach mothers who continue to abuse alcohol during pregnancy (see Chapter 14).

REFERENCES

Alcoholic Beverage Labeling Act of 1988, PL 100-690, 27 U.S.C. 213 § *et seq.*

Blumhagen, J.M. (1985). PHP training for nonphysicians. *Alcohol Health and Research World, 10*(1), 48–49, 75.

Bolario, R., Nanson, J., & Chapman, S. (1994). *Programming for prevention of fetal alcohol syndrome: The Saskatchewan experience.* Paper presented at the NIAAA FAS Prevention Conference, Detroit, MI.

Casiro, O.G., Stanwick, R.S., Pelech, A., & Taylor, V. (1994). Public awareness of the risks of drinking alcohol during pregnancy: The effects of a television campaign. *Canadian Journal of Public Health, 85*(1), 23–27.

Center for Science in the Public Interest. (1991). *Alcohol warning posters: How to get legislation passed in your city.* Washington, DC: Author. (Available from Center for Science in the Public Interest, 1875 Connecticut Avenue, NW, Suite 300, Washington, DC 20009-5728.)

Clarren, S., & Astley, S. (1997). The FAS diagnostic and prevention network in Washington State. In A. Streissguth & J. Kanter (Eds.), *The challenge of fetal alcohol syndrome: Overcoming secondary disabilities* (pp. 38–49). Seattle: University of Washington Press.

Donovan, C.L. (1991). Factors predisposing, enabling and reinforcing routine screening of patients for preventing fetal alcohol syndrome: A survey of New Jersey physicians. *Journal of Drug Education, 21*(1), 35–42.

Dufour, M.C., Williams, G.D., Campbell, K.E., & Aitken, S.S. (1994). Knowledge of FAS and the risks of heavy drinking during pregnancy, 1985 and 1990 (NIAAA Epidemiologic Bulletin No. 33). *Alcohol Health and Research World, 18*(1), 86–92.

Funkhouser, J.E., & Denniston, R.W. (1985). Preventing alcohol-related birth defects: Suggestions for action. *Alcohol Health and Research World, 10*(1), 54–59, 75–76.

Handmaker, N.S. (1993). *Motivating pregnant drinkers to abstain: Prevention in prenatal care clinic.* Unpublished doctoral dissertation, University of New Mexico, Albuquerque.

Institute of Medicine, Stratton, K.R., Howe, C.J., & Battaglia, F.C. (Eds.). (1996). *Fetal alcohol syndrome: Diagnosis, epidemiology, prevention and treatment.* Washington, DC: National Academy Press.

James Bowman Associates. (1994). *Washington State needs assessment survey on fetal alcohol syndrome/effects.* Seattle: Washington State Department of Health, Office of Maternal/Infant Health and Genetics.

Kaskutas, L., & Graves, K. (1994). Relationship between cumulative exposure to health messages and awareness and behavior-related drinking during pregnancy. *American Journal of Health Promotion, 9*, 115–124.

Little, R.E., Streissguth, A.P., & Guzinski, G.M. (1980). Prevention of fetal alcohol syndrome: A model program. *Alcoholism: Clinical and Experimental Research, 4*(2), 185–189.

Little, R.E., Streissguth, A.P., Guzinski, G.M., Grathwohl, H.L., Blumhagen, J.M., & McIntyre, C.E. (1983). Change in obstetrician advice following a two-year community educational program on alcohol use and pregnancy. *American Journal of Obstetrics and Gynecology, 146*(1), 23–28.

Little, R.E., Streissguth, A.P., Guzinski, G.M., Uhl, C.N., Paulozzi, L., Mann, S.L., Young, A., Clarren, S.K., & Grathwohl, H.L. (1985). An evaluation of the pregnancy and health program. *Alcohol Health and Research World, 10*(1), 44–53, 75.

Little, R.E., Streissguth, A.P., Uhl, C.N., Young, A., & Durand, S.R. (1981). *5-HEALTH: The operation of an information and crisis telephone line for alcohol and pregnancy* (Tech. Report No. 81-01). Seattle: University of Washington, Fetal Alcohol and Drug Unit, Pregnancy and Health Programs.

Little, R.E., Young, A., Streissguth, A.P., & Uhl, C.N. (1984). Preventing fetal alcohol effects: Effectiveness of a demonstration project. In R. Porter, M. O'Connor, & J. Whelan (Eds.), *CIBA Foundation Symposium 105: Mechanisms of alcohol damage in utero* (pp. 254–274). London: Pitman.

Masis, K.B., & May, P.A. (1991). A comprehensive local program for the prevention of fetal alcohol syndrome. *Public Health Reports, 106*(5), 484–489.

May, P.A., & Hymbaugh, K.J. (1989). A macro-level fetal alcohol syndrome prevention program for Native Americans and Alaska Natives: Description and evaluation. *Journal of Studies on Alcohol, 50*(6), 508–518.

Miller, W.R. (1989). Increasing motivation for change. In R.K. Hester & W.R. Miller (Eds.), *Handbook of alcoholism treatment approaches: Effective alternatives* (pp. 67–80). Elmsford, NY: Pergamon.

Morse, B.A., Idelson, R.K., Sachs, W.H., Weiner, L., & Kaplan, L.C. (1992). Pediatricians' perspectives on fetal alcohol syndrome. *Journal of Substance Abuse, 4*(2), 187–195.

National Institute on Alcohol Abuse and Alcoholism (NIAAA). (1987). *Program strategies for preventing fetal alcohol syndrome and alcohol related birth defects* (DHHS Publication No. ADM 87-1482). Washington, DC: U.S. Government Printing Office, Department of Documents.

Olegård, R. (1988). The prevention of fetal alcohol syndrome in Sweden. In J.C. Robinson & R.W. Armstrong (Eds.), *Alcohol and child/family health: Proceedings of a conference with particular reference to the prevention of alcohol-related birth defects* (pp. 73–82). Vancouver, British Columbia, Canada: B.C. FAS Resource Group. (Available from the B.C. FAS Resource Group, UBC Department of Pediatrics, Sunny Hill Hospital for Children, Vancouver, B.C. V5M 3E8, CANADA.)

Robinson, J.C., & Armstrong, R.W. (Eds.). (1988). *Alcohol and child/family health: Proceedings of a conference with particular reference to the prevention of alcohol-related birth defects.* Vancouver, British Columbia, Canada: B.C. FAS Resource Group. (Available from the B.C. FAS Resource Group, UBC Department of Pediatrics, Sunny Hill Hospital for Children, Vancouver, B.C. V5M 3E8, CANADA.)

Rogan, A. (1985). 5-HEALTH: A vital link. *Alcohol Health and Research World, 10*(1), 52–53, 75.

Ronan, L. (1985). State strategies for prevention of alcohol-related birth defects. *Alcohol Health and Research World, 10*(1), 60–63, 65, 76–77.

Rosett, H.L., Ouelette, E.M., Weiner, L., & Owens, E. (1977). The prenatal clinic: A site for alcoholism prevention and treatment. In F.A. Seixas (Ed.), *Currents in alcoholism* (Vol. 1, pp. 419–430). New York: Grune & Stratton.

Rosett, H.L., Ouelette, E.M., Weiner, L., & Owens, E. (1978). Therapy of heavy drinking during pregnancy. *Obstetrics and Gynecology, 51*(1), 41–46.

Rosett, H.L., Weiner, L., & Edelin, K.C. (1981). Strategies for prevention of fetal alcohol effects. *Obstetrics and Gynecology, 57*(1), 1–7.

Scharling, J.B. (1993). The prevention of prenatal alcohol use: A critical analysis of intervention studies. *Journal Studies on Alcohol, 54,* 261–267.

Smith, D.W. (1979). Fetal drug syndromes: Effects of ethanol and hydantoins. *Pediatrics in Review, 1*(6), 165–172.

Smith, I.E., & Coles, C.D. (1991). Multilevel intervention for prevention of fetal alcohol syndrome and effects of prenatal alcohol exposure. *Recent Developments in Alcoholism, 9,* 165–182.

Streissguth, A.P., & Little, R.E. (1994). *Alcohol, pregnancy, and the fetal alcohol syndrome: Unit 5. Biomedical education: Alcohol use and its medical consequences* (slide lecture series, 2nd ed.). Hanover, NH: Dartmouth Medical School, Project Cork. (Available by calling 1-800-432-8433.)

Surgeon General's Advisory on Alcohol and Pregnancy. (1981). *FDA Drug Bulletin, 11*(2), 9–10. Rockville, MD: U.S. Department of Health and Human Services.

Washington State Legislation. (1995). Substitute Senate Bill 5688 Chapter 54.

Washington State Liquor Control Board. (1993). Washington Administrative Code 314–12–195.

Weiner, L., Rosett, H.L., & Mason, E.A. (1985). Training professionals to identify and treat pregnant women who drink heavily. *Alcohol Health and Research World, 10(1),* 32–35, 70–71, 74.

14

Effective Prevention Programs for High-Risk Mothers

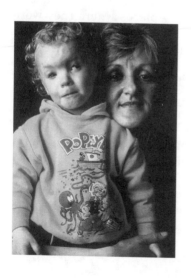

On a fine spring day in 1994, I went to King County Superior Court House to testify on behalf of Christine, a young mother who was addicted to alcohol and heroin. After 1½ years in our Birth to 3 program, which includes more than 1 full year of sobriety and steady growth toward realistic goals of effective parenting; stable, supervised living; and participation in a job-skills training program, Christine was sentenced to the Washington State Prison for Women for several years for some earlier felonies. (There were several counts of forgery committed during her pregnancy to fund her habit.)

At the trial, Christine spoke eloquently on her own behalf. She had learned from her mistakes and was working toward achieving reasonable goals by using available community supports. The judge was convinced of her sincerity and sentenced Christine to 2 years of community supervision instead—a triumph for her advocate, for her community support team, and, most of all, for Christine.

This young mother, at high risk for producing a child with FAS, was effectively on the road to rehabilitation. Her success, along with many others like her, contributed to the data show-

ing that there is something that works with these highest-risk mothers—the Seattle Paraprofessional Advocacy Model: Birth to 3 program.

I have never met a mother who drank during pregnancy because she wanted to hurt her child or because she didn't care. Women whose children are affected by prenatal alcohol exposure are usually those who, for various reasons, were not able to make better choices. Some gave birth to children before anyone suspected that prenatal alcohol exposure was harmful. Others may have received advice from well-meaning but uninformed clinicians who gave them ambiguous messages or failed to respond in a forthright fashion to their timid questions. Others simply did not think of themselves as abusing alcohol, having alcohol problems, or otherwise drinking at risky levels. Some thought of themselves as drug addicts, without considering that their alcohol consumption might be particularly harmful. Others wanted to stop drinking during pregnancy and were tormented by their inability to do so but did not have the resources or know-how to obtain treatment, or they were involved in interpersonal situations that made it impossible to stop drinking without external support, which was unavailable.

Alcohol is an addictive drug (National Institute on Alcohol Abuse and Alcoholism, 1990). People who are addicted to alcohol and other drugs require treatment; however, treatment is not always available, especially for women who live in poverty and stand to lose their children if they go into residential treatment and for the working poor who lack medical coverage. In 1980, Washington State had scarcely any adequate facilities for treating female alcoholics that respected their special needs as women—places where they were able to bring their children, be in separate treatment groups from men, and deal with special addiction-related women's issues such as battering and abuse. Although as of 1997 the situation has now improved in Washington State, a study by Geshan (1993) of the 17 southern states and Washington, D.C., San Juan, Puerto Rico, and the Virgin Islands found that there were still many substantial barriers to effective treatment for alcohol- and drug-abusing pregnant and parenting women. Although some progress is beginning, doubtless the problem exists elsewhere as well.

If communities are to prevent fetal alcohol damage to children, they must begin by extending services to high-risk women and mothers that focus on reducing alcohol intake, increasing family planning, advocating for the mothers, and ensuring safety for the children. There exist several working models that can be replicated in any community without excessive cost.

Researchers at the University of Washington School of Medicine have been involved in two major efforts to prevent FAS by direct intervention with the heaviest drinking mothers. Our first effort, the Pregnancy and Health Program (PHP) (1978–1981), developed methods to identify and work with pregnant women at high risk for abusing alcohol. The Birth to 3 program (1991–1996) developed methods to identify women at high risk upon delivery and work with them until their children reached 3 years of age.

INTERVENING IN ALCOHOL ABUSE DURING PREGNANCY

The Pregnancy and Health Program

The PHP provided many important services to women who abused alcohol; it also effectively circumvented many but not all barriers to care. We successfully developed a two-stage screening process to first identify women at potential risk and then determine which of those were at genuine risk. But we failed in our attempts to develop a detoxification program for pregnant, alcohol-abusing women. In the 1970s, neither obstetricians nor alcoholism treatment programs wanted this responsibility. The two-stage screening process involved 1) a short questionnaire administered in the waiting room of obstetricians' offices, and 2) a brief intervention interview. After the interview, 11% of those individuals who were screened (more than 1,300 Seattle women) were considered to be at genuine risk, and 2.6% were thought to have a current drinking problem. Women were identified as being at genuine risk when they ingested an average of one or more drinks per day, consumed five or more drinks on a single occasion, or showed evidence of a past or present problem with alcohol as determined clinically by a nurse or counselor.

We concluded that a very brief questionnaire could alone determine genuine risk. By asking if 1) the individual ever consumes five or more drinks on any occasion, and 2) she ever feels that she should cut down on drinking, clinicians could detect 92% of the women identified as being at genuine risk by the intervention interview. This simple screening device identified four times as many risk-level drinkers as were documented in the women's obstetrical records.

Once identified, those thought to be at risk were invited to meet with a PHP staff member to discuss their drinking. The purpose of this "brief intervention" was to provide information on alcohol and pregnancy, to recommend abstaining from alcohol during the remainder of the pregnancy, and to help each woman work out an individual plan of action. Many of the women took advantage of this offer. Some individuals seemed able to cut down or stop drinking based on this brief intervention alone, whereas others needed several intervention sessions. Some women, including those who had tried unsuccessfully to cut down, were referred to alcohol treatment specialists trained to deal with issues involving pregnancy. Although terminations were not recommended to women as a function of their alcohol intake, referrals were available upon request.

The service delivery component of the PHP was very successful, as demonstrated by the clear decrease in alcohol use during pregnancy among women who used the program (see Figure 14.1). Three fourths of the women who were drinking moderately to heavily were able to either stop drinking with the brief intervention or to significantly reduce their alcohol use; 86% were judged by independent raters to have improved (Little et al., 1985). Using an index of infant abnormalities and neurological findings previously associated with maternal drinking (Little, Uhl, Palouzzi, et al., 1981), we also found a significant decreasing linear trend in fetal alcohol effects (FAE) among children when mothers decreased their length of alcohol exposure. Mean scores on the FAE index among infants of mothers still drinking at risk levels in the third trimester tripled scores for those infants whose mothers reduced their drinking in

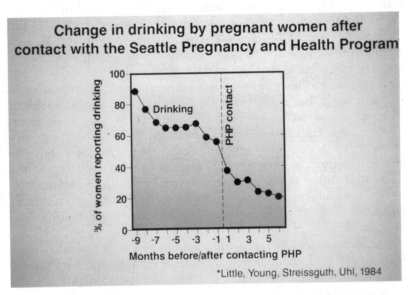

Figure 14.1.   Decrease in maternal alcohol use after intervention during pregnancy. (From Little et al., 1984, p. 264; reprinted by permission.)

the first trimester (Little, Young, Streissguth, & Uhl, 1984). Mothers continuing to drink at high-risk levels also had more pregnancy complications. (See Little & Streissguth, 1981; Little, Streissguth, & Guzinski, 1980; Little et al., 1985; Little, Uhl, Paulozzi, et al., 1981; Little, Uhl, Streissguth, & Guzinski, 1981; Little, Young, Streissguth, & Uhl, 1984; and Uhl, Little, Streissguth, & Guzinski, 1981; for further details of the program and the results.)

There was a sense of exhilaration about preventing prenatal alcohol damage in those early days. It was thrilling to be able to mount such outcome-specific programs against a known agent of mortality and morbidity. Once alcohol was recognized as a teratogen, prevention programs sprang up to protect our children from this assault.

Other Pregnancy Intervention Programs

By the mid-to-late 1970s, Atlanta, Boston, France, and Stockholm, Sweden, had also developed early prevention outcome-specific programs based in the prenatal clinic. Not all of these programs used the combination screening method used by the PHP. Some programs used the 10-Question Drinking History developed by Rosett, Weiner, and Edelin (1983), whereas others based their screening processes purely on alcohol problems and tolerance, using measures such as the T-ACE questions (Sokol, Martier, & Ager, 1989; Sokol, Miller, & Martier, 1991) or the TWEAK test (Russell, 1994).

Results from these programs indicated that reducing prenatal alcohol use leads to better infant outcomes, including higher birth weights, fewer stillbirths, fewer babies with congenital anomalies, and healthier newborns. (For further details, see Aronson & Olegård, 1987; Dehaene, 1995; Halmesmäki, 1988; Handmaker, 1993; Larsson & Bohlin, 1987; Masis & May, 1991; Rosett & Weiner, 1981; Smith, 1991; Smith & Coles, 1991; Smith, Coles, Lancaster, Fernoff, & Falek, 1986; and Weiner & Larsson, 1987).

Almost all of these programs found that many women are able to eliminate or reduce their alcohol intake during pregnancy when they are approached in a nonjudgmental manner and provided a supportive and caring atmosphere. Two thirds of the heavy drinkers in the Boston program stopped drinking after three or more counseling sessions (Weiner & Larsson, 1987). In the Stockholm program, all "excessive drinkers" and 78% of "alcohol abusers" reduced their alcohol intake (Weiner & Larsson, 1987). In Tuba City, Arizona, 85% of the alcohol-abusing pregnant women who participated in the FAS counseling and intervention program carried out by the

Indian Medical Center remained abstinent for the rest of their pregnancies. This service was a hospital-based component of a massive multilevel community effort to prevent FAS that had high visibility and focus in this isolated Native American community (Masis & May, 1991).

In Atlanta, 50 women (34% of an inner-city African American sample) who were given a simple intervention in the prenatal clinic (usually during the second trimester) were able to stop drinking for the remainder of their pregnancies. This intervention consisted of asking women about their alcohol use, telling them about the harmful effects of alcohol during pregnancy, and advising them not to drink. Those with alcohol problems and those with anxiety about their drinking were referred to a psychiatric obstetrics clinic for additional counseling or to community alcohol treatment programs. The 96 women who continued to drink throughout pregnancy had started drinking at an earlier age; had a higher tolerance for alcohol; had more family members with alcohol problems, especially their mothers; and were more likely to drink with family members (Smith, 1991; Smith & Coles, 1991; Smith, Lancaster, Moss-Wells, Coles, & Falek, 1987).

Incorporating Interventions During Pregnancy into Existing Service Systems

Prenatal alcohol and other drug programs can be built into existing service delivery systems at little extra cost. For example, obstetrical nurses can be trained to take on these responsibilities as a routine part of prenatal care. The key components of such a program are as follows:

- Ask each pregnant woman about her alcohol use during and prior to her pregnancy.
- Tell all women (regardless of their reported drinking levels) of the risks associated with drinking during pregnancy.
- Recommend abstinence for the remainder of the pregnancy to all women (regardless of their reported drinking levels).
- Discuss with all drinking women whether they think they will be able to stop or significantly decrease their alcohol use during the remainder of the pregnancy.
- Make appropriate referrals for women who are drinking at risky levels or who feel they will be unable to stop or reduce their drinking during pregnancy.
- Maintain adequate follow-up at prenatal visits and evaluate the need for further help.

- Offer postpartum support to every mother with an alcohol problem, even those who have reduced or eliminated their use of alcohol (e.g., providing a referral for a public health nurse, a social worker, or a paraprofessional advocate).

It is important that each woman be approached with the attitude of helpfulness and support. The goal for heavy-drinking pregnant women is to motivate behavior change, not to punish or to shame. Miller and Rollnick (1991) discuss emphathetic motivational interviewing strategies associated with long-term behavior change (Handmaker, 1993). Jessup and Green (1987) discuss special substance abuse treatment issues for pregnant women.

One of the most critical ingredients for the success of these programs is the conviction of the health care provider that abstinence is the best policy to recommend. When professionals convincingly recommend abstinence from alcohol during pregnancy to all women in prenatal care, there is no room for ambiguity.

I'll never forget the sadness of meeting with an upper–middle-class family whose first young child was born with FAS, almost 10 years after the Surgeon General had recommended not drinking during pregnancy. The attractive mother, with her husband seated beside her and her son scampering about the room, recounted this story:

"Sure I knew about FAS, but I thought you had to drink throughout pregnancy to have a child with FAS. We'd been married a long time, and we partied regularly on weekends with our friends. I was probably drunk when I got pregnant. I tried not to drink during my pregnancy. When I asked my doctor about drinking during pregnancy, he said it was okay to drink a little: "Just don't overdo it," he said. I only really drank five times during my pregnancy—seven or eight beers each time. Another four times, I had two beers. It's okay to use my story to help other families and to help doctors know that they need to be really clear about what they say to their patients about not drinking during pregnancy."

INTERVENING AFTER DELIVERY

Despite the general effectiveness of pregnancy-based intervention programs, there are always a few heavy drinkers who are not persuaded. For example, 10% of the women approached by the PHP did not modify their alcohol use. Women who come from alcoholic households themselves and have long histories of alcohol abuse and failed treatment attempts are often difficult to reach. In addition, those women who fail to obtain prenatal care (many of whom are abusing alcohol and other drugs) are inaccessible to fetal alcohol prevention programs targeted to pregnant women. (This problem is exacerbated in states where women who abuse drugs during pregnancy are prosecuted for child abuse.) Although some states are establishing women-oriented treatment programs, the women most in need of such services are often unable to utilize them effectively. These women are at the highest risk of producing children with FAS/FAE.

To help remedy this problem, the Seattle Paraprofessional Advocacy Program, known locally as Birth to 3, was created to identify mothers at high risk at delivery, to intervene with these mothers after the births of their children, and to help this population of women who so often "slip through the cracks." The birth of a child is the one time even the highest risk mothers touch the health care system.

The Inception of the Birth to 3 Project

In the course of screening more than 7,000 Seattle-area mothers at delivery for a study of cocaine use during pregnancy, we found what we had suspected: An overwhelming majority of those who used cocaine during pregnancy also used alcohol (Carmichael Olson, Grant, Martin, & Streissguth, 1995). Furthermore, the amount of alcohol they used was often substantial and clearly put their children at risk of prenatal alcohol effects. Yet, being involved in obtaining and using an illegal substance put the everyday lives of cocaine-using pregnant women at risk and alienated them from community services. This problem demanded a solution. Rather than continue our research on the impact of prenatal cocaine exposure on children's development, we decided to focus on developing a method to intervene in the destructive lifestyle that kept these drug-abusing women from obtaining prenatal care. With funding from the Center for Substance Abuse Prevention, we undertook the job of identifying and helping the highest-risk mothers in the Seattle community, those who were abusing alcohol and other drugs during their pregnancies but who were not connected to community resources and who received little or no prenatal care.

The Birth to 3 Program

The breadth of the Birth to 3 program went far beyond interventions for pregnant or parenting women (Grant, Ernst, & Streissguth, 1996, 1997; Grant, Ernst, Streissguth, Phipps, & Gendler, 1996; Streissguth

& Grant, 1996). The primary intervention target had to be the mothers' alcohol and other drug abuse and not just for the duration of the pregnancy. Most of these women had already tried alcohol and other drug treatments; but their lives were out of control on all fronts, far beyond the scope of even the female-oriented treatment programs available in Washington State. Children in these homes were often unsafe—part of our responsibility had to be to monitor the health and safety of the target baby and the other children in the household in a much more intense fashion than Children's Protective Services (CPS) was able to undertake. We witnessed in action the "replacement child" phenomenon: When CPS takes one child away, the mother has another. Clearly, effective birth control/family planning issues were essential components of our intervention. We also had to cope with the mothers' unreasonable expectations of getting all of their children back the day they finished treatment. Finally, having learned a bitter lesson from the speedy dissolution of our PHP after the federal demonstration grant funds disappeared, we were determined to find a way to institutionalize Birth to 3 in the community after the 5 years of federal funding were over. If our program was obviously cost-effective, state or county governments might take it on.

We had three basic aims: 1) to help those mothers who abuse alcohol and other drugs to obtain treatment, stay in recovery, address their other problems, and plan any further children; 2) to teach community agencies how to meet the needs of these mothers at high risk who often alienate professionals or fail to use services already available; and 3) to provide the strongest possible motive for another source of funding, public or private, to provide the necessary financial resources once federal funding expired.

Screening Process   In two Seattle hospitals, known to serve a majority of these women at high risk, mothers were approached the day after delivery and given a one-page screening questionnaire by a woman who identified herself as a researcher not part of the hospital staff. Mothers were assured that the information they supplied was confidential and anonymous and would not become part of their hospital or medical records. Those who reported heavy use of illicit drugs or alcohol during pregnancy, who had received little or no prenatal care, and who were unconnected to service providers were invited to participate in a special program for the next 3 years; 92% accepted the offer and were assigned an advocate. It is important to note that this self-report screening process was more sensitive than urine screenings in detecting mothers in need of services. Of the 83% of the mother–child pairs who were screened for illegal drugs, only 60% tested positive. Furthermore, the procedures used here produced clients who had been willing to reveal in a confidential setting that they were abusing alcohol or other drugs, or both, during pregnancy and thus were more likely to be good treatment risks.

Because of the level of community advocacy involved with the program, Birth to 3 soon became so widely known that professionals began referring women whom they had heard were in need of its services. Within a year of its inception, half of the participants had been referred to Birth to 3 by professionals in the community.

The Participants   Over the 18-month recruitment phase, Birth to 3 staff members enrolled 65 women from differing ethnicities (31 African American, 19 Caucasian, 10 Native American, 4 Hispanic, and 1 Asian). Compared with the screening populations of mothers from the study hospitals, Birth to 3 mothers were more likely to be African American or Native American and to have already had several children and were less likely to be legally married or hold high school diplomas. As a group, they were polydrug abusers. Their primary drugs of abuse were tobacco, cocaine, alcohol, and marijuana, although some also used heroin and other drugs. Of the 65 women, 62 were not using birth control at all or were using it only sporadically.

At the time of delivery, 55 received public assistance; 36 were homeless or living in transitional housing; none were employed. Excluding their newborns, these mothers had, collectively, 131 children, 63% of whom were no longer in their care. Research showed that 49 of the mothers had themselves had at least one parent who had abused alcohol or other drugs; 40 had experienced physical or sexual abuse; 38 were raised in foster families for at least part of their childhood. Half of the mothers had considered terminating their most recent pregnancy but were unable to follow through because they did not know how to gain access to services or were unable to obtain or keep appointments.

Advocates in the Birth to 3 Program   The Birth to 3 program provided each mother at high risk with an advocate to guide, supervise, inspire, and teach her with respect to treatment programs, child safety, parenting, shelter, relationships with spouse or partner, and all other fronts on which her life was out of control. Because women like these have been resistant in the past to intervention, advocacy would begin with goals the women themselves selected. In this way, they would have a personal investment in the outcome from the very start. Although terminating alcohol and other drug abuse and achieving effective birth control are programmatic goals, a mother's acknowledging such goals is in no way a requirement to entry into Birth to 3. Gradually, after small successes, trust develops between the mother and her advocate; this, in turn, becomes a springboard for effective change toward a greater range of goals.

Advocates provide hands-on emotional support and practical assistance to the mothers that cannot be duplicated by overworked child welfare workers or public health nurses with high caseloads, other agendas, and time constraints. Through such help, the mothers learned to trust their advocates and to believe in the effectiveness of the advocacy.

Our advocates were paraprofessionals, meaning there were no professional requirements for the position—they didn't have to be nurses, social workers, health aides, or even college graduates. They did have to possess excellent problem-solving skills, high energy, a commitment to helping, and empathy. The advocates received on-the-job training as well as regular and intensive bi-weekly case supervision. They also participated in weekly strategy meetings, in which they supported each other and interacted with community professionals whose services were used by the mothers.

The work of advocacy takes place in the community. Our advocates used state cars to make frequent home visits and to taxi clients. They developed working networks of professionals from child welfare, public health, alcohol and other drug treatment programs, child development programs, mental health, education, and judicial and corrections systems. Through their work with mothers, advocates routinely identified service barriers and met with service providers to lift them. For instance, CPS referred many families to our program in lieu of removing the infants from their mothers' custody at birth. A contract with CPS, drawn up with input from both the mothers and their advocates, stipulated conditions under which the mothers could maintain custody of their children. In these cases, the advocates were responsible for supervising the household and for the well-being of the children. Depending on the capabilities and strengths of the mother, advocates strove to either gradually distance themselves and their services, rendering more power, autonomy, and independence to the mother, or arranged an ongoing, appropriate support network to compensate for each mother's level of functioning.

Results Results from the Birth to 3 program have been overwhelmingly positive. During the first 2 years (1991–1993) of receiving Birth to 3 services, 80% of the women had obtained alcohol and/or drug abuse treatment; 60% of the women had remained abstinent from drugs for at least 6 months; 62% were using long-term family planning methods (including tubal ligations, Norplant, and Depo Provera); 76% of the target children were living with their own families; and 93% of children were receiving well-child care. The Birth to 3 program costs $3,680 per year for each mother served. This figure includes salaries, administrative costs, and operating costs. Incarcerating one of these same mothers for a year would cost $43,950—$36,750 in prison costs and $7,200 in foster care costs. This savings far exceeds an advocate's yearly salary; and considering that each advocate works with 13 to 15 individuals, there is no doubt that Birth to 3 is a cost-effective and lasting solution to a problem that often, left untreated, repeats itself in generation after generation. Studies have shown that the long-term societal costs of children prenatally exposed to alcohol can often multiply as the years pass. As Chasnoff (1991) noted, "Pay now, or pay later."

The following data illustrate the cost effectiveness of Birth to 3's efforts: After 24 months of advocacy, 11 Birth to 3 individuals, with an average of 4 children each, had chosen to have a tubal ligation or Norplant therapy. If each of these women had one more child, the health care costs alone of the pregnancy and the baby's first year for these 11 women would be $170,380, which exceeds the combined annual salaries of 5 advocates who work with 65 such women (Streissguth & Grant, 1996).

Continuing the Birth to 3 Program   In 1996, an anonymous philanthropist, so touched by the work of the advocates, provided the funding to continue Birth to 3 once the official demonstration funding from the federal government ended. Governor Michael Lowry could see the wisdom of intervening in prevention as well. He used money from his emergency fund for a second Birth to 3 program in another city with a high-risk population of alcohol- and drug-abusing mothers. Models for preventing FAS/FAE have been developed and demonstrated to be effective in reducing human suffering and the associated economic costs, especially those associated with secondary disabilities. The technology to solve this problem exists, but to bring the solution to fruition will require a determined populace willing to pay a little extra now to save larger costs in the future—a populace willing to work harder now to ensure that fewer children are born with the brain damage associated with FAS/FAE. Instead of becoming angry with mothers who produce children with FAS/FAE, citizens should invest their time and effort to ensure that the situation never has the opportunity to repeat itself or recycle itself in future generations. Following is a letter that one successful and grateful mother in the Birth to 3 program wrote to her advocate:

I would like to express how important and necessary the Birth to 3 program is and thank Carryn Johnson for her tremendous effort in helping me change my life. Once a person is involved in drugs of any kind, it is hard to change the situation. I found myself confused and distressed when I decided I wanted to turn my life around. Everyone I was associated with took drugs, and people who were clean and sober wanted nothing to do with me.

I had my second child, and I refused to let her be placed in a foster home. My first child had been placed in a home and died of crib death, so I clung to my second child. This time I was blessed. My CPS worker was aware of a program through the University of Washington [Birth to 3]. She set up an interview for me.

When I first met Carryn, I was skeptical. I had to trust someone who could steer me in the "right" direction. I, like most addicts, seek instant gratification, but after more than 15 years of taking drugs, getting clean doesn't happen overnight. Carryn stuck with me. She knew it was going to take time.

Carryn was always (and I mean ALWAYS!) there to answer questions, listen when I needed to talk, and drive me to our appointments. She believed in me when I wasn't sure I could even believe in myself. When I had a problem with welfare, she found the time to drop in on the welfare office and clear up the problem. After her visit, they never tried to have me sign away what was rightfully mine.

Carryn visited my daughter and me when I was in treatment. Just knowing she would come and check on us gave me more incentive to continue striving to improve myself. She made me feel and know I wasn't alone. She would acknowledge my efforts and praise my progress. She helped me gain enough self-confidence that I decided to go back to school.

Once I could see how much I had changed and that people did care about me, there was no stopping my progress. I am now finishing my second year at South Seattle Community College and maintaining a 3.88 grade point average. I would like to eventually work with people.

Without all the hard work Carryn and the Birth to 3 program did for me, I wouldn't be standing on my own. I have now been clean and sober for 3 years (as of next month), and my daughter has been with me since the minute she was born. Thanks to the program, she has a great start in life.

I feel that without their assistance, I would never have known where to begin, let alone how to achieve, staying clean. I wish all women that were in my situation would have the same chance at recovery as I did. I am privileged to have been chosen to take part in it and want to thank all the women who helped.

Thank you, Maureen

REFERENCES

Aronson, M., & Olegård, R. (1987). Children of alcoholic mothers. *Pediatrician, 14,* 57–61.

Carmichael Olson, H., Grant, T.M., Martin, J.C., & Streissguth, A.P. (1995). A cohort study of prenatal cocaine exposure: Addressing methodological concerns. In M. Lewis & M. Bendersky (Eds.), *Mothers, babies, and cocaine: The role of toxins in development* (pp. 129–162). Hillsdale, NJ: Lawrence Erlbaum Associates.

Chasnoff, I.J. (1991). Drugs, alcohol, pregnancy, and the neonate: Pay now or pay later (Editorial). *Journal of the American Medical Association, 266*(11), 1567–1568.

Dehaene, P. (1995). La grossesse et l'alcool [Alcohol and pregnancy]. *Que Sais-Je?, 2934.* Paris: Presses Universitaires de France.

Geshan, S. (1993). *A step toward recovery: Improving access to substance abuse treatment for pregnant and parenting women.* Washington, DC: Southern Regional Project on Infant Mortality. (Call 1-800-800-1910 for more information.)

Grant, T.M., Ernst, C.C., & Streissguth, A.P. (1996). An intervention with high risk mothers who abuse alcohol and drugs: The Seattle advocacy model. *American Journal of Public Health, 86*(12), 1816–1817.

Grant, T.M., Ernst, C.C., & Streissguth, A.P. (1997). *Reaching out to alcohol and drug abusing mothers: A guide for change using paraprofessionals* (Technical Report, No. 97-01). Seattle: University of Washington, Fetal Alcohol and Drug Unit.

Grant, T.M., Ernst, C.C., Streissguth, A.P., Phipps, P., & Gendler, B. (1996). When case management isn't enough: A model of paraprofessional advocacy for drug- and alcohol-abusing mothers. *Journal of Case Management, 5*(1), 3–11.

Halmesmäki, E. (1988). Alcohol counseling of 85 pregnant problem drinkers: The effect on drinking and fetal outcome. *British Journal of Obstetrics and Gynecology, 95,* 243–247.

Handmaker, N.S. (1993). Motivating pregnant drinkers to abstain: Prevention in prenatal care clinics. *Unpublished doctoral dissertation,* University of New Mexico, Albuquerque.

Jessup, M., & Green, J.R. (1987). Treatment of the pregnant alcohol-dependent woman. *Journal of Psychoactive Drugs, 19*(2), 193–203.

Larsson, G., & Bohlin, A.B. (1987). Fetal alcohol syndrome and preventative strategies. *Pediatrician, 14,* 51–56.

Little, R.E., & Streissguth, A.P. (1981). Effects of alcohol on the fetus: Impact and prevention. *Canadian Medical Association Journal, 125,* 159–164.

Little, R.E., Streissguth, A.P., & Guzinski, G.M. (1980). Prevention of fetal alcohol syndrome: A model program. *Alcoholism: Clinical and Experimental Research, 4,* 185–189.

Little, R.E., Streissguth, A.P., Guzinski, G.M., Uhl, C.N., Paulozzi, L., Mann, S.L., Young, A., Clarren, S.K., & Grathwohl, H.L. (1985). An evaluation of the Pregnancy and Health Program. *Alcohol Health and Research World, 10*(1), 44–53, 75.

Little, R.E., Uhl, C.N., Paulozzi, L., Streissguth, A.P., Guzinski, G.M., Clarren, S.K., & Altman, G. (1981). *The pregnancy and health program: III. Pregnancy outcome and its relation to intervention in maternal drinking in a prenatal population* (Tech. Report No. 81–04). Seattle: University of Washington, Pregnancy and Health Programs.

Little, R.E., Uhl, C.N., Streissguth, A.P., & Guzinski, G.M. (1981) *The pregnancy and health program: II. Treatment for alcohol-related problems in pregnant women* (Tech. Report No. 81–03). Seattle: University of Washington, Pregnancy and Health Programs.

Little, R.E., Young, A., Streissguth, A.P., & Uhl, C.N. (1984). Preventing fetal alcohol effects: Effectiveness of a demonstration project. In R. Porter, M. O'Connor, & J. Whelan (Eds.), *CIBA Foundation Symposium 105: Mechanisms of alcohol damage in utero* (pp. 254–274). London: Pitman.

Masis, K.B., & May, P.A. (1991). A comprehensive local program for the prevention of fetal alcohol syndrome. *Public Health Reports, 106,* 484–489.

Miller, W.R., & Rollnick, S. (1991). *Motivational interviewing: Preparing people to change addictive behaviors.* New York: Guilford Press.

National Institute on Alcohol Abuse and Alcoholism (NIAAA). (1990, January). *Seventh special report to the U.S. Congress on Alcohol and Health.* Washington, DC: U.S. Department of Health and Human Services.

Rosett, H.L., & Weiner, L. (1981). Identifying and treating pregnant patients at risk from alcohol. *Canadian Medical Association Journal, 125,* 149–154.

Rosett, H.L., Weiner, L., & Edelin, K.C. (1983). Treatment experience with pregnant problem drinkers. *Journal of the American Medical Association, 249,* 2029–2033.

Russell, M. (1994). New assessment tools for risk drinking during pregnancy. *Alcohol Health and Research World, 18,* 55–61.

Smith, I.E. (1991). *Preventing fetal alcohol syndrome: An ecological approach. Healthy Roots.*

Smith, I.E., & Coles, C.D. (1991). Multilevel intervention for prevention of fetal alcohol syndrome and effects of prenatal alcohol exposure. *Recent Developments in Alcoholism, 9,* 165–180.

Smith, I.E., Coles, C.D., Lancaster, J., Fernoff, P.M., & Falek, A. (1986). The effect of volume and duration of prenatal alcohol exposure on neonatal physical and behavioral development. *Neurobehavioral Toxicology and Teratology, 8,* 375–381.

Smith, I.E., Lancaster, J.S., Moss-Wells, S., Coles, C.D., & Falek, A. (1987). Indentifying high-risk pregnant drinkers: Biological and behavioral correlates of continuous heavy drinking during pregnancy. *Journal of Studies on Alcohol, 48,* 304–309.

Sokol, R.J., Martier, S.S., & Ager, J.W. (1989). The T-ACE Questions: Practical prenatal detection of risk drinking. *American Journal of Obstetrics and Gynecology, 160,* 863–868.

Sokol, R.J., Miller, S.I., & Martier, S.S. (1991). *Identifying the alcohol-abusing obstetric/gynecologic patient: A practical approach* (ADM Publication No. 81-1163). Washington, DC: U.S. Department of Health and Human Services, National Institute on Alcohol Abuse and Alcoholism.

Streissguth, A.P., Grant, T.L., & Ernst, C.C. (1996/1997). *The Birth to 3 program: A plan of action for Washington State.* Paper presented to the House of Representatives Committee on Children and Family Services, Olympia, WA.

Uhl, C.N., Little, R.E., Streissguth, A.P., & Guzinski, G.M. (1981). *The Pregnancy and Health Program: I. Screening for alcohol use in a prenatal clinic* (Tech. Report No. 81-02). Seattle: University of Washington, Pregnancy and Health Programs.

Weiner, L., & Larsson, G. (1987). Clinical prevention of fetal alcohol effects: A reality: Evidence for the effectiveness of intervention. *Alcohol Health and Research World, 11*(4), 60–63, 92–94.

Epilogue

In 1980, when I first gathered researchers together from around the world to address scientific questions about alcohol's effect on prenatal development, I viewed the challenge as both scientific and educational. Through science, the answers would be found; through education, the necessary policies would emerge.

After 25 years of direct work with the long-term consequences that fetal alcohol syndrome (FAS) and fetal alcohol effects (FAE) have on adolescents and adults with the syndrome, the issues for me have changed. As I view the dramatic consequences FAS/FAE has on individual children, as I realize how poorly our society is equipped for helping them, and as I see each generation repeating the cycle, I realize that science and education alone are not enough to solve this tragic problem.

It is essential that we reach a level of public knowledge that will fuel tremendous change—change of a magnitude we have only now begun to appreciate. Research is still needed—but research of a different sort: not just on causes but on lives and specifically on the

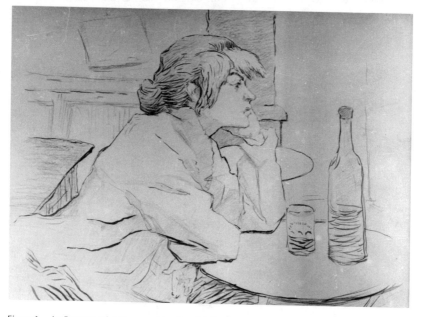

Figure 1.   *La Buveuse* [The Hangover] by Henri de Toulouse-Lautrec. (From Musée Toulouse-Lautrec; reprinted by permission.)

type of help children and adults affected by fetal alcohol exposure need to lead productive lives and to control costly and painful secondary disabilities. We need programs to identify and help those mothers unable to stop drinking based on informational education alone. We need public policies and public campaigns that continue to educate and warn each new generation of young people in order to protect them from habits and lifestyles that can insidiously cripple their children. Drinking during pregnancy is linked with disaster—personal disaster for the "bright-eyed ones," disaster for their families and their hopes for their young, and disaster for all segments of our society as we struggle to pay the huge price of this destruction. We, as a society, suffer when we produce children with disabilities, and we as a society pay the costs—more than a million dollars across the lifetime of each affected child—when we fail to prevent FAS.

There should be no doubt. It is *alcohol*, not the other associated risk factors; it is *alcohol*, not the other drugs, legal or illegal, that a mother might also be taking; it is *alcohol* that causes FAS and the other effects of prenatal alcohol exposure described in this book. If women did not drink alcohol during pregnancy, no more children would be born with FAS/FAE.

Everyone who reads this book can be part of the solution.

Resource Appendix

VIDEOS/SLIDES

Alcohol, Pregnancy, and the Fetal Alcohol Syndrome

Streissguth, A.P., & Little, R.E. (1994). *Alcohol, pregnancy, and the fetal alcohol syndrome* (slide lecture series, 2nd ed.). Hanover, NH: Dartmouth Medical School, Project Cork. Teaching unit with 79 slides and 62 pages of accompanying text that gives comprehensive overview of the effects of maternal drinking on the fetal development of the central nervous system; also explains facial and behavioral characteristics of individuals with FAS/FAE and outlines current research and public health issues. (Available by calling 1-800-432-8433.)

David with FAS

Kanata Productions & National Film Board of Canada and CBC. (1996). *David with FAS* [Film]. Princeton, NJ: Films for the Humanities and Sciences. 45-minute video about David Vandenbrink, a 21-year-old man with FAS whose condition went undiagnosed for 18 years. (Available from Films for the Humanities and Sciences, Post Office Box 2053, Princeton, NJ 08543-2053, or call 1-800-257-5126.)

The Fabulous FAS Quiz Show

March of Dimes Foundation, Washington State Department of Health, and State Superintendent of Public Instruction. (1994). *The fabulous FAS quiz show.* Seattle: March of Dimes Foundation, Western Washington Chapter. Emmy Award–winning video and teachers' guide. Targets middle school students to help them make the right choices regarding alcohol and reproduction and promotes the prevention of babies born with FAS birth defects. (Available by calling 206-624-1373.)

The Honour of All

Alkali Lake Indian band. (1986). *The honour of all* [video recording]. Williams Lake, British Columbia, Canada: Micro-Video Productions. Documents the journey of a small Canadian Indian Reserve as it moves from an extremely high alcoholism rate to establishing nearly 100% sobriety. (Available from the North American Public Broadcasting Consortium, Post Office Box 8311, Lincoln, NE 68501.)

What's Wrong with My Child?

Wenner, K. (Executive Producer). (1992, November 27). *What's wrong with my child? 20/20.* New York: American Broadcasting Company. Features clips of writer Michael Dorris and his adoptive son with FAS, also interviews other children with FAS and experts on the syndrome. (Available by calling 1-800-CALL-ABC.)

ORGANIZATIONS

Access to Respite Care and Help (ARCH)

ARCH National Resource Center, 800 Eastowne Drive, Suite 105, Chapel Hill, NC 27514 (1-800-473-1727). Provides support services to service providers and families of children with disabilities through training, technical assistance, evaluation, and research.

Alcohol and Drug 24-Hour Help Line

(1-800-562-1240). Sponsored by the Washington State Substance Abuse Coalition (1-800-662-9111). (Look inside front of your telephone book for local alcohol/drug help lines.)

American Association of University Affiliated Programs

8630 Fenton Street, Suite 410, Silver Spring, MD 20910 (301-588-8252). Provides listing of federally established programs for service, research, and training in the field of developmental disabilities. Includes 60 university affiliated programs and 14 mental retardation/developmental disabilities research centers, which can provide information on state resources for people of all ages who are suspected of having FAS/FAE.

American Montessori Society (AMS)

281 Park Avenue South, 6th floor, New York, NY 10010 (212-358-1250). Nonprofit organization dedicated to stimulating the use of the Montessori teaching approach in private and public schools. Montessori's holistic curriculum promotes the development of social skills, emotional growth, and physical coordination, as well as cognitive preparation.

The Arc of the United States

500 East Border Street, S-300, Arlington, TX 76010 (817-261-6003). Private, nonprofit organization devoted to improving the lives of

people with mental retardation and fostering research and education for the prevention of mental retardation in babies and young children; local chapters offer services as well as a *Family Handbook on Future Planning*, FAS campaign kits, brochures, booklets, posters and public service advertisements, and action plans for legislative advocacy.

Association of Waldorf Schools of North America (AWSNA)

3911 Bannister Road, Four Oaks, CA 95628 (916-961-0927). Supports and encourages Waldorf schools, which take a holistic educational approach that seeks to address the full and harmonious development of children's spiritual, emotional, and physical capabilities; provides information for those interested in Waldorf schools.

Center for Science in the Public Interest (CSPI)

1875 Connecticut Avenue, NW, Suite 300, Washington, DC 20009 (202-332-9110). Nonprofit education and advocacy organization that focuses on reducing damage caused by alcohol; seeks to promote health and well-being by educating the public about nutrition and alcohol; represents citizens' interests before legislative, regulatory, and judicial bodies.

Family Empowerment Network (FEN)

University of Wisconsin, 610 Langdon Street, Madison, WI 53703 (1-800-462-5254). National, nonprofit organization that exists to empower families affected by FAS and other drug-related birth defects through education and support; also publishes newsletter *FenPen*.

FAS/FAE Information Service, Canadian Centre on Substance Abuse

75 Albert Street, Suite 300, Ottawa, Ontario, Canada K1P 5E7 (1-800-559-4514 in Canada; 613-235-4048 outside of Canada). Bilingual information and links to support groups, prevention projects, resource centers, and experts on FAS/FAE.

FAS/FAE Support Network of British Columbia

14326 Currie Drive, Surrey, British Columbia, Canada V3R BA4 (604-589-1854). Aids in and advocates for the development of home-, school-, and community-based services that will meet the needs of individuals with FAS/FAE, their families, and associated professionals.

FAS Family Resource Institute (FAS*FRI)

Post Office Box 2525, Lynnwood, WA 98036 (1-800-999-3429). Nonprofit organization that advocates for individuals with FAS/FAE and their families; offers training for parents and professionals, organizes support groups, makes referrals, provides written materials, and publishes the newsletter *FAS Times.*

Federation of Families for Children's Mental Health (FFCMH)

1021 Prince Street, Alexandria, VA 22314 (703-684-7710; Internet Web site: http://www.ffcmh.org). Puts callers in touch with local offices that assist in locating community resources for emotional, behavioral, or mental disorders.

Fetal Alcohol and Drug Unit (FADU)

University of Washington, 180 Nickerson Street, Suite 309, Seattle, WA 98109 (206-543-7155). Conducts research, offers clinical service, and disseminates information on FAS/FAE.

Fetal Alcohol Education Program (FAEP)

Boston University, School of Medicine, 1975 Main Street, Concord, MA 01742 (508-369-7713). Provides training and individual consultation to health care professionals, parents, and educators; develops and distributes teaching packages, articles, books, and brochures.

Fetal Alcohol Information Service (FASIS)

Post Office Box 95597, Seattle, WA 98145-2597. Nonprofit organization that publishes newsletter *Iceberg* and provides reprints (write for a sample copy).

Healthy Mothers, Healthy Babies (HMHB)

National Headquarters, 409 12th Street, SW, Washington, DC 20024 (202-863-2458). Promotes public awareness and education about prenatal health, develops networks for sharing information, and distributes public and professional education materials.

March of Dimes Birth Defects Foundation (MOD)

National Headquarters, 1275 Mamaroneck Avenue, White Plains, NY 10605 (1-888-MO-DIMES). National, nonprofit organization dedicated to healthier babies through prevention of birth defects; provides financial support and conducts programs of research, education, and community services; also offers award-winning video and interactive teachers' guide, *The Fabulous FAS Quiz Show,* that targets middle school students. (Available by calling 206-624-1373).

National Alliance for the Mentally Ill (NAMI)

200 North Glebe Road, Suite 1015, Arlington, VA 22203-3754 (703-524-7600). Nonprofit, self-help, support, and advocacy organization of families and friends of people with brain disorders. Provides education and supports increased funding for research.

National Association for Family and Addiction Research and Education (NAFARE)

200 North Michigan Avenue, Suite 300, Chicago, IL 60601 (312-541-1272). Nonprofit organization that develops training programs, curricula, articles, and brochures on prenatal substance abuse.

National Association of Protection and Advocacy Systems (NAPAS)

900 2nd Street, NE, Suite 211, Washington, DC 20002 (call for local state chapter). Federally mandated organization that works to protect the rights of people with disabilities, including mental illness. Handles discrimination, neglect, and abuse issues. Provides information, referrals, and resource materials.

National Organization of Social Security Claimants' Representatives (NOSSCR)

6 Prospect Street, Midland Park, NJ 07432 (1-800-431-2804). Association of more than 3,000 attorneys and paralegals who represent Social Security and Supplemental Security Income claimants; provides quality representation and advocates for beneficial changes in the disability determination and adjudication process.

National Organization on Fetal Alcohol Syndrome (NOFAS)

1819 H Street, NW, Suite 750, Washington, DC 20006 (1-800-66-NOFAS). Nonprofit organization that works to raise public awareness, implement strategies for prevention and intervention, and influence public policy decisions on FAS/FAE; also provides informative literature regarding FAS.

North American Council on Adoptable Children (NACAC)

970 Raymond Avenue, Suite 106, St. Paul, MN 55114 (612-644-3036). National, nonprofit organization that provides education, outreach, and research information; holds annual conference and offers resource list of parent support groups.

P.A.R.E.N.T.S

540 West International Airport Road, Suite 200, Anchorage, AK 99518 (907-563-2246; in Alaska, call 1-800-770-5437). Parent information organization that empowers Alaskan families who experience disabilities by providing resources, training, and support statewide. Educational packets are sent nationally. Packets that deal specifically with FAS are available for parents, educators, and the legal community.

Parents Are Vital in Education (PAVE)

6316 South 12th Street, Tacoma, WA 98465 (206-565-2266). Private, nonprofit organization that informs parents of children with special needs of their legal rights to education and services; also provides workshops and informational packets.

Project II/GOARC (GOARC)

3610 Dodge Street, Suite 101, Omaha, NE 68131 (402-346-5220). Member agency of the United Way of the Midlands. Provides brochure detailing what people with developmental disabilities should say if picked up by the police.

Public Interest Law Center of Philadelphia (PILCOP)

125 South 9th Street, Suite 700, Philadelphia, PA 19107 (215-627-7100). National advisory group for justice for people with developmental disabilities. (For additional assistance in legal matters, contact your local County Public Defender's Office.)

Society of Counsel Representing Accused Persons (SCRAP)

1401 East Jefferson, Suite 200, Seattle, WA 98122 (1-800-275-1445). King County Public Defender's Office. Local organization that provides legal advice, suggestions, and support nationwide for people criminally accused and their families.

Society of Special Needs Adoptive Parents (SNAP)

United Kingdom Building, Suite 150, 409 Granville Street, Vancouver, British Columbia, Canada V3T 3E3 (604-687-3114). Nonprofit organization that offers support, education, information, and advocacy for families of children with special needs; also distributes newsletter and runs a resource library.

PARENT SUPPORT GROUPS

Alaska

Anchorage Parent Education Group, contact Carolyn (907) 694-6644 or Cheri (907) 277-3710.

Canada

FAS/FAE Information Service, Canadian Centre on Substance Abuse in Ottawa, Ontario. Contact Carole Julian (800) 559-4514 in Canada; (613) 235-4048 outside of Canada.

Peer Support Group for Women Parenting Children with FAS/NAS, contact YWCA Crabtree Corner (604) 689-2808 in Vancouver, British Columbia.

Support Group for Caregivers of Individuals with FAS/FAE, contact Jan Lutke (604) 589-1854 in Surrey, British Columbia.

Yellowknife, Northwest Territories, contact Helen White (403) 873-5785.

California

Contact Liz Zemke, PHN, MS (209) 432-6035 or FAX (209) 432-8942.

Contact Lynn Bilke (619) 589-1257 or Karen Aquiree (619) 430-8170.

Colorado

Fetal Alcohol and Substance Abuse Coalition, contact Karen Riley (303) 764-8361.

Illinois

Contact Kelly King-Shaw (309) 691-3800 or Colleen Matarelli (309) 682-2024.

Indiana

Contact Lisa Smith (765) 737-6430.

Iowa

FAS/FAE Prime Time Two Support Group, contact Leslie Schmalzried (515) 961-8830 in Indianola.

Kentucky

FAS Support Group, contact Easter Seals (606) 491-1171.

Michigan

Catholic Human Services, contact Martie Manty, M.A., CSW (616) 947-8110 in Traverse City.

Parents Supporting Parents, contact Barbara Wybrecht (313) 662-7231, Betsy Soden (313) 662-2906 in Ann Arbor, or Pam O'Briant (810) 736-8099 in Flint.

Minnesota

Thunderspirit Lodge Support Group, contact Joyce Glass (612) 290-9920.

Missouri

The Family Information Network, contact Peggy Oba (816) 361-7589 in Kansas City, or Jenni Loynd (314) 993-4882 or Pat Krippner (314) 962-6397 in St. Louis.

Nevada

Contact Cindy Kuhn (702) 459-4303.

New Jersey

Support Network for Adoptive and Foster Parents, contact Ronnie Jacobs (201) 261-2183 in Paramus.

Ohio

Columbus Central Area Ohio FAS/FAE Support Group, contact Phil Petrosky (614) 755-4803 or Marge Schaim (513) 931-2116.

Pennsylvania

FAS Parents and Caregivers Support Group, contact Diane (717) 769-6092 or JoAnne (717) 769-6289 in Woolrich.

Texas

Contact Sandy Shidler at The Arc (214) 317-1206 in Dallas.

Virginia

FAS/FAE Kid Connection, contact Mary Ann Lee (804) 520-2201 in Chester.

Washington

Eastern Washington Biological Mothers Support Group, contact Kathy Dunham (509) 337-6911 or (509) 522-0622.

Eastern Washington Fetal Alcohol Support Group, contact Janet Vernon (509) 684-3772.

Tri-Cities Support Group, contact Kathy Dodson (509) 545-2207, Karen Reep (509) 627-6104, or the Neurological Center (509) 943-8455.

Southwest Washington, contact Joanne Roberts (360) 896-6147 or (360) 696-8444 in Vancouver.

Snohomish County FAS Parent Support Group, contact Jocie DeVries (206) 775-9598.

Contact Marceil Ten Eyck (206) 827-1773 in Bellevue; Vickie McKinney (206) 531-2878 in Tacoma; Dorthy Beckwith (509) 663-3793 in Chelan/Douglas County; or Nina Burks (206) 842-5129 on Bainbridge Island.

West Virginia

Contact Florence Kanter (304) 452-8862.

Wisconsin

National Family Empowerment Network, contact Moira Chamberlain (800) 462-5254 in Madison.

Permissions

Permission to reprint the following materials is gratefully acknowledged:

Photographs, pages ii (top left) and 53 (left and middle): From Hanson, J.W., Jones, K.L., & Smith, D.W. (1976). Fetal alcohol syndrome: Experience with 41 patients. *Journal of the American Medical Association, 235*(14), 1459; reprinted by permission of the American Medical Association, copyright 1976.

Photograph, page ii (top right): From Streissguth, A.P., Barr, H.M., & Martin, B.C. (1984). Alcohol exposure in utero and functional deficits in children during first few years of life. In R. Porter, M. O'Connor, & J. Whelan (Eds.), *Mechanics of alcohol damage in utero* (pp. 176–196). London: Pitman; reprinted by permission of the Ciba Foundation.

Photographs, page ii (bottom middle), 95, and 263: by George Steinmetz; reprinted by permission.

Photographs, pages ii (top middle) and 1 (middle and right): From Streissguth, A.P., Clarren, S.K., & Jones, K.L. (1985). Natural history of fetal alcohol syndrome: Ten year follow-up of eleven patients. *Lancet, 2,* 85–91; © by The Lancet, Ltd. 1985; reprinted by permission.

Photograph, page xv: by Rob Casey; reprinted by permission.

Photographs, pages 1 (left) and 35: From Jones, K.L., Smith, D.W., Ulleland, C.N., & Streissguth, A.P. (1973, June 9). Pattern of malformation in offspring of chronic alcoholic mothers. *Lancet, 2,* 1267–1271; © by The Lancet, Ltd. 1973; reprinted by permission.

Photographs, pages 3 and 247 (left, middle, and right): From Streissguth, A.P., Aase, J.M., Clarren, S.K., Randels, S.P., Ladue, R.A., & Smith, D.F. (1991, April 17). Fetal alcohol syndrome in adolescents and adults. *Journal of the American Medical Association, 265,* 1961–1967; reprinted by permission of the American Medical Association, copyright 1991.

Vignettes, pages 119, 145, and 165: From Streissguth, A.P. (1994). A long-term perspective of FAS. *Alcohol Health and Research World, 18*(1), 74–81; reprinted by permission.

Photograph, page 119: From LaLoo, M. (1993, November). When alcohol hurts children: Fetal alcohol syndrome and fetal alcohol effects with Marceil Ten Eyck. *Journey Press*; reprinted by permission.

Extract, page 174: From Dorris, M. (1989). *The broken cord* (pp. 11–14, 45, 264). New York: HarperCollins; reprinted by permission.

Vignettes, pages 234, 235, and 236: From Streissguth, A.P., Moon-Jordan, A., & Clarren, S.K. (1995). Alcoholism in four patients with fetal alcohol syndrome: Recommendations for treatment. *Alcoholism Treatment Quarterly, 13*(2), 89–103; reprinted by permission of Hayworth Press, Inc.

Index

Page numbers followed by "f" indicate figures; numbers followed by "t" indicate tables.

Abstracting difficulty, 152t
  advocate strategies for handling, 155
Activities, solitary, 193
ADHD, *see* Attention-deficit/ hyperactivity disorder
Adolescents, 136–138
  narratives, 208
  psychosocial needs of, 123, 124t–125t
  see also Students
Adoptive parents, 174–177
  narratives, 175–176
Adult life, 138–140
  narratives, 138, 139, 185–186, 187, 233–234
  preparing children for, 185–205
  problems encountered in, 185–187
  psychosocial needs in, 123, 125t
Advisory panels, 259
Advocacy, 145–163
  for advocates, 162
  establishing, 222
  group, 200–201
  guidelines for school, 222–225
  individual, 201–202
  with mental health system, 238
  narratives, 145–146, 149, 150, 156–157, 157–159, 202–203
  ongoing, 202–203
  preventing secondary disabilities through, 159–162
  strategies for, 160, 160t–161t
Advocates
  advocating for, 162
  basic facts about, 149
  definition of, 147–148
  fathers as, 173–174
  narratives, 207–208
  school-based, 214
  tasks of, 214, 215t

strategies for handling behavioral and emotional effects, 149–159, 152t—153t
  who can be, 148–149
After-care, 232–234
Age-related changes, 25–27
Alaska, 258
Alaskan Natives, 256
Alcohol
  equivalencies, 20, 20f
  impact on children, 71–94
    narratives, 71–72
  neurobehavioral effects of narrative, 55
  teratology, 61–67
  pregnancy and
    animal findings, 65–67
    myths about, 255
    public policy, 35–52
    Surgeon General's Advisory on Alcohol and Pregnancy, 48, 249, 257
    warning signs, 258, 259f
  teratogenic effects of, 55–70
    animal studies of, 58–61, 59f
    research implications, 65–67
    see also Fetal alcohol effects (FAE); Fetal alcohol syndrome (FAS)
Alcohol abuse
  advocacy strategies for preventing, 160t
  among women of childbearing age, 83, 84f
  in individuals with FAS/FAE, 110
  treatments for, 234–237
    intervening during pregnancy, 265–269
    vignettes, 234–235, 236
  see also Alcoholism
Alcohol and Brain Development (West), 43

Alcohol awareness campaigns, 47
Alcohol problems
  measuring during pregnancy, 80
  in people with FAS, 110, 234
Alcohol-related birth defects
    (ARBD), 29
  categorization of, 30
Alcohol-related effects, 30
Alcohol-related neurodevelop-
    mental disorder (ARND), 5
  categorization of, 30
  diagnosis of, 27–30, 28f
  narrative, 27–28
  see also Fetal alcohol effects
    (FAE)
Alcoholic Beverage Labeling Act of
    1988 (PL 100-90), 249, 257
Alcoholism
  families with, 72
    children of, 81–83
    narrative, 72–73
  maternal, 36–37
    birth weight of offspring of, 78f,
      78–79
    children of, 73–77
    effects of, 77–81
    husbands with, 173–174
    narrative, 72–73
    recognition of, 172–173
  paternal, 81–83
  see also Alcohol abuse
Alcoholism counselors, 255
American Medical Association, 47
Anti-Drug Abuse Act of 1988
    (PL 100-690), 48
Apprenticeships, 200–202
ARBD, see Alcohol-related birth
    defects
Arc, see The Arc
Arithmetic disability, 152t, 155
Arizona, 258
ARND, see Alcohol-related neuro-
    developmental disorder
Asperger syndrome, 74
Association for Retarded Citizens,
    see The Arc
Atlanta, Georgia, 267, 268
Attention problems, 126, 134
  Attention-deficit/hyperactivity
    disorder (ADHD), 108

advocate strategies for handling,
    152t
and the corpus callosum, 100

BACs, see Blood-alcohol
    concentrations
Bancroft School, 203–204
BATF, see Bureau of Alcohol,
    Tobacco, and Firearms
Bayley Scales of Infant
    Development, 131
Behavior(s)
  adaptive, 31, 217
  advocate strategy for inferring
    needs from, 150–151
  brain–behavior relationships
    narratives, 67
    research implications, 66–67
    that contribute to primary
      disabilities, 100–102
  inappropriate sexual, 110
    advocacy strategies for
      preventing, 160t
  averting, 193
  monitoring and modifying, 223
  maladaptive, 103, 104t
  mother–infant interaction, 130
  social, 127
  socially appropriate, 191–193
Behavior problems
  misconceptions about, 121
  questions for evaluating, 151
Behavioral effects
  advocate strategies for handling,
    149–150, 152t–153t
  in humans and animals, 65, 65t
  lifelong, 123–125
Behavioral phenotype, 127
  common items in, 126–127
  identifying, 126–127
Behavioral therapy, cognitive, 193
Berlin, Germany, 75
Binge drinking, see Social drinking
Birth defects, alcohol-related, 29
  categorization of, 30
Birth parents, 74, 229
Birth to 3 program, 265, 270–275
  advocates in, 272–273
  continuing, 274–275

narrative, 263–264, 275
participants, 272
project inception, 270
results, 273–274
screening process, 271–272
Birth weight, 78*f*, 78–79
Blood-alcohol concentrations (BAC), 60
Boston, Massachusetts, 267
Boston University, 256
Brain damage, 96–100
advocate strategies for behavioral manifestations of, 149–150
functional, 99–100
electroencephalograms (EEGs), 99
positron emission tomography (PET) scans, 100
misconceptions about, 121
organic, 122–123
primary disabilities from, 96–100
research implications, 66
structural, 97–99
structure via autopsies, 97–98
structure via magnetic resonance imaging (MRI), 98*f*, 98–99
traumatic injury, 197
Brain–behavior relationships
narratives, 67
research implications, 66–67
that contribute to primary disabilities, 100–102
British Columbia, Canada, 48
The Broken Cord (Dorris), 44–45, 48
Bureau of Alcohol, Tobacco, and Firearms (BATF), 47, 257

California
alcohol and pregnancy warning signs in, 258
alcohol awareness campaign in, 47
Capacity Building Project for the Prevention of Primary and Secondary Disabilities, 259
Case management, 202–203
Case/comparison group study, 41–42

CDC, *see* Centers for Disease Control and Prevention
Center for Substance Abuse Prevention, 270
Centers for Disease Control and Prevention (CDC), 45–46, 105
Central nervous system (CNS), alcohol-related effects, 18–19, 19*t*
advocate strategies for handling, 152*t*
measuring, 30–31
in neonates, 84–85
Children
of alcoholic fathers and families, 81–83
outcomes of, 82–83
research in Kauai, Hawaii, 82
of alcoholic mothers, 73–77
description, 77–81
narratives, 77–78
research in Berlin, Germany, 75
research in Göteborg, Sweden, 73–74
research in Helsinki, Finland, 77
research in Nantes, France, 75–76
alcohol's impact on, 71–94
narratives, 71–72
early school-age, neurobehavioral findings in, 86–87
FAS facial characteristics in, 23–24, 24*f*
narratives, 185–187
preparing for adulthood, 185–205
preschool, 132–134
neurobehavioral findings in, 86–87
psychosocial needs, 123, 124*t*
school-age, 134–136
narratives, 207–208
neurobehavioral findings in, 86–87
of women who drink socially, 83–87
see also Students
Children's Protective Services (CPS), 271

Classroom teachers
FAS overview for, 218–222
guidelines for, 221, 221*t*
Clinical recognition
in France and Seattle, 38–40, 39*f*,
40*f*
history of, 36–40
CNS, *see* Central nervous system
Cognitive behavioral therapy, 193
Cognitive impairments, 106, 106*t*
Collaborative Perinatal Project
(National Institute on
Neurologic Diseases and
Stroke), 41
Communication problems, 126, 146
Community, sense of, 203–204
Community life
preparing for, 183–245
recommended social provisions
for, 199
Community services, 229–234
intake, 229–231
narratives, 233–234
Coordinators, state, 258
Corrections, 238–242
advocacy strategies for
preventing, 161*t*
incarceration, 109
vignettes, 241–242
CPS, *see* Children's Protective
Services
Criminality
advocacy strategies for
preventing, 161*t*
incarceration, 109
juvenile justice and corrections,
238–242
Crippled Children's Services, 170

DAMP, *see* Deficits in attention,
motor control, and perception
DDD, *see* Division of Develop-
mental Disabilities
Deficits in attention, motor control,
and perception (DAMP), 74
Delancey House, 204
Delaware, 258
*A Demonstration Grant to Prevent
Fetal Alcohol Syndrome and
Intervene in Female Alcohol*

Abuse During Pregnancy,
251
Demonstration projects, 47
see also specific projects
Denial
family, 166–169
narratives, 168, 169–172
professional, 169–172
Department of Health, Genetics
Office, 231
Detour learning test, 62, 62*f*
Diagnosis, 17–33
in adolescents and adults, 230
clinics for, 268
criteria for, 18–19
early, 189
helping to understand, 224–225
misconceptions about, 122
narratives, 7–8, 17, 22
and parenting, 174–177
problems with getting, 6–8
process, 20–23
*Diagnostic and Statistical Manual
of Mental Disorders, Fourth
Edition* (DSM-IV), 228
Diagnostic services, 199–200
Disabilities
hidden, 146
learning, 146
recognizing and accepting,
187–188
see also Primary disabilities;
Secondary disabilities;
specific impairments
Disorientation, 153*t*, 155, 157
Disrupted school experiences, 109
advocacy strategies for
preventing, 161*t*
Division of Developmental
Disabilities (DDD), 161, 201,
231
Documenting fetal alcohol
exposure, 19–20
Dose–response relationship, 57
Drinking
maternal, 178–179
during pregnancy
public policy on, 46–48
Seattle Pregnancy and Health
Program (PHP), 266*f*,
266–267

socially, 83–87
see also Alcohol abuse; Alcoholism
Drug abuse
advocacy strategies for
preventing, 160t
among women of childbearing
age, 83, 84f
in individuals with FAS/FAE, 110
treatments for, 234–237
vignette, 234–235
DSM-IV, see Diagnostic and Statistical Manual of Mental Disorders, Fourth Edition

Early school-age children
neurobehavioral findings in, 86–87
see also Children
Education, public, 251–254
programs, 256–257
see also School(s)
Educators
classroom teachers
FAS overview for, 218–222
guidelines for, 221, 221t
guidelines for, 220–222
EEGs, see Electroencephalography
Electroencephalography (EEGs), 84
of functional brain damage,
99–100
Emotional effects, 151–154,
152t–153t
Employment, see Jobs; Work
experiences
Executive function tasks, 102
Exencephaly, 58–59, 60f
Expectations, realistic, 156–157
Experimental animal research, see
Animal studies

FABS, see Fetal Alcohol Behavior
Scale
Facial effects, 59, 61f
age-related changes in, 25–27
Facilitating appropriate
supervision, 224
Facilitating practical work skills,
224
FAE, see Fetal alcohol effects
Failure to thrive, 38
Families, 165–181

alcoholic, 72
children of, 81–83
building personal strengths in,
190–199
diversity of, 165–166
listening to, 180
narratives, 72–73, 165–166,
166–167, 172–173, 177–178,
193
needs of, 177–180
providing information to,
179–180
questions to ask, 178–179
supporting and providing
opportunities for sharing
in, 177–178
teamwork between school and,
224
Fantastic Antone Succeeds, 219
FAS, see Fetal alcohol syndrome
FAS Family Resources Institute
(FAS-FRI), 201
FAS-FRI, see FAS Family Resources
Institute
FAS Times, 218
Fathers
as advocates, 173–174
alcoholic, 81–83
narratives, 173–174
see also Parents
FenPen, 218
Fetal Alcohol and Drug Unit, 43–44
Fetal Alcohol Behavior Scale
(FABS), 107, 126
Fetal alcohol effects (FAE), 5, 18
behavioral phenotype of, 126–127
cognitive impairments associated
with, 106, 106t
denial of
family, 166–169
professional, 169–172
diagnosis of, 27–30, 28f
misconceptions about, 122
narrative, 27–28
diagnostic services, 199–200
IQ distribution for, 103, 103f
life-span approach to, 127–140
lifelong behavioral, 123–125
maladaptive behaviors and
symptoms of, 103, 104t
misconceptions about, 120–123

Fetal alcohol effects
(FAE)—*continued*
preventing, 247–278
primary disabilities, 95–115
problems and concerns of,
123–125
psychosocial needs associated
with, 123, 124t–125t
recommendations, 123–125
secondary disabilities, 95–115,
108f
most prevalent, 228
services to help people with,
199–204
treatment approach, 122
see also Alcohol-related neurodevelopmental disorder
(ARND); Fetal alcohol
syndrome (FAS)
Fetal alcohol exposure, documenting, 19–20
Fetal alcohol syndrome (FAS)
age-related changes in features
of, 25–27
behavioral phenotype of, 126–127
brain damage in, 96–100
categorization of, 29
cause of, 4, 5f
classification of, 19
clinical recognition of
in France and Seattle, 38–40,
39f, 40f
history of, 36–40
cognitive impairments, 106, 106t
denial of
family, 166–169
professional, 169–172
diagnosis of, 17–33
at birth, 39, 39f
misconceptions about, 122
narratives, 7–8, 17, 22
and parenting, 174–177
problems with getting, 6–8
process for, 20–23
diagnostic criteria for, 18–19
diagnostic services for, 199–200
early studies, 36–37
facial characteristics of, 23–24, 24f
incidence of, 8–9
IQ distribution for, 103, 103f

life-span approach to, 117–181,
127–140
living with, 119–143
long-term effects of, 43–46
maladaptive behaviors and
symptoms in, 103, 104t
management of
advocacy model for, 145–163
misconceptions about, 122
narrative, 13–15
misconceptions about, 120–123
mothers with, 165
narratives, 3–4
overview of, 3–16
for classroom teachers,
218–222
physical findings in, 23–25
preparing for community life
with, 183–245
prevention of
demonstration projects, 47
efforts, 48
primary disabilities, 95–115
problems and concerns of,
123–125
problems with studying, 9–11
psychosocial needs associated
with, 123, 124t–125t
public awareness of, 35–52
recommendations for, 123–125
science of, 53–115
scientific validation of, 40–43
secondary disabilities, 95–115,
108f
most prevalent, 228
services to help people with,
199–204
Finland, 77
5-HEALTH (hot line), 252
Florida, 258
Foster parents, 174–177
France
clinical recognition of fetal
alcohol syndrome (FAS) in,
38–40, 40f
pregnancy intervention
programs, 267
prevention efforts, 48
research on children of alcoholic
mothers in, 75–76

Friends, 191–193
Functional skills, 223

Georgia, 258
Germany, 75
Göteborg, Sweden, 73–74
Group advocacy, 200–201
Growth deficiency effects, 58–59,
    59*f*

Habituation problems, 85, 126
    advocate strategies for handling,
    152*t*
Handbook of Teratology (Riley and
    Vorhees), 43
Head Start, 132
*Health Caution on Fetal Alcohol
    Syndrome* (U.S. Department
    of Health, Education and
    Welfare), 47
Health effects, 77–81
    narratives, 77–78
Healthy Mothers–Healthy Babies,
    253
Helsinki, Finland, 77
Hidden disabilities, 146
High school, 196, 197
High-risk mothers, 263–278
Hockeystick crease, 25
Home, *see* Families
Hot lines, 252
Housing, 203–204
"How Alcohol Affects the Body"
    (Yale Center for Alcohol), 46
Human services, *see* Services
Hyperactivity, *see* Attention-deficit/
    hyperactivity disorder

Iceberg, 218
Illinois, 258
Impulsivity problems, 126, 152*t*
Inappropriate sexual behaviors,
    110
    advocacy strategies for
    preventing, 160*t*
    averting, 193
    monitoring and modifying, 223
Incarceration, 109, 238–242

advocacy strategies for
    preventing, 161*t*
Indian Health Service, 200, 256
    *Manual on Adolescents and
    Adults with FAS/FAE, with
    Special Reference to
    American Indians*, 44
Indian Medical Center, 268
Individual advocacy, 201–202
Infants, 128–132
    CNS dysfunction in, 84–85
    mental and motor impairments,
    85–86
    mother–infant interaction, 130
    narrative, 129
    psychosocial needs, 123, 124*t*
Information processing
    impairments, 85–86
Information sharing, 179–180
Institute of Medicine (IOM), 5
    categorization of fetal alcohol
    syndrome (FAS), 29–30
    classification of fetal alcohol
    syndrome (FAS), 19
Institutional responsibilities, 243
Intake, 229–231
    brief examination, 230
    interpreting data and taking
    action, 230–231
    interview, 229–230
Intelligence Quotient, *see* IQ
    testing
*International Classification of
    Diseases* (World Health
    Organization), 20
Interventions
    brief, 265–266
    after delivery, 269–275
    during pregnancy, 265–269
        incorporating into existing
        service systems, 268–269
        narrative, 269
        programs, 267–268
    see also specific programs
Interviewing
    intake, 229–230
    Life History Interview (LHI),
    107, 186
    motivational, 254–255
IOM, *see* Institute of Medicine

IQ testing, 31
   scores, 103, 103*f*, 131, 217*f*

Job placements
   narrative, 227
   ongoing supervision in, 202–203
Job training, 197–198, 200–202
Jobs
   facilitating practical skills for,
      224
   learning to enjoy, 194–199
   learning to work, 194–199
   narratives, 194–195, 195–196,
      196–197, 198–199
   transition to, 196, 197
   see also Work experiences
Judgment problems, 153*t*
Juvenile justice, 238–242
   see also Law, trouble with

Kallikak, Pauline (vignette), 36–37,
   37*f*
Kauai, Hawaii, 82
Kentucky, 258
Keys to Caregiving (video series), 130

Lancet, 39
Law, trouble with, 109
   advocacy strategies for
      preventing, 161*t*
   corrections, 238–242
   incarceration, 109
Learning disabilities, 146
Learning socially appropriate
   behavior, 191–193
Learning to be alone, 193
Learning to be friends, 191–193
Learning to enjoy working, 194–199
Learning to work, 194–199
Learning-to-learn skills, 132
LHI, *see* Life History Interview
Life History Interview (LHI), 107,
   186
Life-span approach, 117–181,
   127–140
   narratives, 127, 128
Limitations
   advocate strategies for helping
      define, 154–156

methods of compensating for,
   157–159
   see also Disabilities; *specific
   impairments*
Listening to families, 180
Long-term effects
   behavioral, 123–125
   misconceptions about, 121–122
   narrative, 67
   research implications, 67
   tracking, 43–46
Longitudinal prospective study,
   42–43
Lowry, Michael, 259

Magnetic resonance imaging, 98*f*,
   98–99
Magnetoencephalography (MEG),
   102
Maine
   alcohol and pregnancy warning
      signs in, 258
   public education campaign in,
      253
Maladaptive behaviors, 103, 104*t*
Malformation, 58–59, 59*f*
Management or treatment plan,
   232
   see also Interventions
*Manual on Adolescents and Adults
   with FAS/FAE, with Special
   Reference to American
   Indians* (Indian Health
   Service), 44
March of Dimes, 47
   Western Washington Chapter,
      253
Maternal alcoholism, 36–37
   children who live with, 73–77
   birth weight of, 78*f*, 78–79
   effects of, 77–81
   in medical records, 178–179
      documenting prenatal alcohol
         exposure, 23, 178
   importance of disclosing, 179
   narrative, 72–73
   questions to ask about, 178–179
   recognition of, 172–173
Meetings, periodic, 222–223
MEG, *see* Magnetoencephalography

Memory problems, 153t, 155, 157
Mental health impairments, 109
    advocacy model for, 238
    preventive strategies, 161t
    in infancy, 85–86
    treatment of, 237–238
Mental retardation, 146
    misconceptions about, 121
Michigan, 258
Minnesota, 258
Misconceptions, 120–123
Missouri, 258
Monitoring
    inappropriate sexual behaviors,
        223
    see also Supervision
Montessori Schools, 132
Mother–infant interaction, 130
Mothers
    alcoholic, 36–37
    birth weight of offspring of, 78f,
        78–79
    children of, 73–77, 77–81, 78f,
        83–87
    effects of, 77–81
    husbands of, 173–174
    narrative, 72–73
    questions to ask about,
        178–179
    recognition of, 172–173
    with fetal alcohol syndrome
        (FAS), 165
    prevention programs for, 263–278
    support for, 172–173
    who drink socially, 83–87
    see also Parents
Motivational interviewing,
    254–255
Motor functioning impairments,
    85–86
Motor perception dysfunction
    (MPD), 74
MPD, see Motor perception
    dysfunction

NAMI, see National Association on
    Mental Illness
Nantes, France, 75–76
National Association on Mental
    Illness (NAMI), 202

National Council on Alcoholism, 253
National Health Survey (1990), 10
National Institute on Alcohol Abuse
    and Alcoholism (NIAAA), 8,
    39, 58, 83
    demonstration projects, 47, 251
    public education campaign, 253
National Institute on Neurologic
    Diseases and Stroke
    Collaborative Perinatal
    Project, 41
National Organization of Social
    Service Claimants Represen-
    tatives (NOSSCR), 202
Native Americans, 256
Nebraska
    alcohol and pregnancy warning
        signs in, 258
    public education campaign in,
        253
Needs
    advocate strategy for inferring
        from behaviors, 150–151
    families', 177–180
Neonatal Behavioral Assessment
    Scale, 130
Neonates
    central nervous system (CNS)
        dysfunction in, 84–85
    see also Infants
Neurobehavioral effects
    findings in preschool and early
        school-age children, 86–87
    narrative, 55
Neurobehavioral teratogens,
    61–62
    alcohol, 61–67
    animal studies, 62, 62f
Neuropsychological impairments,
    100–102
New Jersey, 258
New Mexico, 258
New York, 258
NIAAA, see National Institute on
    Alcohol Abuse and
    Alcoholism
North Carolina, 253
NOSSCR, see National
    Organization of Social
    Service Claimants
    Representatives

Organizational skills, problems
    with, 126
Overstimulation, 126

Parenting, 174–177
Parents
    advocacy, 168–169, 201
    adoptive and foster, 174–177
    narratives, 175–176, 188–189,
        215–217, 217–218
    school–parent collaboration,
        215–218
    support groups, 177
Parent–teacher associations (PTA),
    212
Partial fetal alcohol syndrome, 29
Paternal alcoholism, 81–83
Patient history, 23
Peer groups, 137
Perseveration, 153t, 155
PET, see Positron emission
    tomography
PFAE, see Possible fetal alcohol
    effects
Phenotype, behavioral, 126–127
PHP, see Pregnancy and Health
    Program
Physical examination, 22–23
    brief intake examination, 230
Physical findings, 23–25
Planning
    early, 188–190
    10-step school plan, 214–215,
        216t
Planning beyond school, 224
Positron emission tomography
    (PET), 100
Possible fetal alcohol effects
    (PFAE), 5
    diagnosis of of, 29
    lifelong behavioral effects,
        123–125
Pregnancy and alcohol
    animal findings, 65–67
    myths about, 255
    public policy on, 35–52
        history of, 46–48
    Surgeon General's Advisory on
        Alcohol and Pregnancy, 48,
        249, 257

warning signs, 258, 259f
Pregnancy and Health Program
    (PHP) (Washington State),
    13, 13f, 249, 251, 265–267
    brief intervention, 265–266
    change in drinking by pregnant
        women after contact with,
        266f, 266–267
    professional training, 254,
        255–256
    public education efforts, 252
    screening process, 265
    service delivery, 266–267
Pregnancy care workers, 255
Pregnancy interventions, 265–269
    incorporating into existing
        service systems, 268–269
    narrative, 269
    programs, 267–268
    see also specific programs
Prenatal alcohol and other drug
    programs, 268
    key components of, 268–269
Prenatal alcohol exposure
    central nervous system (CNS)
        effects of, 18–19, 19t
    effects of, 4–6, 5f, 18
        behavioral, 65, 65t
        brain damage, 66
        exencephaly, 58–59, 60f
        facial, 59, 61f
        long-term, 67
        malformation and growth
            deficiency, 58–59, 59f
        research implications, 66–67
        topics for retrospective history,
            20, 21f
        wishes for people affected by,
            140–141
    see also Fetal alcohol effects
        (FAE)
Preschool children, 132–134
    neurobehavioral findings in,
        86–87
    see also Children
Prevention, 247–278
    demonstration projects, 47
    efforts, 48
    five Ps of, 250
    program for Native Americans
        and Alaskan Natives, 256

programs for high-risk mothers, 263–278
of secondary disabilities, 159–161
Swedish program, 257
see also specific programs, projects
Primary disabilities, 95–115, 146–147
brain–behavior relationships that contribute to, 100–102
measuring, 102–103
narratives, 95
from organic brain damage, 96–100
see also specific disabilities
Professional denial, 169–172
Professional training, 254–257
narratives, 254
programs, 256–257
Prostitutes, 243, 243f
Protective factors, 110–112
Psychosocial needs, 123, 124t–125t
PTAs, see Parent–teacher associations
Public awareness, 35–52
Public education, 47, 251–254
Pregnancy and Health Program (PHP) efforts, 252
programs, 256–257
see also School(s)
PL 100-90, see Alcoholic Beverage Labeling Act of 1988
PL 100-690, see Anti-Drug Abuse Act of 1988
Public policy, 35–52, 249–262, 257–258
history of, 46–48
narratives, 35

Reasoning, 127
Recognizable Patterns of Human Malformations, 20
Rehabilitation, vocational, 201
Rent subsidy, 158
Replacement child phenomenon, 271
Research, 43, 53–115
animal studies, 43, 59f
of alcohol teratogenesis, 58–61, 59f
of behavioral effects of prenatal alcohol exposure, 65, 65t
of exencephaly effects of prenatal alcohol exposure, 58–59, 60f
of facial effects of prenatal alcohol exposure, 59, 61f
of neurobehavioral teratology of alcohol, 62, 62f
relevance for humans, 65–67
case/comparison group study, 41–42
on children of alcoholic fathers and families, 82
on children of alcoholic mothers
in Berlin, Germany, 75
in Göteborg, Sweden, 73–74
in Helsinki, Finland, 77
in Nantes, France, 75–76
on children of women who drink socially, 83–87
early studies, 36–37
on functional brain damage, 99–100
long-term follow-up studies, 43–46
longitudinal prospective study, 42–43
new, 186–187
on structural brain damage, 97–99
on teratogenic effects of alcohol, 65–67
Residential facilities, 203–204
Response inhibition, 63
Rhode Island, 258
Risk factors, 110–112
Roubaix, France, 48

Safe housing, 203–204
San Juan, Puerto Rico, 264
School(s)
fetal alcohol syndrome (FAS) support teams at, 213–214
guidelines for, 207–226
guidelines for advocacy model at, 222–225
teamwork between home and, 224
10-step plan for students, 214–215, 216t

School advocates, 214
   tasks of, 214, 215t
School-age children, 134–136
   narratives, 207–208
   neurobehavioral findings in,
      86–87
   see also Children; Students
School districts
   FAS/FAE plan for, 210–215
   FAS task forces, 212–213
   recommendations for, 212
School experiences
   disrupted, 109
      advocacy strategies for
         preventing, 161t
   helping make pleasurable, 224
School–parent collaboration,
      215–218
   narrative, 215–217
Science, 53–115
Scientific validation, 40–43
Seattle, Washington, 38–40, 39f
Seattle Paraprofessional Advocacy
      Model: Birth to 3 program,
      270–275
   advocates in, 272–273
   continuing the, 274–275
   narratives, 263–264, 275
   participants in, 272
   project inception, 270
   results of, 273–274
   screening process, 271–272
Secondary disabilities, 95–115, 108,
      108f
   advocacy strategies for preventing,
      159–162, 160t–161t
   measuring, 104–110
   most prevalent, 228
   narratives, 95, 107
   protective factors, 110–111
   risk factors, 110–111
   see also specific disabilities
Self-reflection problems, 153t
Self-regulation problems, 152t
Services, 199–204
   community, 229–234
   guidelines for, 227–245
   incorporating pregnancy
      interventions into, 268–269
   narrative, 227
   recommended, 199

Sexual behaviors, inappropriate,
      110
   advocacy strategies for
      preventing, 160t
   averting, 193
   monitoring and modifying, 223
Sharing information, 179–180
   opportunities for, 177–178
Shelter, 203–204
Skills
   functional, 223
   practical work, 224
Sobriety, 172–173
Social behavior, 127
Social drinking, 83–87
Social institutions, 243
Social Security Administration, 201
Social Services Disability system,
      231
Socially appropriate behavior,
      191–193
Solitary activities, 193
Solitude, 193
South Dakota, 258
Space disorientation, 153t, 155, 157
Special Olympics, 193
SSI, see Supplemental Security
      Income
State FAS coordinators, 258
State Genetics Office, 231
Stockholm, Sweden, 267
Strengths
   advocate strategies for helping
      identify, 154–156
   personal, 190–199
Students
   building relationships with,
      222–223
   guidelines for advocacy model
      with, 222–225
   guidelines for educators of,
      220–222
   helping complete school and plan
      beyond, 224
   narratives, 221–222
   needs of, 209, 209t
   school-based advocates for,
      214–215
   tasks of, 214, 215t
   10-step school plan for, 214–215,
      216t

see also Adolescents; Children
Supervision
  facilitating, 224
  monitoring inappropriate sexual
    behaviors, 223
  narratives, 202–203
  ongoing, 202–203
Supplemental Security Income
  (SSI), 199, 201
Support for families, 177–178
Support teams, 213–214
Surgeon General's Advisory on
  Alcohol and Pregnancy, 48,
  249, 257
Survival skills, 198
Sweden
  pregnancy intervention
    programs, 267
  prevention efforts, 48, 257
  research on children of alcoholic
    mothers in, 73–74

T-ACE questions, *see* Tolerance,
  Annoyed, Cut Down, Eye
  Opener questions
Task forces, 259
  district-level, 212–213
TBI, *see* Traumatic brain injury
Teachers
  FAS overview for, 218–222
  guidelines for, 221, 221t
Teaching functional skills, 223
Teamwork
  establishing, 224
  support teams, 213–214
10-Question Drinking History, 267
Teratology, 56–61
  alcohol, 58–61, 59f
  neurobehavioral, 61–62
  outcomes in exposed offspring,
    56, 57t
The Arc, 202, 253
Time disorientation, 153t, 155,
  157
Toddlers, 132–134
Tolerance, Annoyed, Cut Down, Eye
  Opener (T-ACE) questions,
  267
Tolerance, Worry about drinking,
  Eye opener, Amnesia, Cut

down on drinking (TWEAK)
  test, 267
Training
  job, 197–198
  professional, 254–257
  programs, 256–257
Traumatic brain injury (TBI), 197
Treatment(s)
  for alcohol and other drug abuse,
    234–237
    vignettes, 234–235, 236
  mental health, 237–238
  misconceptions about, 122
  see also Interventions
Treatment plan, 232
Troubleshooting, 223
Tuba City, Arizona, 267–268
TWEAK test, *see* Tolerance, Worry
  about drinking, Eye opener,
  Amnesia, Cut down on drinking test
20/20 (television program), 48

University of Washington, 200
University of Washington FAS
  Diagnostic Clinic, 259
University of Washington Medical
  School, 103
  demonstration program, 47
U.S. Department of Health,
  Education and Welfare,
  *Health Caution on Fetal
  Alcohol Syndrome*, 47
Utah, 258

VABS, *see* Vineland Adaptive
  Behavior Scales
VABS Maladaptive Behavior Scale,
  105
Vermont, 253
Vineland Adaptive Behavior Scales
  (VABS), 105
  scores, 217f
Virgin Islands, 264
Vocational rehabilitation (VR), 201
VR, *see* Vocational rehabilitation

Waldorf Schools, 132
Warning labels, 257–258

Warning signs, 258, 259*f*
Washington, D.C., 264
Washington State, 264
  alcohol and pregnancy warning
    signs, 258, 259*f*
  Department of Health, 258
  Division of Alcohol and
    Substance Abuse, 252–253,
    258
  FAS coordinators, 258
  FAS prevention activities, 259
  hot line, 258
  Pregnancy and Health Program
    (PHP), 13, 13*f*, 249, 251, 252,
    254, 255–256, 265–267
"Washington State Needs
    Assessment Survey on Fetal
    Alcohol Syndrome/Effects,"
    259
Wide Range Achievement Test–
    Revised (WRAT–R) scores,
    217*f*

Wisconsin General Test Apparatus,
    60
Women of childbearing age
  alcohol and other drug use
    among, 83, 84*f*
  see also Mothers
Work experiences
  facilitating practical skills, 224
  learning to work and to enjoy
    working, 194–199
  narratives, 194–195, 195–196,
    196–197, 198–199, 227
  placements, 227
  transition to work, 196, 197
  see also Jobs
World Health Organization, 20
WRAT–R, *see* Wide Range
    Achievement Test–Revised

Yale Center for Alcohol, "How
    Alcohol Affects the
    Body," 46

46